Practice *Planner*

Arthur E. Jongsma, Jr., Series Editor

Helping therapists help their clients...

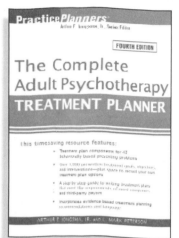

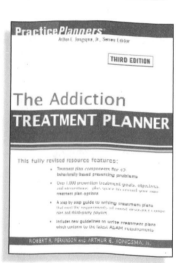

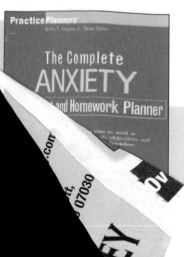

Treatment Planners cover all the necessary elements for developing formal treatment plans, including detailed problem definitions, long-term goals, short-term objectives, therapeutic interventions, and DSM-IV™ diagnoses.

❑ The Complete Adult Psychotherapy Treatment Planner, Fourth Edition........978-0-471-76346-8 / $55.00
❑ The Child Psychotherapy Treatment Planner, Fourth Edition ....978-0-471-78535-4 / $55.00
❑ The Adolescent Psychotherapy Treatment Planner, Fourth Edition ....978-0-471-78539-2 / $55.00
❑ The Addiction Treatment Planner, Third Edition..978-0-471-72544-2 / $55.00
❑ The Couples Psychotherapy Treatment Planner ....978-0-471-24711-1 / $55.00
❑ The Group Therapy Treatment Planner, Second Edition ....978-0-471-66791-9 / $55.00
❑ The Family Therapy Treatment Planner ....978-0-471-34768-2 / $55.00
❑ The Older Adult Psychotherapy Treatment Planner ....978-0-471-29574-7 / $55.00
❑ The Employee Assistance (EAP) Treatment Planner ....978-0-471-24709-8 / $55.00
❑ The Gay and Lesbian Psychotherapy Treatment Planner ....978-0-471-35080-4 / $55.00
❑ The Crisis Counseling and Traumatic Events Treatment Planner ....978-0-471-39587-4 / $55.00
❑ The Social Work and Human Services Treatment Planner ....978-0-471-37741-2 / $55.00
❑ The Continuum of Care Treatment Planner ....978-0-471-19568-9 / $55.00
❑ The Behavioral Medicine Treatment Planner..978-0-471-31923-8 / $55.00
❑ The Mental Retardation and Developmental Disability Treatment Planner ...978-0-471-38253-9 / $55.00
❑ The Special Education Treatment Planner..978-0-471-38872-2 / $55.00
❑ The Severe and Persistent Mental Illness Treatment Planner, Second Edition ...978-0-470-18013-6 / $55.00
❑ The Personality Disorders Treatment Planner ....978-0-471-39403-7 / $55.00
❑ The Rehabilitation Psychology Treatment Planner ....978-0-471-35178-8 / $55.00
❑ The Pastoral Counseling Treatment Planner..978-0-471-25416-4 / $55.00
❑ The Juvenile Justice and Residential Care Treatment Planner ....978-0-471-43320-0 / $55.00
❑ The School Counseling and School Social Work Treatment Planner ....978-0-471-08496-9 / $55.00
❑ The Psychopharmacology Treatment Planner ....978-0-471-43322-4 / $55.00
❑ The Probation and Parole Treatment Planner..978-0-471-20244-8 / $55.00
❑ The Suicide and Homicide Risk Assessment & Prevention Treatment Planner..978-0-471-46631-4 / $55.00
❑ The Speech-Language Pathology Treatment Planner..978-0-471-27504-6 / $55.00
❑ The College Student Counseling Treatment Planner ....978-0-471-46708-3 / $55.00
❑ The Parenting Skills Treatment Planner ....978-0-471-48183-6 / $55.00
❑ The Early Childhood Education Intervention Treatment Planner ....978-0-471-65962-4 / $55.00
❑ The Co-Occurring Disorders Treatment Planner ....978-0-471-73081-1 / $55.00
❑ The Sexual Abuse Victim and Sexual Offender Treatment Planner ....978-0-471-21979-8 / $55.00
❑ The Complete Women's Psychotherapy Treatment Planner ....978-0-470-03983-0 / $55.00

The **Complete Treatment and Homework Planners** series of books combines our bestselling *Treatment Planners* and *Homework Planners* into one easy-to-use, all-in-one resource for mental health professionals treating clients suffering from the most commonly diagnosed disorders.

❑ The Complete Depression Treatment and Homework Planner ....978-0-471-64515-3 / $48.95
❑ The Complete Anxiety Treatment and Homework Planner ....978-0-471-64548-1 / $48.95

ePlanners® sold ...

Ⓦ **WILEY**

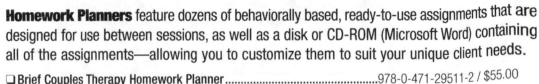
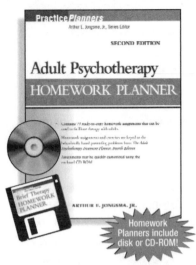
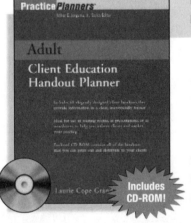
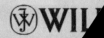

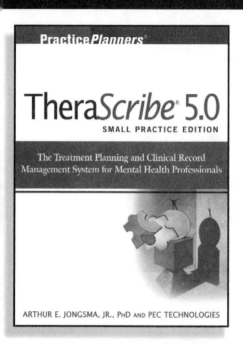
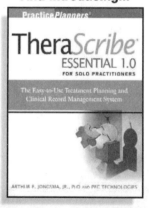
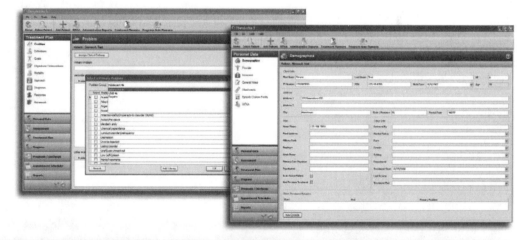
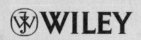

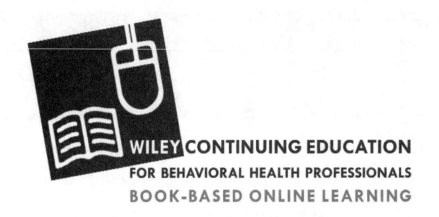
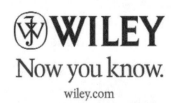

The Severe and Persistent Mental Illness Progress Notes Planner

Practice*Planners*® Series

Treatment Planners

The Complete Adult Psychotherapy Treatment Planner, Fourth Edition
The Child Psychotherapy Treatment Planner, Fourth Edition
The Adolescent Psychotherapy Treatment Planner, Fourth Edition
The Addiction Treatment Planner, Third Edition
The Continuum of Care Treatment Planner
The Couples Psychotherapy Treatment Planner
The Employee Assistance Treatment Planner
The Pastoral Counseling Treatment Planner
The Older Adult Psychotherapy Treatment Planner
The Behavioral Medicine Treatment Planner
The Group Therapy Treatment Planner
The Gay and Lesbian Psychotherapy Treatment Planner
The Family Therapy Treatment Planner
The Severe and Persistent Mental Illness Treatment Planner
The Mental Retardation and Developmental Disability Treatment Planner
The Social Work and Human Services Treatment Planner
The Crisis Counseling and Traumatic Events Treatment Planner
The Personality Disorders Treatment Planner
The Rehabilitation Psychology Treatment Planner
The Special Education Treatment Planner
The Juvenile Justice and Residential Care Treatment Planner
The School Counseling and School Social Work Treatment Planner
The Sexual Abuse Victim and Sexual Offender Treatment Planner
The Probation and Parole Treatment Planner
The Psychopharmacology Treatment Planner
The Speech-Language Pathology Treatment Planner
The Suicide and Homicide Treatment Planner
The College Student Counseling Treatment Planner
The Parenting Skills Treatment Planner
The Early Childhood Intervention Treatment Planner
The Co-Occurring Disorders Treatment Planner
The Complete Women's Psychotherapy Treatment Planner

Progress Note Planners

The Child Psychotherapy Progress Notes Planner, Third Edition
The Adolescent Psychotherapy Progress Notes Planner, Third Edition
The Adult Psychotherapy Progress Notes Planner, Third Edition
The Addiction Progress Notes Planner, Second Edition
The Severe and Persistent Mental Illness Progress Notes Planner
The Couples Psychotherapy Progress Notes Planner
The Family Therapy Progress Notes Planner

Homework Planners

Brief Couples Therapy Homework Planner
Brief Employee Assistance Homework Planner
Brief Family Therapy Homework Planner
Grief Counseling Homework Planner
Group Therapy Homework Planner
Divorce Counseling Homework Planner
School Counseling and School Social Work Homework Planner
Child Therapy Activity and Homework Planner
Addiction Treatment Homework Planner, Third Edition
Adolescent Psychotherapy Homework Planner II
Adolescent Psychotherapy Homework Planner, Second Edition
Adult Psychotherapy Homework Planner, Second Edition
Child Psychotherapy Homework Planner, Second Edition
Parenting Skills Homework Planner

Client Education Handout Planners

Adult Client Education Handout Planner
Child and Adolescent Client Education Handout Planner
Couples and Family Client Education Handout Planner

Complete Planners

The Complete Depression Treatment and Homework Planner
The Complete Anxiety Treatment and Homework Planner

Practice*Planner*®

Arthur E. Jongsma, Jr., Series Editor

The Severe and Persistent Mental Illness Progress Notes Planner Second Edition

David J. Berghuis

Arthur E. Jongsma, Jr.

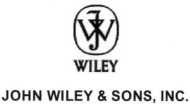

WILEY

JOHN WILEY & SONS, INC.

To my father, Donald W. Berghuis, with love.

—D. J. B.

To Justin David De Graaf and Carter Warren De Graaf, my grandsons, gifts from God, filled with promise.

—A. E. J.

CONTENTS

PRACTICE*PLANNERS*® SERIES PREFACE

The practice of psychotherapy has a dimension that did not exist 30, 20, or even 15 years ago—accountability. Treatment programs, public agencies, clinics, and even group and solo practitioners must now justify the treatment of patients to outside review entities that control the payment of fees. This development has resulted in an explosion of paperwork. Clinicians must now document what has been done in treatment, what is planned for the future, and what the anticipated outcomes of the interventions are. The books and software in this Practice*Planners*® series are designed to help practitioners fulfill these documentation requirements efficiently and professionally.

The Practice*Planners*® series is growing rapidly. It now includes not only the original *Complete Adult Psychotherapy Treatment Planner*, Fourth Edition, *The Child Psychotherapy Treatment Planner*, Fourth Edition, and *The Adolescent Psychotherapy Treatment Planner*, Fourth Edition, but also *Treatment Planners* targeted to specialty areas of practice, including: women, addictions, juvenile justice/residential care, couples therapy, employee assistance, behavioral medicine, therapy with older adults, pastoral counseling, family therapy, group therapy, psychopharmacology, neuropsychology, therapy with gays and lesbians, special education, school counseling, probation and parole, therapy with sexual abuse victims and offenders, and more.

Several of the *Treatment Planner* books now have companion *Progress Notes Planners* (e.g., Adult, Adolescent, Child, Addictions, Severe and Persistent Mental Illness, Couples). More of these planners that provide a menu of progress statements that elaborate on the client's symptom presentation and the provider's therapeutic intervention are in production. Each *Progress Notes Planner* statement is directly integrated with "Behavioral Definitions" and "Therapeutic Interventions" items from the companion *Treatment Planner*.

The list of therapeutic *Homework Planners* is also growing from the Homework Planner for Adults, to Adolescent, Child, Couples, Group, Family, Addictions, Divorce, Grief, Employee Assistance, and School Counseling/School Social Work Homework Planners. Each of these books can be used alone or in conjunction with their companion *Treatment Planner*. Homework assignments are designed around each presenting problem (e.g., Anxiety, Depression, Chemical Dependence, Anger Management, Panic, Eating Disorders) that is the focus of a chapter in its corresponding *Treatment Planner*.

Client Education Handout Planners, another branch in the series, provides brochures and handouts to help educate and inform adult, child, adolescent, couples, and family clients on a myriad of presenting problems mental health issues, as well as life skills techniques. The list of presenting problems for which information is provided mirrors the list of presenting problems in the *Treatment Planner* of the title similar to that of the *Handout Planner*. Thus, the problems for which educational material is provided in the *Child and Adolescent Client Education Handout Planner* reflect the presenting problems listed in *The Child* and *The Adolescent Psychotherapy*

Treatment Planner books. The handouts are included on CD-ROMs for easy printing from your computer and are ideal for use in waiting rooms, at presentations, as newsletters, or as information for clients struggling with mental illness issues.

In addition, the series also includes Thera*Scribe*®, the latest version of the popular treatment planning, clinical record-keeping software. Thera*Scribe* allows the user to import the data from any of the *Treatment Planner, Progress Notes Planner,* or *Homework Planner* books into the software's expandable database. Then the point-and-click method can create a detailed, neatly organized, individualized, and customized treatment plan along with optional integrated progress notes and homework assignments.

Adjunctive books, such as *The Psychotherapy Documentation Primer*, and *Clinical, Forensic, Child, Couples and Family, Continuum of Care,* and *Chemical Dependence Documentation Sourcebook,* contain forms and resources to aid the mental health practice management. The goal of the series is to provide practitioners with the resources they need in order to provide high-quality care in the era of accountability—or, to put it simply, we seek to help you spend more time on patients and less time on paperwork.

ARTHUR E. JONGSMA JR.
Grand Rapids, Michigan

ACKNOWLEDGMENTS

We need to thank many people who helped make this book a reality. The professional community that found these books to be so helpful has made it necessary for the series to be expanded, and this is the latest installment, making the Practice*Planners* a complete treatment package. So we thank the clinicians who find our books helpful. A special nod goes to the staff at Newaygo County Mental Health and Ionia County Community Mental Health Services, both in Michigan. We are indebted to the clients who have taught us so much about how to work with severe and persistent mental illness, and we thank them as well.

D. J. B.
A. E. J.

INTRODUCTION

ABOUT PRACTICE*PLANNERS*® PROGRESS NOTES

Progress notes are not only the primary source for documenting the therapeutic process, but also one of the main factors in determining the client's eligibility for reimbursable treatment. The purpose of the *Progress Notes Planner* series is to assist the practitioner in easily and quickly constructing progress notes that are thoroughly unified with the client's treatment plan.

Each *Progress Notes Planner:*

- Saves you hours of time-consuming paperwork.
- Offers the freedom to develop customized progress notes.
- Features over 1,000 prewritten progress notes summarizing patient presentation and treatment delivered.
- Provides an array of treatment approaches that correspond with the behavioral problems and *DSM-IV* diagnostic categories in the corresponding companion *Treatment Planner*.
- Offers sample progress notes that conform to the requirements of most third-party payors and accrediting agencies, including The Joint Commission (TJC), the Council on Accreditation (COA), the Commission Accreditation of Rehabilitation Facilities (CARF), and the National Committee for Quality Assurance (NCQA).

HOW TO USE THIS PROGRESS NOTES PLANNER

This *Progress Notes Planner* provides a menu of sentences that can be selected for constructing progress notes based on the behavioral definitions (or client's symptom presentation) and therapeutic interventions from its companion *Treatment Planner*. All progress notes must be tied to the patient's treatment plan. Session notes should elaborate on the problems, symptoms, and interventions contained in the plan.

Each chapter title is a reflection of the client's potential presenting problem. The first section of the chapter, "Client Presentation," provides a detailed menu of statements that may describe how that presenting problem manifested itself in behavioral signs and symptoms. The numbers in parentheses within the Client Presentation section correspond to the numbers of the Behavioral Definitions from the *Treatment Planner*.

The second section of each chapter, "Interventions Implemented," provides a menu of statements related to the action that was taken within the session to assist the client in making progress. The numbering of the items in the Interventions Implemented section follows exactly the numbering of Therapeutic Intervention items in the corresponding *Treatment Planner*.

All item lists begin with a few keywords. These words are meant to convey the theme or content of the sentences that are contained in that listing. The clinician may peruse the list of keywords to find content that matches the client's presentation and the clinician's intervention.

It is expected that the clinician may modify the prewritten statements contained in this book to fit the exact circumstances of the client's presentation and treatment. To maintain complete client records, in addition to progress note statements that may be selected and individualized from this book, the date, time, and length of a session; those present within the session; the provider; provider's credentials' and a signature must be entered in the client's record.

A FINAL NOTE ABOUT PROGRESS NOTES AND HIPAA

Federal regulations under the Health Insurance Portability and Accountability Act (HIPAA) govern the privacy of a client's psychotherapy notes, as well as other protected health information (PHI). PHI and psychotherapy notes must be kept secure, and the client must sign a specific authorization to release this confidential information to anyone beyond the client's therapist or treatment team. Further, psychotherapy notes receive other special treatment under HIPAA; for example, they may not be altered after they are initially drafted. Instead, the clinician must create and file formal amendments to the notes if he or she wishes to expand, delete, or otherwise change them. Our Thera*Scribe* software provides functionality to help clinicians maintain the proper rules concerning handling PHI, by giving the ability to lock progress notes once they are created, to acknowledge patient consent for the release of PHI, and to track amendments to psychotherapy notes over time.

Does the information contained in this book, when entered into a client's record as a progress note, qualify as a "psychotherapy note" and therefore merit confidential protection under HIPAA regulations? If the progress note that is created by selecting sentences from the database contained in this book is kept in a location separate from the client's PHI data, then the note could qualify as psychotherapy note data that is more protected than general PHI. However, because the sentences contained in this book convey generic information regarding the client's progress, the clinician may decide to keep the notes mixed in with the client's PHI and not consider it psychotherapy note data. In short, how you treat the information (separated from or integrated with PHI) can determine if this progress note planner data is psychotherapy note information. If you modify or edit these generic sentences to reflect more personal information about the client or you add sentences that contain confidential information, the argument for keeping these notes separate from PHI and treating them as psychotherapy notes becomes stronger. For some therapists, our sentences alone reflect enough personal information to qualify as psychotherapy notes, and they will keep these notes separate from the client's PHI and require specific authorization from the client to share them with a clearly identified recipient for a clearly identified purpose.

ACTIVITIES OF DAILY LIVING (ADL)

CLIENT PRESENTATION

1. Substandard Grooming and Hygiene (1)*

A. The client came to the session poorly groomed.

B. The client displayed poor grooming, as evidenced by strong body odor, disheveled hair, or dirty clothing.

C. Others have noted that the client displays substandard grooming and hygiene.

D. The client has begun to show an increased focus on his/her hygiene and grooming.

E. The client's hygiene and grooming have been appropriate, with clean clothing and no strong body odor.

2. Failure to Use Basic Hygiene Techniques (2)

A. The client gave evidence of a failure to use basic hygiene techniques, such as bathing, brushing his/her teeth, or washing his/her clothes.

B. When questioned about his/her basic hygiene techniques, the client reported that he/she rarely bathes, brushes his/her teeth, or washes his/her clothes.

C. The client has begun to bathe, brush his/her teeth, and dress himself/herself in clean clothes on a regular basis.

D. The client displayed increased personal care through the use of basic hygiene techniques.

3. Medical Problems (3)

A. The client's poor hygiene has caused specific medical problems.

B. The client is experiencing dental difficulties due to his/her poor hygiene.

C. Due to the client's poor personal hygiene, he/she is experiencing medical problems that put others at risk.

D. As the client has improved his/her personal hygiene, his/her medical problems have decreased.

4. Poor Diet (4)

A. Due to the client's inability to cook meals properly, he/she has experienced deficiencies in his/her diet.

B. The client makes poor food selections, which has caused deficiencies in his/her diet.

C. The client has displayed an increased understanding of and willingness to use a healthier diet.

D. As the client's diet has improved, his/her overall level of physical functioning has improved.

5. Impaired Reality Testing (5)

A. The client's impaired reality testing and bizarre behaviors cause problems with his/her performance of activities of daily living (ADL).

---

* The numbers in parentheses correlate to the number of the Behavioral Definition statement in the companion chapter with the same title in *The Severe and Persistent Mental Illness Treatment Planner,* 2nd ed. (Berghuis and Jongsma) by John Wiley & Sons, 2008.

B. The client's decreased reality testing causes him/her to have a decreased motivation to perform ADLs.

C. As the client has become more reality focused, his/her completion of ADLs has increased.

6. Social Skills Deficits (6)

A. The client displayed poor social interaction skills.

B. The client displayed poor eye contact, insufficient interpersonal attending, and awkward social responses.

C. As the client's severe and persistent mental illness symptoms have stabilized, his/her interaction skills have increased.

D. The client now displays more appropriate eye contact, interpersonal attending skills, and social responses.

7. Others Excuse Poor ADLs (7)

A. The client described a history of others excusing his/her poor performance on ADLs.

B. The client's family and friends rarely confront him/her on his/her poor performance on ADLs, as they believe this to be an inevitable component of his/her mental illness.

C. Friends and family members have become more direct with the client about giving feedback regarding his/her performance on ADLs.

D. The client's performance on ADLs has increased, as others have expected increased responsibility from him/her.

8. Inadequate Knowledge Regarding ADLs (8)

A. The client displayed an inadequate level of knowledge or functioning in basic skills around the home.

B. The client indicated that he/she has little experience in doing basic ADLs around the home (e.g., cleaning floors, washing dishes, disposing of garbage, keeping fresh food available).

C. As the client has gained specific knowledge about how to perform basic duties around the home, his/her ADLs have become more appropriate.

9. Losses Due to Poor Hygiene (9)

A. The client described that he/she has experienced loss of relationship, employment, or other social opportunities due to his/her poor hygiene and inadequate attention to grooming.

B. The client's family, friends, and employer have all indicated a decreased desire to be involved with him/her due to his/her poor hygiene and inadequate attention to grooming.

C. As the client's hygiene and grooming have improved, he/she has experienced improvement in relationships, employer acceptance, and other social opportunities.

INTERVENTIONS IMPLEMENTED

1. Prepare an Inventory of ADLs (1)*

A. The client was assisted in preparing an inventory of positive and negative functioning regarding his/her ADLs.

B. The client's inventory of positive and negative functioning regarding ADLs was reviewed within the session.

C. The client was given positive feedback regarding his/her accurate inventory of positive and negative functioning regarding ADLs.

D. The client has prepared his/her inventory of positive and negative functioning regarding ADLs but needed additional feedback to develop an accurate assessment.

E. The client has not prepared an inventory of positive and negative functioning regarding ADLs and was redirected to do so.

2. Assign Obtaining Feedback (2)

A. The client was asked to identify a trusted individual from whom he/she can obtain helpful feedback regarding daily hygiene and grooming.

B. The client has received helpful feedback regarding his/her daily hygiene and grooming, and this was reviewed within the session.

C. The client has declined to seek or use any feedback regarding his/her daily hygiene and grooming and was redirected to complete this assignment.

3. Review Diet (3)

A. The client's diet was reviewed.

B. The client was referred to a dietician for an assessment regarding basic nutritional knowledge and skills, usual diet, and nutritional deficiencies.

C. The client reported that he/she has met with the dietician, and the results of his/her assessment were reviewed.

D. The client displayed an understanding of his/her nutritional functioning as the assessment was reviewed.

E. The client displayed a lack of understanding about the information contained in the nutritional assessment and was provided with additional feedback in this area.

F. The client has not followed through on his/her referral to a dietician and was redirected to do so.

4. Review Rejection (4)

A. The client was asked to identify painful experiences in which rejection was experienced due to the lack of performance of basic ADLs.

B. The client was provided with empathy as he/she identified painful experiences in which rejection was experienced due to the lack of performance of basic ADLs.

C. The client's broken relationships, loss of employment, and other painful experiences were reviewed within the session.

---

* The numbers in parentheses correlate to the number of the Therapeutic Intervention statement in the companion chapter with the same title in *The Severe and Persistent Mental Illness Treatment Planner,* 2nd ed. (Berghuis and Jongsma) by John Wiley & Sons, 2008.

D. The client could not identify painful experiences related to poor performance of basic ADLs and was asked to continue to focus in these areas.

5. Review Medical Risks (5)

A. Specific medical risks associated with poor hygiene and nutrition or lack of attention to other ADLs were reviewed.

B. Medical risks (e.g., dental problems, risk of infection, lice, and other health problems) were identified and discussed.

C. The client was assisted in developing an understanding about the medical risks associated with poor nutrition and hygiene or lack of attention to other ADLs.

D. The client agreed that he/she is at a higher medical risk due to poor nutrition and hygiene or lack of attention to other ADLs and was focused on remediation efforts.

E. The client rejected the identified concerns regarding medical risks.

6. Facilitate Expressing Emotions (6)

A. The client was assisted in expressing his/her emotions related to impaired performance in ADLs.

B. The client was assisted in identifying specific emotions regarding impaired performance in ADLs (e.g., embarrassment, depression, and low self-esteem).

C. Empathy was provided to the client as he/she expressed his/her emotions regarding impaired performance in ADLs.

D. The client was reluctant to admit to any negative emotions regarding impaired performance of ADLs and was provided with feedback about likely emotions that he/she may experience.

7. Identify Secondary Gain (7)

A. The possible secondary gain associated with decreased ADL functioning was reviewed.

B. The client identified specific secondary gains that he/she has attained for decreased functioning in ADLs (e.g., less involvement in potentially difficult social situations), and these were reviewed within the session.

C. The client denied any pattern of secondary gain related to decreased functioning in his/her ADLs and was provided with hypothetical examples of the secondary gains.

8. Refer for Psychological Testing (8)

A. The client was referred for an assessment of cognitive abilities and deficits.

B. Objective psychological testing was administered to the client to assess his/her cognitive strengths and weaknesses.

C. The client cooperated with the psychological testing, and he/she received feedback about the results.

D. The psychological testing confirmed the presence of specific cognitive abilities and deficits.

E. The client was not compliant with taking the psychological evaluation and was encouraged to participate completely.

9. Recommend Remediating Programs (9)

A. The client was referred to remediating programs that are focused on removing deficits for performing ADLs, including skill-building groups, token economies, or behavior-shaping programs.

B. The client was assisted in remediating his/her deficits for performing ADLs through the use of skill-building groups, token economies, and behavior-shaping programs.

C. As specific programs have assisted the client in removing deficits for performing ADLs, his/her ADLs have gradually increased.

10. Educate about Mental Illness and Decompensation (10)

A. The client was educated about the expected or common symptoms of his/her mental illness, which may negatively impact basic ADL functioning.

B. As his/her symptoms of mental illness were discussed, the client displayed an understanding of how these symptoms may affect his/her ADL functioning.

C. The client's poor performance on ADLs was interpreted as an indicator of psychiatric decompensation.

D. The client's pattern of poor ADLs and psychiatric decompensation was shared with the client, caregivers, and medical staff.

E. The client acknowledged his/her poor performance on ADLs as prodromals of his/her psychiatric decompensation, and this was supported during the session.

F. The client, caregivers, and medical staff concurred regarding the client's general psychiatric decompensation.

G. The client denied psychiatric decompensation, despite being told that his/her poor performance on ADLs is an indication of psychiatric decompensation.

11. Refer to a Physician (11)

A. The client was referred to a physician for an evaluation for a prescription of psychotropic medications.

B. The client was reinforced for following through on a referral to a physician for an assessment for a prescription of psychotropic medications, but none were prescribed.

C. The client has been prescribed psychotropic medications.

D. The client declined evaluation by a physician for a prescription of psychotropic medications and was redirected to cooperate with this referral.

12. Educate about Psychotropic Medications (12)

A. The client was taught about the indications for and the expected benefits of psychotropic medications.

B. As the client's psychotropic medications were reviewed, he/she displayed an understanding about the indications for and expected benefits of the medications.

C. The client displayed a lack of understanding of the indications for and expected benefits of psychotropic medications and was provided with additional information and feedback regarding his/her medications.

13. Monitor Medications (13)

A. The client was monitored for compliance with his/her psychotropic medication regimen.

B. The client was provided with positive feedback about his/her regular use of psychotropic medications.

C. The client was monitored for the effectiveness and side effects of his/her prescribed medications.

D. Concerns about the effectiveness and side effects of the client's medications were communicated to the physician.

E. Although the client was monitored for side effects from the medications, he/she reported no concerns in this area.

14. Organize Medications (14)

A. The client was provided with a pillbox for organizing and coordinating each dose of his/her medications.

B. The client was taught about the proper use of the medication compliance packaging/reminder system.

C. The client was tested on his/her understanding of the use of the medication compliance packaging/reminder system.

D. The client was provided with positive feedback about his/her regular use of the pillbox to organize his/her medications.

E. The client has not used the pillbox to organize his/her medications and was redirected to do so.

15. Coordinate Medication Compliance Oversight (15)

A. Family members and/or caregivers were instructed on how to regularly dispense and/or monitor the client's medication compliance.

B. Family members and/or caregivers indicated an understanding of how to monitor the client's medication compliance.

C. The client's medication compliance was reviewed, and family members and/or caregivers indicated that he/she is regularly medication compliant.

D. Family members and/or caregivers indicated that the client is not medication compliant, and this was reviewed with the client.

16. Arrange for a Physical Examination (16)

A. A full physical examination was arranged for the client, and the physician was encouraged to prescribe remediation programs to aid the client in performing ADLs.

B. A physician examined the client, and specific negative medical effects of low functioning on ADLs were identified.

C. The physician has identified specific recommendations to help remediate the effects of the client's poor ADL skills.

D. The physician has not identified any physical effects related to the client's poor performance on ADLs.

E. Specific ADL remediation behaviors were reviewed with the client.

17. Refer to a Dentist (17)

A. The client was referred to a dentist to determine dental treatment needs.

B. Specific dental treatment needs were identified, and ongoing dental treatment was coordinated.

C. No specific dental treatment needs were identified, but a routine follow-up appointment was made.

D. The client has not followed through on the referral for dental services and was redirected to do so.

18. Provide Educational Material (18)

A. The client was provided with educational material to help him/her learn basic personal hygiene skills.

B. The client was referred to specific portions of books and videos on the topic of personal hygiene.

C. The client was referred to written material such as *The Complete Guide to Better Dental Care* (Taintor and Taintor) or *The New Wellness Encyclopedia* (Editors of University of California-Berkeley).

D. The client has surveyed the educational material, and important points were reviewed within the session.

E. The client has not reviewed the educational material and was requested to do so.

19. Refer for One-to-One Training (19)

A. The client was referred to the agency medical staff for one-to-one training in basic hygiene needs and techniques.

B. The client has reviewed specific hygiene needs and techniques with the agency medical staff and was supported for this.

C. The client has not yet met with agency medical staff for one-to-one training in basic hygiene needs and techniques and was redirected to do so.

20. Refer to a Psychoeducational Group (20)

A. The client was referred to a psychoeducational group focused on teaching personal hygiene skills.

B. The psychoeducational group was used to help the client learn to give and receive feedback about hygiene skill implementation.

C. The client has attended a psychoeducational group and received feedback about hygiene skill implementation, which was processed within the session.

D. The client was verbally reinforced for using the group feedback about hygiene skill implementation.

E. The client has not attended the psychoeducational group for hygiene skill implementation and was redirected to do so.

21. Encourage Scheduled Hygiene Performance (21)

A. The client was encouraged to perform basic hygiene skills on a regular schedule (e.g., the same time and in the same order each day).

B. The client was reinforced for his/her pattern of performing basic hygiene skills on a regular schedule.

C. The client has not performed his/her personal hygiene skills on a scheduled basis and was redirected to do so.

22. Refer to Behavioral Treatment (22)

A. The client was referred to a behavioral treatment specialist to develop and implement a program to monitor and reward the regular use of ADL techniques.

B. An individualized behavioral treatment plan has been developed to monitor and reward the client's regular use of ADL techniques.

C. As the client has increased his/her regular use of ADL techniques, he/she has earned rewards within the behavioral treatment plan.

D. The client's increased completion of ADLs through the use of a behavioral treatment plan was reviewed.

E. The client was assisted in developing a self-monitoring program for performing his/her ADLs.

F. The client has resisted compliance with a behavioral treatment plan to monitor and reward the regular use of his/her ADL techniques and was redirected to do so.

23. Provide Feedback (23)

A. The client was provided with feedback about progress in his/her use of self-monitoring to improve personal hygiene.

B. The client appeared to react positively to the feedback that was given regarding his/her progress in the use of self-monitoring to improve performance of ADLs.

C. The client accepted the negative feedback that was given regarding his/her lack of use of self-monitoring to improve personal hygiene.

24. Review Community Resources (24)

A. A list of community resources was reviewed with the client to assist him/her in improving his/her personal appearance (e.g., laundromat/dry cleaner, hair salon/barber).

B. As community resources were reviewed, the client displayed an understanding and commitment to use appropriate community resources.

C. The client has not used community resources to improve his/her personal appearance and was provided with additional encouragement to do so.

25. Arrange for a Tour of Community Resources (25)

A. Arrangements were made for the client to tour community facilities for cleaning and pressing clothes, cutting and styling hair, or purchasing soap and deodorant.

B. As the community resources were reviewed, the client showed an increased understanding of how these resources can be used to improve performance of ADLs.

C. The client continued to display a lack of understanding about the use of community facilities to assist in performing ADLs, and this information was reiterated.

26. Assess for Substance Abuse (26)

A. The client was assessed for substance abuse that may exacerbate poor performance in ADLs.

B. The client was identified as having a concomitant substance abuse problem.

C. Upon review, the client does not display evidence of a substance abuse problem.

27. Refer for Substance Abuse Treatment (27)

A. The client was referred to a 12-step recovery program (e.g., Alcoholics Anonymous or Narcotics Anonymous).

B. The client was referred to a substance abuse treatment program.

C. The client has been admitted to a substance abuse treatment program and was supported for this follow-through.

D. The client has refused the referral to a substance abuse treatment program, and this refusal was processed.

28. Teach Housekeeping Skills (28)

A. The client was taught about basic housekeeping skills through references to books on this subject.

B. As the client has been taught basic housekeeping skills, he/she has displayed an increased understanding of these needs and techniques.

C. The client continues to display a lack of understanding of basic housekeeping skills, and this information was presented again in a different fashion.

29. Provide Cleaning Feedback (29)

A. The client was given feedback about the care of his/her personal area, apartment, or home.

B. The client appeared to be reinforced by the positive feedback that he/she has received about his/her personal area, apartment, or home.

C. The client was given negative feedback, which prompted him/her to pledge to improve his/her personal area, apartment, or home.

30. Encourage Family Members and/or Caregivers to Assign Chores (30)

A. The client's family members and/or caregivers were encouraged to provide regular assignment to the client of basic chores around the home.

B. Family members and/or caregivers were reinforced for having provided regular assignment of basic chores around the home.

C. Family members and/or caregivers have not provided regular assignment of basic chores around the home and were redirected to do so.

31. Teach Cooking Techniques (31)

A. The client was taught some basic cooking techniques.

B. Cookbooks were used to teach the client basic cooking techniques.

C. As the client has been taught about basic cooking techniques, he/she has displayed an increased understanding of food preparation.

D. The client displayed a lack of understanding of food preparation procedures and was provided with additional remedial information in this area.

32. Refer/Conduct a Dietary Group (32)

A. The client was referred to a psychoeducational group focused on teaching cooking skills and dietary needs.

B. The client displayed an increased understanding of dietary needs and cooking skills as a result of involvement in the psychoeducational group.

C. The client has not attended the psychoeducational group focused on teaching cooking skills and dietary needs and was redirected to do so.

33. Facilitate a Community Education Class (33)

A. The client's enrollment in a community education cooking class or seminar was facilitated.

B. The client was supported for his/her regular attendance to a community education cooking class or seminar.

C. The client has not regularly attended the community education class or seminar, and his/her irregular attendance was processed to resolution.

34. Review for Safety Hazards (34)

A. The client's living situation was inspected for potential safety hazards.

B. The client has identified potential safety hazards and these were reviewed.

C. The client was assisted in remediating his/her potential safety hazards in his/her home.

D. The client has not remediated his/her potential home safety hazards and was redirected to do so.

35. Assist in Advocating Resolution of Safety Hazards (35)

A. The client was assisted with requests to the appropriate parties (landlord, home providers, or family members) to remediate home safety hazards.

B. The client was supported in his/her advocacy to remediate home safety hazards, insect infestations, and other concerns that would confound ADLs.

C. The client has not appropriately advocated for himself/herself regarding seeking resolution of home safety hazards, and he/she was given additional direction in this area.

36. Facilitate Involvement in Programs for Safety Equipment (36)

A. Arrangements were made for the client to become involved in programs that assist him/her in procuring safety equipment (e.g., free smoke or carbon monoxide detectors).

B. The client was provided with support for his/her pursuit of programs that assist with procuring safety equipment.

C. The client has not used programs to assist himself/herself with procuring needed safety equipment and was directed to follow up on this.

37. Teach about High-Risk Sexual Behaviors (37)

A. The client was taught about high-risk sexual behaviors.

B. The client was referred to a free condom program to decrease the risk in his/her sexual behaviors.

C. The client's understanding of his/her high-risk sexual behaviors and how to remediate these concerns was reviewed.

D. The client has implemented precautions to decrease his/her risk of sexually transmitted disease and was provided with positive feedback for these changes.

E. The client does not appear to understand or use appropriate precautions regarding his/her high-risk sexual behaviors and was reeducated about these issues.

38. Teach Remediation of High-Risk Drug Use Behaviors (38)

A. The client was taught about the serious risk that is involved with sharing needles for drug abuse.

B. The client was referred to a needle exchange program.

C. The client was referred to a substance abuse treatment program.

D. The client reported a decreased pattern of high-risk drug abuse behaviors and was provided with positive reinforcement for this change.

E. The client has not used techniques to decrease his/her high-risk drug abuse behaviors and was redirected to do so.

39. Assist in Developing Intervention Plans (39)

A. The client was assisted in developing intervention plans to avoid injury, poisoning, or other self-care problems during periods of mania, psychosis, or other decompensation.

B. The client reiterated specific procedures to obtain assistance when decompensating, including calling a treatment hotline, contacting a therapist or physician, or going to the hospital emergency department, and was supported for his/her plan.

C. The client displayed an understanding of his/her crisis intervention plan and was provided with positive feedback and reminders in this area.

D. The client has not developed a crisis intervention plan and was provided with more direct information in this area.

AGING

CLIENT PRESENTATION

1. Advanced Age (1)*

A. As the client has grown older, he/she has become more dependent on others.

B. The client's advanced age has exacerbated his/her severe and persistent mental illness concerns.

C. The client displayed denial regarding the effects of aging on his/her ability to function independently.

D. The effects of the client's advanced age have been ameliorated through the use of an enhanced support network and greater supervision.

2. Decreased Intensity of Symptoms (2)

A. As the client has advanced in age, he/she has reported a gradual decrease in the intensity of his/her severe and persistent mental illness symptoms.

B. The client's overall level of functioning has gradually increased as he/she has aged.

C. As the client has aged, he/she displays less intense thought disorder symptoms and more ability to control his/her symptoms.

3. Cognitive Decline (3)

A. The client presented with clear evidence of impaired abstract thinking and a tendency to think in a rather concrete manner.

B. The client showed evidence of short- and long-term memory deficits.

C. The client displayed periods of confusion.

D. The client has struggled to learn new information.

E. As the client has complied with treatment approaches, he/she has reported an amelioration of his/her cognitive difficulties.

4. Loss of Social Support System (4)

A. The client reported that he/she has been losing his/her support system due to the infirmity or death of members of his/her family of origin and friends.

B. Individuals whom the client has regularly relied upon have been less capable of providing support to the client.

C. The client has begun to develop a new social support system.

5. Little Interest from Offspring (5)

A. The client reported that he/she receives little or no support or attention from his/her children.

B. The client's children identified that they struggle with providing support for the client due to his/her long history of severe and persistent mental illness.

---

* The numbers in parentheses correlate to the number of the Behavioral Definition statement in the companion chapter with the same title in *The Severe and Persistent Mental Illness Treatment Planner,* 2nd ed. (Berghuis and Jongsma) by John Wiley & Sons, 2008.

C. As the client has improved the relationship with his/her children, he/she has enjoyed increased support from them.

6. Serious Medical Condition (6)

A. The client presented with serious medical problems related to his/her advanced age that are having a negative impact on daily living.

B. The client has pursued treatment for his/her medical condition.

C. The client has refused treatment for his/her medical condition.

D. The client has not sought treatment for his/her medical condition because of a lack of insurance and financial resources.

E. The client's serious medical condition is now under treatment and is showing signs of improvement.

7. Medication Side Effects (7)

A. The client displayed specific physical deficits due to long-term use of psychotropic medications (e.g., tardive dyskinesia).

B. The client displayed tremors, grimaces, twitches, and involuntary vocal tics due to the long-term use of psychotropic medications.

C. The client expressed concern about continued use of psychotropic medications due to the long-term physical deficits he/she has experienced.

D. Medication adjustment has assisted in reducing the effects of the long-term use of psychotropic medications.

8. Spiritual Confusion (8)

A. The client reported concerns about spiritual confusion due to uncertainty about the meaning or purpose in life and fears surrounding mortality issues.

B. The client's severe and persistent mental illness issues have confounded his/her attempts to find meaning or purpose in life.

C. The client has sought out spiritual guidance to help resolve concerns about mortality issues and the meaning and purpose of his/her life.

D. The client reported that he/she has become more at peace due to involvement in spiritual activities.

9. Decreased ADLs/IADLs (9)

A. The client has displayed a decreased ability to perform activities of daily living (ADLs) (e.g., personal hygiene needs, caring for home, meal preparation) due to his/her advanced age.

B. The client reported that he/she has had to decrease his/her independent activities of daily living (IADLs); (e.g., grocery shopping, other activities within the community) due to his/her age-related infirmities.

C. As treatment has progressed, the client has identified ways to modify his/her performance of ADLs/IADLs and is now performing these more regularly.

D. The client has received support for his/her performance of ADLs/IADLs and is performing these more regularly.

10. Suicidal Ideation (10)

A. The client reported experiencing recent suicidal ideation but denied having any specific plan to implement suicidal urges.

B. The client reported ongoing suicidal ideation and has developed a specific plan for suicide.

C. The frequency and intensity of the client's suicidal urges have diminished.

D. The client was admitted to a psychiatric facility because he/she had a specific suicide plan and strong suicidal urges.

E. The client stated that he/she has not experienced any recent suicidal ideation.

11. Abuse Vulnerability (11)

A. The client displayed increased vulnerability to sexual, physical, and psychological abuse due to his/her age-related limitations.

B. The client reported an increased exposure to sexual, physical, or psychological abuse.

C. The client's vulnerability to abuse has declined as he/she has developed better coping mechanisms.

D. The client reported feeling safer regarding the potential of being subjected to sexual, physical, or psychological abuse.

12. Anger Outbursts (12)

A. The client has displayed anger outbursts due to his/her frustration over age-related declining abilities.

B. The client often vents his/her anger in an inappropriate manner when he/she experiences the effects of his/her aging.

C. As treatment has progressed, the client has developed better frustration coping mechanisms and has decreased his/her pattern of anger outbursts.

D. The client does not often display anger outbursts.

INTERVENTIONS IMPLEMENTED

1. Identify Aging Issues and Fears (1)*

A. The client was requested to identify negative situations that have occurred due to aging issues.

B. The client was requested to list fears about concerns related to aging issues.

C. Empathic listening was used as the client discussed his/her fears about concerns related to aging issues.

D. The client received support and encouragement as he/she identified some of the concerns that have occurred due to his/her advancing age.

E. The client did not clearly identify concerns or fears related to aging issues and was redirected to review these areas.

2. Provide Aging Information (2)

A. The client was provided with general information regarding the aging process.

---

* The numbers in parentheses correlate to the number of the Therapeutic Intervention statement in the companion chapter with the same title in *The Severe and Persistent Mental Illness Treatment Planner,* 2nd ed. (Berghuis and Jongsma) by John Wiley & Sons, 2008.

B. The client was encouraged to read books on the aging process (e.g., *The Practical Guide to Aging* by Cassel or *Alzheimer's and Dementia: Questions You Have . . . Answers You Need* by Hay).

C. The client has read material regarding the aging process, and this was discussed within the clinical contact.

D. The client has not read material regarding the aging process and was redirected to do so.

3. Clarify Emotions (3)

A. The client was encouraged to share his/her emotions regarding aging issues (e.g., fear of abandonment, sadness regarding loss of abilities).

B. The client has continued to share his/her feelings and has been assisted in identifying causes for them.

C. Distorted cognitive messages contribute to the client's emotional response.

D. The client demonstrated a sad affect and tearfulness when describing his/her feelings.

E. As the client has developed better coping mechanisms, he/she reports a decrease in his/her feelings of abandonment and sadness.

4. Teach Healthy Anger Expression (4)

A. The client was taught about healthy ways to express anger (e.g., using writing, drawing, or the empty-chair technique).

B. Writing, drawing, and the empty-chair technique have been helpful in allowing the client to express feelings of anger, hurt, or sadness.

C. The client appeared uncomfortable with the use of anger expression techniques, had difficulty verbalizing his/her angry emotions, and was provided with additional encouragement in this area.

5. Coordinate Caregiver Training (5)

A. Training was coordinated for caregivers in techniques of physical management and diffusion of the client's anger.

B. The caregivers have been trained in physical management and anger diffusion techniques.

C. Caregivers have used physical management and anger diffusion techniques to assist the client in decreasing his/her angry outbursts.

6. List Benefits of Aging Process (6)

A. The client was asked to prepare a list of benefits that are related to the aging process.

B. The client was provided with support and feedback as he/she shared his/her list of benefits that are related to the aging process (e.g., decreased work expectations, new residential opportunities).

C. The client denied any benefits that are related to the aging process and was redirected to these areas.

7. Provide Information Regarding Aging and Mental Illness (7)

A. The client was provided with specific information about the impact of the aging process on his/her mental illness.

B. The tendency for severe and persistent mental illness symptoms to decrease in intensity as an individual ages was presented and discussed.

C. The client described his/her own pattern of decreased mental illness symptoms as he/she has aged.

D. The client denied that he/she has experienced a pattern of decreased mental illness symptoms as he/she has aged.

8. Referral for a Physical Evaluation (8)

A. The client was referred for a complete physical evaluation by a medical professional who is knowledgeable in both geriatric and mental illness concerns.

B. The client has completed his/her physical evaluation, and the results of this evaluation were processed.

C. The client has not submitted to a physical evaluation and was redirected to do so.

9. Support and Monitor Physical Evaluation Recommendations (9)

A. The client was supported in following up on the recommendations from the medical evaluation.

B. The client's follow-up on the recommendations from the medical evaluation have been monitored.

C. The client was reinforced for following up on the recommendations from the medical evaluation.

D. The client has not regularly followed up on his/her medical evaluation recommendations and was redirected to do so.

10. Assist in Physical Health Needs Expression (10)

A. The client was taught how to express his/her physical health needs to the medical staff.

B. The client's bizarre descriptions of his/her physical health problems were "translated" to the medical staff to assist in providing more clear communication.

C. Role playing was used to practice asking questions of or reporting concerns to the medical staff.

D. The client has provided more information to the medical staff as a result of more assertive and clear expression of needs.

E. The client continues to fail to express his/her physical health needs to the medical staff and was given additional direction.

11. Interpret and Investigate Decompensation (11)

A. The client's psychiatric decompensation was interpreted as a possible reaction to medical instability and the stress that is associated with it.

B. As the client has decompensated psychiatrically, inquiries have been made about his/her medical needs.

C. The client accepted the interpretation that he/she is struggling with medical concerns, feels more stressed, and has been decompensating psychiatrically due to these problems.

D. The client denied any medical difficulties that have led to his/her psychiatric decompensation, and he/she was given further education in this area.

12. Obtain and Review Physical Health Information (12)

A. Having procured the necessary authorization from the client to release confidential material, information was obtained about the physical health concerns that he/she experiences.

B. The physician has provided information about the client's physical health, and this was reviewed with him/her.

C. The client's physical health report has not been received from the physician, so an additional request for information was sent.

D. Health concerns and recovery needs were reviewed with the client on a regular basis.

E. The client was asked specific questions about his/her understanding of his/her recovery needs and health concerns.

F. The client was provided with positive feedback as he/she displayed understanding of his/her physical health concerns.

G. The client has continued to display poor understanding of his/her physical health concerns, and these data were reviewed again.

13. Refer to a Physician (13)

A. The client was referred to a physician for an evaluation for a prescription of psychotropic medications.

B. The client was reinforced for following through on a referral to a physician for an assessment for a prescription of psychotropic medications, but none were prescribed.

C. The client has been prescribed psychotropic medications.

D. The client declined evaluation by a physician for a prescription of psychotropic medications and was redirected to cooperate with this referral.

14. Educate about Psychotropic Medications (14)

A. The client was taught about the indications for and the expected benefits of his/her psychotropic medications.

B. As the client's psychotropic medications were reviewed, he/she displayed an understanding about the indications for and expected benefits of the medications.

C. The client displayed a lack of understanding of the indications for and expected benefits of psychotropic medications and was provided with additional information and feedback regarding his/her medications.

D. The client was monitored for compliance with his/her psychotropic medication regimen.

E. The client was provided with positive feedback about his/her regular use of psychotropic medications.

F. Concerns about the effectiveness and side effects of the client's medications were communicated to the physician.

G. Although the client was monitored for side effects from the medications, he/she reported no concerns in this area.

15. Assess Ability to Adhere to Medication Regimen (15)

A. The client was assessed regarding his/her ability to regularly adhere to his/her medication regimen.

B. The client was asked about the times, dosages, and types of medications he/she should be taking.

C. The client's ongoing use of his/her medications was closely monitored to make certain that he/she was adhering to his/her medication regimen.

D. The client was provided with positive feedback as he/she displayed the ability to adhere to his/her medication regimen.

E. The client displayed a lack of understanding about his/her medications, has failed to adhere to his/her medication regimen, and was directed to have others dispense his/her medications to him/her.

16. Organize and Monitor Medications (16)

A. The client was provided with a pillbox for organizing and coordinating each dose of his/her medications.

B. The client was taught about the proper use of the medication compliance packaging/reminder system; he/she was tested on his/her understanding of the use of the medication compliance packaging/reminder system.

C. The client was provided with positive feedback about his/her regular use of the pillbox to organize his/her medications.

D. The client has not used the pillbox to organize his/her medications and was redirected to do so.

E. The number of pills left in the client's prescription of psychotropic medications was counted and compared with the expected amount that should remain.

F. Discrepancies within the expected and actual amounts of medications remaining were reviewed with the client and medical staff.

G. The client's remaining medications correspond with the amount expected to remain, and this was reviewed with the client.

17. Coordinate/Facilitate Multiple Physicians' Communication (17)

A. Authorizations from the client to release confidential information were obtained so that multiple physicians can communicate with each other regarding the medications that are prescribed.

B. The client's physicians were contacted regarding the use of multiple medications and encouraged to consult with each other regarding the client's overall medication needs.

C. The client declined to provide authorizations to release confidential information for his/her multiple physicians.

D. The client's multiple physicians worked together to provide a coordinated review of his/her complete medication regime.

E. Specific changes in the client's medication regime were instituted after his/her multiple physicians conferred.

F. No changes have been made subsequent to the client's multiple physicians conferring.

G. The client's multiple physicians have not been in regular contact to review his/her variety of medications.

18. Evaluate and Develop Support for ADLs/IADLs (18)

A. The client's overall level of functioning in ADLs and IADLs were evaluated, identifying strengths, weaknesses, and expected future levels of functioning.

B. Concerns about the client's ability to perform his/her ADLs and IADLs in the future were identified.

C. Specific supports were developed for helping the client to maintain his/her ADLs and IADLs.

D. Contact was made with the family, community resources, and staff to assist them in developing support treatment for the client's ADLs and IADLs.

19. Review Hearing and Vision Needs (19)

A. An increase in the client's auditory and visual hallucinations was noted, not accompanied by other severe and persistent mental illness symptoms, which triggered a review of his/her hearing and vision needs.

B. The client reported difficulties relating to hearing and vision, and exams in these areas were coordinated.

C. Upon inquiry, the client denied any pattern of hearing or vision concerns.

20. Refer for Vision/Hearing Exams (20)

A. The client was referred to an audiologist for a clinical assessment of his/her hearing abilities.

B. The client was referred to an ophthalmologist for a specific evaluation of his/her vision needs.

C. Expert clinical review of the client's hearing and vision indicated deficits in these areas, as well as suggestions for remediation.

D. No concerns were identified through the expert clinical evaluations of hearing and vision.

21. Refer to Supervised Residence (21)

A. The client was referred to an appropriate supervised residential care center.

B. The client agreed with the referral to a supervised residential care center.

C. The client has been accepted at a supervised residential care center.

D. The client has refused to accept a referral to an appropriate residential care center and was given additional encouragement to do so.

22. Advocate with Housing Programs (22)

A. Advocacy was performed with age-appropriate housing programs to assist the housing program in accepting the client and to provide needed adaptations for him/her.

B. Training was provided to the housing program staff to assist them in adapting to the client's needs.

C. Housing staff were trained about the client's symptoms, prodromals, and treatment techniques used for him/her.

D. Housing staff displayed an increased understanding and comfort level with the client after receiving training.

E. Despite advocacy, the housing program has been reluctant to accept the client.

23. Differentiate Hospitalization and Age-Appropriate Residence (23)

A. The client's history of institutionalization was reviewed with him/her.

B. The client was taught the difference between his/her previous psychiatric hospitalizations and a relatively restrictive residential placement due to aging concerns.

C. The client's hard-won independence from restrictive psychiatric settings was acknowledged, and the restrictive residence due to aging was differentiated from the restrictive psychiatric setting.

D. The client displayed understanding and acceptance of the more restrictive residential placement due to aging concerns.

E. The client continues to balk at the suggestion of a more restrictive residential placement due to aging concerns and was redirected in this area.

24. Empathize Regarding Losses (24)

A. The client's history of significant losses due to death, geographical move, aging, or physical/mental disability was reviewed.

B. The client was provided with support and empathy as he/she expressed feelings regarding his/her history of losses.

C. The client was reluctant to express his/her emotions regarding his/her pattern of loss but was encouraged to do so.

25. Educate about Grief and Mental Illness (25)

A. The client was educated about the typical pattern of grief.

B. The client was educated about how the grief process may impact his/her severe and persistent mental illness symptoms.

C. The client failed to understand the effect of the grief process on his/her severe and persistent mental illness symptoms, and this information was reviewed again.

26. Refer for Individual/Group Therapy (26)

A. The client was referred for individual therapy to work through the grief associated with his/her losses.

B. The client has followed through on participating in individual therapy focused on grief and was provided with reinforcement for this.

C. The client was referred to a support group for grief and loss issues.

D. The client was referred to a support group for chronic mental illness concerns.

E. The client has become involved in a support group and reports that this is helpful.

F. The client has not followed through on the referral to therapy and was encouraged to do so.

27. Develop Social Skills (27)

A. The client was assisted in developing social skills.

B. The client was provided with positive support as he/she displayed increased social skills.

C. The client has struggled to develop social skills and was provided with additional feedback in this area.

28. Coordinate Social Activities (28)

A. The client was linked to age-appropriate social activities.

B. The client has become more involved in age-appropriate social activities and was given positive reinforcement for these choices.

C. The client has refused involvement in age-appropriate social activities and was redirected to investigate available options.

29. Refer to a Recreational Therapist (29)

A. The client was referred to a recreational therapist for an evaluation of recreational abilities, needs, and opportunities.

B. The client has followed through with the recommendation to see a recreational therapist, and the results of this evaluation have been shared with the client.

C. The client has not followed through on the referral to a recreational therapist and was redirected to do so.

30. Focus on Self-Regulation (30)

A. The client was focused on the need to regulate his/her own social involvement depending on his/her needs and symptoms.

B. The client identified that he/she varies the frequency and intensity of social contacts in order to modulate his/her stress level and was given feedback about this technique.

C. The client reported a decreased stress level due to his/her modulation of social contact, and the success of this was reviewed.

D. The client reported that he/she does not modulate his/her social involvement depending on his/her needs and symptoms and was redirected to use this technique.

31. Identify New Opportunities (31)

A. The client was assisted in identifying activities in which he/she can now be engaged as his/her psychotic symptoms have gradually abated.

B. The client listed many activities in which he/she wishes to engage as psychotic symptoms have gradually abated, and this list was reviewed.

C. The client failed to identify activities in which he/she wishes to engage as his/her mental illness symptoms lessen and was given additional feedback in this area.

32. Identify Relationships to Restore (32)

A. The client was requested to identify important relationships that he/she would like to restore.

B. The client declined to identify any relationships that he/she would like to restore and was given additional feedback in this area.

33. Develop a Plan for Restoring Relationships (33)

A. The client was assisted in developing a specific plan for restoring relationships.

B. The client has implemented his/her plan for restoring relationships, and this was reviewed.

C. The client has struggled to identify how he/she wishes to restore relationships and was given additional feedback in this area.

34. Provide Information to Family and Caregivers (34)

A. The family and caregivers were provided with adequate information and training relative to the client's mental illness, physical health, and aging concerns.

B. The family and caregivers were recommended to read material regarding coping with providing care to someone with severe mental illness.

C. Specific books were recommended to the client's family and caregivers (e.g., *Surviving Schizophrenia* by Torrey or *Helping Someone with Mental Illness* by Carter and Golant).

D. Family members and caregivers were assisted in processing the information and training that has been provided regarding the client's mental illness, physical health, and aging concerns.

E. The family and caregivers continued to struggle with the client's mental illness, physical health, and aging concerns and were provided with additional feedback in these areas.

35. Empathize with the Caregiver (35)

A. The caregiver was allowed to vent about difficulties that are related to supervising the client.

B. Empathy was displayed as the caregiver was focused on making a commitment for continued care.

C. The caregiver was assisted in developing alternative plans for the client's care.

D. The caregiver was confronted when he/she began to deride the client.

36. Educate the Caregiver and Family Members (36)

A. The client's caregivers and family members were educated about programs, techniques, and options for caring for older adults.

B. The client's caregivers and family members were referred to guidebooks regarding caring for older adults.

C. The client's caregivers and family members were referred to specific materials (e.g., *Coping with Your Difficult Older Parent* by Lebow, Cane, and Lebow) regarding caring for older adults.

D. The client's caregivers and family members were assisted in processing key concepts from their reading and learning about how to care for older adults.

37. Assess Elder Abuse (37)

A. The client was assessed for whether he/she has been a victim of elder abuse in any form.

B. Concerns related to abuse of the client were identified, and immediate steps were taken to secure his/her safety.

C. Elder abuse was suspected, and the appropriate adult protective services agency has been informed.

D. There is no evidence that the client has been a victim of elder abuse in any form.

E. The client was gently, empathetically probed for his/her emotional reaction to being the victim of abuse.

F. The client was cautious and defensive about describing his/her emotional reaction to his/her abuse and was provided with support and feedback in this area.

G. The client struggled to identify and coherently express his/her emotions regarding the abuse done to him/her and was provided with support and feedback in this area.

38. Facilitate Changes to Stop Abuse (38)

A. The client was assisted in making specific changes related to his/her residence in order to immediately terminate the abuse he/she has suffered.

B. The client was assisted in making changes in the programs in which he/she is involved to terminate the abuse that has occurred to him/her within those programs.

C. The client was assisted in making any necessary changes to assist in terminating the abuse he/she has been experiencing.

D. The client has failed to make changes to help terminate the abuse and was redirected and assisted to make these changes.

E. Applicable abuse reporting procedures as outlined in local law were followed regarding the suspected or identified elder abuse.

F. Agency guidelines were followed regarding the suspected or identified elder abuse.

G. Peer or supervisory support was obtained regarding reporting suspected or confirmed elder abuse.

39. Educate about Elder Abuse (39)

A. The client and caregivers were assisted in defining and identifying elder abuse.

B. The client and caregivers were provided specific information about steps to take if they identify elder abuse.

C. The client and caregiver were supported for displaying an understanding of the definition and criteria for elder abuse and how to respond.

D. The client and caregiver continue to be confused and uncertain about the concepts related to elder abuse and were provided with additional feedback in this area.

40. Advocate Change in Guardian/Payee (40)

A. The client was urged to request a change in his/her legal guardian or payee procedures in order to stem financial abuse.

B. The court was petitioned for a change in the client's legal guardian status in order to stem financial abuse.

C. The client's legal guardian or payee procedures have been changed in an effort to discontinue the financial abuse.

D. The client declined to make any changes in his/her legal guardian or payee procedures and was redirected to do so.

41. Review Specialized Needs Due to Physical Deterioration (41)

A. The focus of today's clinical contact was on the client's specialized needs that he/she will face due to the natural deterioration of physical capabilities that are associated with aging.

B. The client was reinforced for displaying an understanding of the specialized needs that he/she will require due to his/her physical decompensation due to aging.

C. The client does not appear to understand or accept the specialized needs that he/she may experience due to his/her natural deterioration of physical capabilities and was provided with additional feedback in this area.

42. Coordinate Information Regarding Programs (42)

A. The client was provided with information regarding residential or other programs that are available to him/her as he/she ages.

B. The client was assisted with a tour of residential programs that are available to him/her as he/she ages.

C. The client was reinforced for displaying an increased understanding of the options available to him/her as he/she ages.

D. The client struggled to understand the residential programs and other programs that he/she may need as he/she ages and was given additional feedback in this area.

43. Develop a Written Plan for Incapacitation (43)

A. The client was directed to develop a written plan to detail his/her wishes should he/she be legally unable to make his/her own decisions.

B. The client was assisted in developing a written plan to detail his/her wishes should he/she become legally unable to make his/her own decisions.

C. The client was reinforced for developing a plan for guardianship, advanced medical directives, and last will and testament.

D. The client has not developed a plan for his/her possible incapacitation and was redirected to do so.

ANGER MANAGEMENT

CLIENT PRESENTATION

1. Explosive, Destructive Outbursts (1)*

A. The client described a history of loss of temper in which he/she has destroyed property in fits of rage.

B. The client described a history of loss of temper that dates back many years, involving verbal outbursts, as well as property destruction.

C. As treatment has progressed, the client has reported increased control over his/her temper and a significant reduction in incidents of poor anger management.

D. The client has had no recent incidents of explosive outbursts that have resulted in destruction of any property or intimidating verbal assaults.

2. Explosive, Assaultive Outbursts (1)

A. The client described a history of loss of anger control to the point of physical assaults on others who were the target of his/her anger.

B. The client has been arrested for assaultive attacks on others when he/she has lost control of his/her temper.

C. The client has used assaultive acts as well as threats and intimidation to control others.

D. The client has made a commitment to control his/her temper and terminate all assaultive behavior.

E. There have been no recent incidents of assaultive attacks on anyone, in spite of the client having experienced periods of anger.

3. Violent Outbursts Due to Altered Perception of Reality (2)

A. The client described a history of violent actions that have occurred during a psychotic episode of perceived threat.

B. The client reported that his/her pattern of hallucinations and delusions have caused a threatening altered perception of reality, which has led to violent actions.

C. As the client has gained a better reality orientation that is less threatening, his/her violent actions have diminished.

D. The client reported no recent incidents of violent actions committed as a result of threatening hallucinations or delusions.

4. Loss of Inhibition or Regard for Consequences (3)

A. The client reported a pattern of impulsive anger outbursts that have occurred when he/she has lost his/her natural inhibition.

---

* The numbers in parentheses correlate to the number of the Behavioral Definition statement in the companion chapter with the same title in *The Severe and Persistent Mental Illness Treatment Planner,* 2nd ed. (Berghuis and Jongsma) by John Wiley & Sons, 2008.

B. The client identified a pattern of impulsive anger outbursts without regard to the painful consequences that occur due to these anger outbursts.

C. As the client has become more stable in his/her mood, he/she has reported a decrease in impulsive anger outbursts.

D. The client reported that he/she is able to inhibit his/her impulses to react in an angry manner and considers the consequences for his/her actions.

E. The client reported that he/she has not engaged in any recent incidents of impulsive anger outbursts.

5. Hostile Overreaction (4)

A. The client described a history of reacting angrily to rather insignificant irritants in his/her daily life.

B. The client indicated that he/she recognizes that he/she becomes too angry in the face of rather minor frustrations and irritants.

C. Minor irritants have resulted in explosive, angry outbursts that have led to destruction of property and/or striking out physically at others.

D. The client has made significant progress at increasing his/her frustration tolerance and reducing explosive overreactivity to minor irritants.

E. The client has not overreacted with anger to minor frustrations or irritants.

6. Paranoid Ideation (5)

A. The client described a history of incidents in which he/she has become easily offended and was quick to anger.

B. The client described a pattern of defensiveness in which he/she feels easily threatened by others and becomes angry with them.

C. The client described periods during which he/she projects threatening motivations onto others, then reacts with irritability, defensiveness, and anger.

D. The client reported a decreased pattern of inappropriate paranoid thought, which has led to fewer anger outbursts.

E. The client has become less defensive and has not shown any recent incidents of unreasonable anger.

7. Intimidation and Control (6)

A. The client identified a pattern of violent actions, threats, or verbally abusive language used to intimidate and control others when feeling threatened.

B. The client presented in a hostile, angry, uncooperative, and intimidating manner during the clinical contact.

C. The client is trying to act in a more cooperative manner within social and employment settings.

D. The client is showing less irritability and argumentativeness.

E. The client displayed a willingness to not have to be in control of all situations.

8. Challenges Authority (7)

A. The client's history shows a consistent pattern of challenging or disrespectful treatment of authority figures.

B. The client acknowledged that he/she becomes angry quickly when someone in authority gives direction to him/her.

C. The client's disrespectful treatment of authority figures has often erupted in explosive, aggressive outbursts.

D. The client has made progress in controlling his/her overreactivity to taking direction from those in authority and is responding with more acts of cooperation.

E. The client now takes direction from authority figures without reacting angrily.

9. Angry, Tense Body Language (8)

A. The client presented with verbalizations of anger as well as tense, rigid muscles and glaring facial expressions.

B. The client expressed his/her anger with bodily signs of muscle tension, clenched fists, and refusal to make eye contact.

C. The client appeared more relaxed, less angry, and did not exhibit physical signs of aggression.

D. The client's family and/or caregiver reported that he/she has been more relaxed within the home setting and has not shown glaring looks or pounded his/her fists on the table.

10. History of Abuse (9)

A. The client has vague memories of inappropriate, abusive verbal, physical, and/or sexual contact.

B. The client recalled clear, detailed memories of experiences of verbal, physical, and/or sexual abuse in his/her childhood or adulthood.

C. The client displayed a pattern of overreaction to stress, due to his/her history of childhood abuse.

D. The client has decreased his/her overreaction to stress as he/she has worked through his/her pattern of childhood verbal, physical, and/or sexual abuse.

11. Self-Directed Anger (10)

A. The client displayed self-directed anger, as evidenced by a history of multiple suicidal gestures and/or threats.

B. The client has engaged in self-mutilating behavior as an expression of his/her anger toward himself/herself.

C. The client has made a commitment to terminate suicidal gestures and threats.

D. The client agreed to stop the pattern of self-mutilating behavior.

E. There have been no recent reports of occurrences of suicidal gestures, threats, or self-mutilating behavior.

INTERVENTIONS IMPLEMENTED

1. Develop Trust (1)*

A. Today's clinical contact focused on building the level of trust with the client through consistent eye contact, active listening, unconditional positive regard, and warm acceptance.

---

* The numbers in parentheses correlate to the number of the Therapeutic Intervention statement in the companion chapter with the same title in *The Severe and Persistent Mental Illness Treatment Planner,* 2nd ed. (Berghuis and Jongsma) by John Wiley & Sons, 2008.

B. Empathy and support were provided for the client's expression of thoughts and feelings during today's clinical contact.

C. The client was provided with support and feedback as he/she described his/her maladaptive pattern of anger expression.

D. As the client has remained mistrustful and reluctant to share his/her underlying thoughts and feelings, he/she was provided with additional reassurance.

E. The client verbally recognized that he/she has difficulty establishing trust because he/she has often felt let down by others in the past, and was accepted for this insight.

2. Assess Anger Dynamics (2)

A. The client was assessed for various stimuli that have triggered his/her anger.

B. The client was helped to identify situations, people, and thoughts that have triggered his/her anger.

C. The client was assisted in identifying the thoughts, feelings, and actions that have characterized his/her anger responses.

3. Arrange More Restrictive Setting (3)

A. The client was judged to be at imminent risk of harm to himself/herself or others, and an admission to a more restrictive treatment setting was coordinated.

B. The client declined voluntary admission to a more restrictive treatment setting and was petitioned to be involuntarily admitted.

C. The client has decreased his/her pattern of angry outbursts as a result of treatment in a more structured setting.

D. The client reacted to the threat of an impending psychiatric hospitalization with a decrease in his/her anger outbursts.

4. Remove Anger-Provoking Stimuli (4)

A. The client's environment was reviewed for possible anger-provoking stimuli.

B. Specific anger-provoking stimuli were removed from the client's environment.

5. Physician Referral (5)

A. The client was referred to a physician to undergo a thorough examination to rule out any organic contributors for anger outbursts and to receive recommendations for further treatment options.

B. The client has followed through on the physician evaluation referral, and specific medical etiologies for anger outbursts were reviewed.

C. The client was supported as he/she is seeking out medical treatment that may decrease his/her anger outbursts.

D. The client has followed through on the physician evaluation referral, but no specific medical etiologies for anger outbursts have been identified.

E. The client declined evaluation by a physician for a prescription of psychotropic medications and was redirected to cooperate with this referral.

6. Review Substance Abuse (6)

A. The client's use of street drugs or alcohol as a contributing factor to anger control problems was reviewed.

B. The client identified that he/she often experiences his/her anger control problems in the context of using street drugs or alcohol, and this pattern was processed.

C. The client denied any pattern of use of street drugs or alcohol as a contributing factor to his/her anger control problems and was directed to monitor this area.

7. Evaluate Substance Abuse (7)

A. The client was evaluated for his/her use of substances, the severity of his/her substance abuse, and treatment needs/options.

B. The client was referred to a clinician knowledgeable in both substance abuse and severe and persistent mental illness treatment in order to accurately assess his/her substance abuse concerns and treatment needs.

C. The client was compliant with the substance abuse evaluation, and the results of the evaluation were discussed with him/her.

D. The client did not participate in the substance abuse evaluation and was encouraged to do so.

8. Refer to a Physician for Psychotropic Medications (8)

A. The client was assessed for the need for psychotropic medication.

B. The client was referred to a physician for an evaluation for a prescription of psychotropic medications.

C. The client has followed through on a referral to a physician and has been assessed for a prescription of psychotropic medications, but none were prescribed.

D. The client has been prescribed psychotropic medications.

E. The client declined an evaluation by a physician for a prescription of psychotropic medication and was redirected to do so.

9. Monitor Medications and Side Effects (9)

A. The client was monitored for compliance with his/her psychotropic medication regimen, as well as possible side effects.

B. The client was provided with positive feedback about his/her regular use of psychotropic medications.

C. The client was monitored for the effectiveness and side effects of his/her prescribed medications.

D. The client identified significant medication side effects, and these were reported to the medical staff.

E. Possible side effects of the client's medications were reviewed, but he/she denied experiencing any side effects.

F. Concerns about the client's medication effectiveness and side effects were communicated to the physician.

G. Although the client was monitored for medication side effects, he/she reported no concerns in this area.

10. Assign Anger Journal (10)

A. The client was educated about triggers for anger.

B. The client was assigned to keep a daily journal in which he/she will document persons or situations that cause anger, irritation, or disappointment.

C. The client was assigned "Anger Journal" in the *Adult Psychotherapy Homework Planner*, Second Edition (Jongsma).

D. The client has kept a journal of anger-producing situations, and this material was processed within the session.

E. The client has become more aware of the causes for and targets of his/her anger as a result of journaling these experiences on a daily basis; the benefits of this insight were reflected to him/her.

F. The client has not kept an anger journal and was redirected to do so.

11.   List Targets of/Causes for Anger (11)

A. The client was assigned to list as many of the causes for and targets of his/her anger that he/she is aware of.

B. The client's list of targets of and causes for anger was processed in order to increase his/her awareness of anger management issues.

C. The client has indicated a greater sensitivity to his/her anger feelings and the causes for them as a result of the focus on these issues.

D. The client has not been able to develop a comprehensive list of causes for and targets of anger and was provided with tentative examples in this area.

12.   Identify Anger (12)

A. The client was assisted in becoming more aware of the frequency with which he/she experiences anger and the signs of it in his/her life.

B. Situations were reviewed in which the client experienced anger but refused to acknowledge it or minimized the experience.

C. The client has acknowledged that he/she is frequently angry and has problems with anger management and was provided with positive feedback about this process.

13.   Identify Anger Expression Models (13)

A. The client was assisted in identifying key figures in his/her life that have provided examples to him/her of how to positively or negatively express anger.

B. The client was reinforced as he/she identified several key figures who have been negative role models in expressing anger explosively and destructively.

C. The client was supported and reinforced for acknowledging that he/she manages his/her anger in the same way that an explosive parent figure had done when he/she was growing up.

D. The client was encouraged to identify positive role models throughout his/her life whom he/she could respect for their management of anger feelings.

E. The client was supported as he/she acknowledged that others have been influential in teaching him/her destructive patterns of anger management.

F. The client failed to identify key figures in his/her life who have provided examples to him/her as to how to positively express his/her anger and was questioned more specifically in this area.

14. List Negative Anger Impact (14)

A. The client was assisted in listing ways that his/her explosive expression of anger has negatively impacted his/her life.

B. The client was supported as he/she identified many negative consequences that have resulted from his/her poor anger management.

C. It was reflected to the client that his/her denial about the negative impact of his/her anger has decreased and he/she has verbalized an increased awareness of the negative impact of his/her behavior.

D. The client has been guarded about identifying the negative impact of his/her anger and was provided with specific examples of how his/her anger has negatively impacted his/her life and relationships (e.g., injuring others or self, legal conflicts, loss of respect from self or others, destruction of property).

15. Identify Bodily Impact of Anger (15)

A. The client was taught the negative impact that anger can have on bodily functions and systems.

B. The client indicated an increased awareness of the stress of his/her anger on such things as heart, brain, and blood pressure; this awareness was applied to his/her own functioning.

C. The client was reinforced as he/she has tried to reduce the frequency with which he/she experiences anger in order to reduce the negative impact that anger has on bodily systems.

16. Reconceptualize Anger (16)

A. The client was assisted in reconceptualizing anger as involving different components that go through predictable phases.

B. The client was taught about the different components of anger, including cognitive, physiological, affective, and behavioral components.

C. The client was taught how to better discriminate between relaxation and tension.

D. The client was taught about the predictable phases of anger, including demanding expectations that are not met, leading to increased arousal and anger, which leads to acting out.

E. The client displayed a clear understanding of the ways to conceptualize anger and was provided with positive reinforcement.

F. The client has struggled to understand the ways to conceptualize anger and was provided with remedial feedback in this area.

17. Identify Positive Consequences of Anger Management (17)

A. The client was asked to identify the positive consequences he/she experienced in managing his/her anger.

B. The client was assisted in identifying positive consequences of managing anger (e.g., respect from others and self, cooperation from others, improved physical health).

C. The client was asked to agree to learn new ways to conceptualize and manage anger.

18. Teach Calming Techniques (18)

A. The client was taught deep-muscle relaxation, rhythmic breathing, and positive imagery as ways to reduce muscle tension when feelings of anger are experienced.

B. The client has implemented the relaxation techniques and reported decreased reactivity when experiencing anger; the benefits of these techniques were underscored.

C. The client has not implemented the relaxation techniques and continues to feel quite stressed in the face of anger; he/she was encouraged to use the techniques.

19. Assign Use of Calming Techniques (19)

A. The client was assigned implementation of calming techniques in his/her daily life when facing anger trigger situations.

B. The client related situations in which he/she has appropriately used calming techniques when facing anger trigger situations; this progress was reinforced.

C. The client described situations in which he/she has not used calming techniques and these failures were reviewed and redirected.

20. Explore Self-Talk (20)

A. The client's self-talk that mediates his/her angry feelings was explored.

B. The client was assessed for self-talk, such as demanding expectations reflected in "should," "must," or "have to" statements.

C. The client was assisted in identifying and challenging his/her biases and in generating alternative self-talk that correct for the biases.

D. The client was taught about how to use correcting self-talk to facilitate a more flexible and temperate response to frustration.

21. Assign Self-Talk Homework (21)

A. The client was assigned a homework exercise in which he/she identifies anger self-talk and generates alternatives that help moderate anger reactions.

B. The client's use of self-talk alternatives was reviewed within the session.

C. The client was reinforced for his/her success in changing angry self-talk to more moderated alternatives.

D. The client was provided with corrective feedback to help improve his/her use of alternative self-talk to moderate his/her angry reactions.

22. Assign Thought-Stopping Technique (22)

A. The client was directed to implement a thought-stopping technique on a daily basis between sessions.

B. The client was assigned "Making Use of the Thought-Stopping Technique" in the *Adult Psychotherapy Homework Planner,* 2nd ed. (Jongsma).

C. The client's use of the thought-stopping technique was reviewed.

D. The client was provided with positive feedback for his/her helpful use of the thought-stopping technique.

E. The client was provided with corrective feedback to help improve his/her use of the thought-stopping technique.

23. Teach Assertive Communication (23)

A. The client was taught about assertive communication through instruction, modeling, and role-playing.

B. The client was referred to an assertiveness training class.

C. The client displayed increased assertiveness and was provided with positive feedback in this area.

D. The client has not increased his/her level of assertiveness and was provided with additional feedback in this area.

24. Teach Conflict Resolution Skills (24)

A. The client was taught conflict resolution skills.

B. The client was taught empathy and active listening skills.

C. "I messages" and respectful communication were taught via role modeling, role-playing, and instruction.

D. Assertiveness without aggression and compromise were emphasized to the client.

E. "Applying Problem-Solving to Personal Conflict" from *Adult Psychotherapy Homework Planner,* 2nd ed. (Jongsma) was assigned to the client.

F. The benefits, successes, and struggles of implementing conflict resolution skills were reviewed.

25. Teach Problem-Solving Skills (25)

A. The client was taught problem-solving skills (e.g., identify the problem, brainstorm all solutions, select best option, implement course of action, and evaluate results).

B. Modeling, role-playing, and behavioral rehearsal were used to help the client use problem-solving skills to work through several current conflicts.

C. The client was reinforced for his/her grasp of problem-solving skills.

D. The client struggled to grasp the use of problem-solving skills and was provided with remedial feedback in this area.

26. Construct Strategy for Managing Anger (26)

A. The client was assisted in constructing a client-tailored strategy for managing his/her anger.

B. The client was encouraged to combine somatic, cognitive, communication, problem-solving, and conflict resolution skills relevant to his/her needs.

C. The client was reinforced for his/her comprehensive anger management strategy.

D. The client was redirected to develop a more comprehensive anger management strategy.

27. Select Challenging Situations for Managing Anger (27)

A. The client was provided with situations in which he/she may be increasingly challenged to apply his/her new strategies for managing anger.

B. The client was asked to identify his/her likely upcoming challenging situations for managing anger.

C. The client was urged to use his/her strategies for managing anger in successively more difficult situations.

28. Consolidate Anger Management Skills (28)

A. The client was assisted in consolidating his/her new anger management skills.

B. Techniques such as relaxation, imagery, behavioral rehearsal, modeling, role-playing, or vivo exposure/behavioral experiences were used to help the client consolidate the use of his/her new anger management skills.

C. The client's use of techniques to consolidate his/her anger management skills were reviewed and reinforced.

29. Monitor/Decrease Outbursts (29)

A. The client's reports of angry outbursts were monitored, toward the goal of decreasing their frequency, intensity, and duration.

B. The client was urged to use his/her new anger management skills to decrease the frequency, intensity, and duration of his/her anger outbursts.

C. The client's progress in decreasing his/her angry outbursts was reviewed.

D. The client was reinforced for his/her success at decreasing the frequency, intensity, and duration of his/her anger outbursts.

E. The client has not decreased his/her frequency, intensity, or duration of anger outbursts and corrective feedback was provided.

30. Encourage Disclosure (30)

A. The client was encouraged to discuss his/her anger management goals with trusted persons who are likely to support his/her change.

B. The client was assisted in identifying individuals who are likely to support his/her change.

C. The client has reviewed his/her anger management goals with trusted persons, and their responses were processed.

D. The client has not discussed his/her anger management goals and was redirected to do so.

31. Educate Support System about Gains (31)

A. The client's family, friends, and caregivers were educated about anger management and the concepts that the client has learned in therapy.

B. The client's family, friends, and caregivers were educated about the specific goals that the subject has developed in regard to his/her anger management needs and how the family can facilitate the client's therapeutic gains.

C. The family members were reinforced for their understanding and support of the client's anger management concerns.

D. Family members have not displayed support and understanding for the client's anger management concerns and were redirected to provide this to the client.

32. Develop Support Network's Safety Plan (32)

A. Members of the client's support network, including family, friends, and caregivers, were educated on how to manage the client's anger episodes.

B. The family members, friends, and caregivers were assisted in developing an understanding of when to contact public safety officials.

C. The client was informed about the support network's safety plan.

D. The safety plan has been used and has helped to contain the client's anger outbursts.

E. The safety plan has not been helpful toward containing the client's anger outbursts, and additional plans were developed in this area.

33. Discuss Management of Lapse Risk Situations (33)

A. The client was assisted in identifying future situations or circumstances in which lapses could occur.

B. The session focused on rehearsing the management of future situations or circumstances in which lapses could occur.

C. The client was reinforced for his/her appropriate use of lapse management skills.

D. The client was redirected in regard to his/her poor use of lapse management skills.

34. Encourage Routine Use of Strategies (34)

A. The client was instructed to routinely use the strategies that he/she has learned in therapy (e.g., calming, adaptive self-talk, assertion, and/or conflict resolution).

B. The client was urged to find ways to build his/her strategies into his/her life as much as possible.

C. The client was reinforced as he/she reported ways in which he/she has incorporated copying strategies into his/her life and routine.

D. The client was redirected about ways to incorporate his/her new strategies into his/her routine and life.

35. Develop a Coping Card (35)

A. The client was provided with a coping card on which specific coping strategies were listed.

B. The client was assisted in developing his/her coping card in order to list his/her helpful coping strategies.

C. The client was encouraged to use his/her coping card when struggling with anger-producing situations.

36. Schedule Maintenance Sessions (36)

A. The client was assisted in scheduling maintenance sessions to help maintain therapeutic gains and adjust to life without anger outbursts.

B. Positive feedback was provided to the client for his/her maintenance of therapeutic gains.

C. The client has displayed an increase in anger symptoms and was provided with additional relapse prevention strategies.

37. Assign Reading Material (37)

A. The client was assigned to read material that educates him/her about anger and its management.

B. The client was directed to read *Overcoming Situational and General Anger: Client Manual* (Deffenbacher and McKay).

C. The client was directed to read *Of Course You're Angry* (Rosselini and Worden).

D. The client was directed to read *The Anger Control Workbook* (McKay).

E. The client has read the assigned material on anger management, and key concepts were reviewed.

F. The client has not read the assigned material on anger management and was redirected to do so

38. Teach Forgiveness (38)

A. The client was taught about the process of forgiveness and encouraged to begin to implement this process as a means of letting go of his/her feelings of strong anger.

B. The client focused on the perpetrators of pain from the past and he/she was encouraged to target them for forgiveness.

C. The advantages of implementing forgiveness versus holding on to vengeful anger were processed with the client.

D. Positive feedback was provided as the client has committed himself/herself to attempting to begin the process of forgiveness with the perpetrators of pain.

E. The client has not been able to begin the process of forgiveness of the perpetrators of his/her pain and was urged to start this process as he/she feels able to.

39. Assign Books on Forgiveness (39)

A. The client was assigned to read books on forgiveness.

B. The client was assigned to read the book *Forgive and Forget* (Smedes) to increase his/her sensitivity to the process of forgiveness.

C. The client has read the book *Forgive and Forget,* and key concepts were processed within the session.

D. The client acknowledged that holding on to angry feelings has distinct disadvantages over his/her beginning the process of forgiveness; he/she was urged to start this process.

E. The client has not followed through with completing the reading assignment of *Forgive and Forget* and was encouraged to do so.

40. Advocate within the Court System (40)

A. Steps were taken to advocate for the client within the court system to assist him/her in receiving assistance, legal representation, leniency, or sentencing that is commensurate with his/her mental illness status.

B. Due to the advocacy provided on behalf of the client, the court has provided appropriate assistance, legal representation, leniency, or sentencing that is commensurate with his/her mental illness status.

C. Although advocacy has been provided for the client within the court system, the court has not accommodated his/her mental illness status.

ANXIETY

CLIENT PRESENTATION

1. Apprehension Due to Severe and Persistent Mental Illness Symptoms (1)*

A. The client identified a pattern of apprehension and nervousness in response to his/her severe and persistent mental illness symptoms.

B. The client identified specific symptoms, such as frightening hallucinations or manic/racing thoughts, which have led to increased anxiety.

C. The client described a general state of nervousness due to his/her severe and persistent mental illness symptoms.

D. As treatment has progressed, the client has reported a decrease in the severity of his/her mental illness symptoms and a decreased level of anxiety.

2. Excessive Worry (2)

A. The client described preoccupation with worry that something dire would happen.

B. The client showed some recognition that his/her excessive worry is beyond the scope of rationality, but he/she feels unable to control the anxiety.

C. The client described that he/she worries about issues related to family, personal safety, health, and employment, among other things.

D. The client reported that his/her worry about life circumstances has diminished and that he/she is living with more of a sense of peace and confidence.

3. Motor Tension (3)

A. The client described a history of restlessness, tiredness, muscle tension, and shaking.

B. The client moved about in his/her chair frequently and sat stiffly.

C. The client said that he/she is unable to relax and is always restless and stressed.

D. The client reported that he/she has been successful in reducing levels of tension and increasing levels of relaxation.

E. The client appeared more relaxed as he/she sat calmly during the clinical contact.

4. Fear Due to Persecutory Delusions (4)

A. The client described a pattern of recurrent or persistent fear due to persecutory delusions or other bizarre beliefs.

B. The client described his/her delusions and bizarre beliefs, as well as the anxiety that he/she experiences due to these beliefs.

C. The client has identified his/her delusions as not based on reality and reports a decreased pattern of anxiety.

---

* The numbers in parentheses correlate to the number of the Behavioral Definition statement in the companion chapter with the same title in *The Severe and Persistent Mental Illness Treatment Planner,* 2nd ed. (Berghuis and Jongsma) by John Wiley & Sons, 2008.

D. As the client's persecutory delusions or other bizarre beliefs have decreased, he/she has also identified a decrease in his/her fear.

5. Hypervigilance (5)

A. The client related that he/she is constantly feeling on edge, sleep is interrupted, and concentration is difficult.

B. The client reported being irritable in interactions with others as his/her patience is thin and he/she worries about everything.

C. The client's family members report that he/she is difficult to get along with, as his/her irritability is high.

D. As new anxiety/coping skills have been implemented, the client's level of tension has decreased, sleep has improved, and irritability has diminished.

6. Concentration Difficulties (6)

A. The client reported an inability to concentrate or maintain his/her train of thought due to anxious preoccupation.

B. The client's lack of ability to concentrate has resulted in poor functioning in his/her social, vocational, and educational needs.

C. The client's ability to concentrate seems to be increasing as he/she reports decreased anxious preoccupation.

INTERVENTIONS IMPLEMENTED

1. Develop Trust (1)*

A. Today's clinical contact focused on building the level of trust with the client through consistent eye contact, active listening, unconditional positive regard, and warm acceptance.

B. Empathy and support were provided for the client's expression of thoughts and feelings during today's clinical contact.

C. The client was provided with support and feedback as he/she described his/her maladaptive pattern of anxiety.

D. As the client has remained mistrustful and reluctant to share his/her underlying thoughts and feelings, he/she was provided with additional reassurance.

E. The client verbally recognized that he/she has difficulty establishing trust because he/she has often felt let down by others in the past and was accepted for this insight.

2. Assess Nature of Anxiety Symptoms (2)

A. The client was asked about the frequency, intensity, duration, and history of his/her anxiety symptoms, fear, and avoidance.

B. *The Anxiety Disorder's Interview Schedule for DSM-IV* (DiNardo, Brown, and Barlow) was used to assess the client's anxiety symptoms.

C. The assessment of the client's anxiety symptoms indicated that his/her symptoms are extreme and severely interfere with his/her life.

---

* The numbers in parentheses correlate to the number of the Therapeutic Intervention statement in the companion chapter with the same title in *The Severe and Persistent Mental Illness Treatment Planner*, 2nd ed. (Berghuis and Jongsma) by John Wiley & Sons, 2008.

D. The assessment of the client's anxiety symptoms indicates that these symptoms are moderate and occasionally interfere with his/her daily functioning.

E. The results of the assessment of the client's anxiety symptoms indicate that these symptoms are mild and rarely interfere with his/her daily functioning.

F. The results of the assessment of the client's anxiety symptoms were reviewed with the client.

3. Develop a Time Line (3)

A. A graphic time line display was used to help the client chart his/her pattern of anxiety symptoms.

B. The client identified his/her precursors, triggers, anxiety symptoms, and effects on a time line to review how he/she experiences and is affected by anxiety.

C. The client displayed a greater understanding of his/her pattern of anxiety problems and was given support and feedback in this area.

D. The client failed to adequately understand his/her pattern of anxiety symptoms and was redirected in this area.

4. Psychological Testing (4)

A. A psychological evaluation was conducted to determine the extent and severity of the client's anxiety symptoms.

B. The Penn State Worry Questionnaire was used to assess the client's level of worry.

C. The client approached the psychological testing in an honest, straightforward manner and was cooperative with any requests presented to him/her.

D. The client was uncooperative and resistant to engage during the evaluation process and was advised to use this testing to discover more about himself/herself.

E. The results of the psychological evaluation were reviewed with the client.

5. Refer for a Physical Evaluation (5)

A. The client was referred to a physician to undergo a thorough examination to rule out any medical etiologies for anger outbursts and to receive recommendations for further treatment options.

B. The client has followed through on the physician evaluation referral, and specific medical etiologies for anger outbursts were reviewed.

C. The client was supported as he/she is seeking out medical treatment that may decrease his/her anger outbursts.

D. The client has followed through on the physician evaluation referral, but no specific medical etiologies for anger outbursts have been identified.

E. The client declined evaluation by a physician and was redirected to cooperate with this referral.

6. Follow Up on Physical Evaluation Recommendations (6)

A. The client was supported in following up on the recommendations from the medical evaluation.

B. The client's follow-up on the recommendations from the medical evaluation has been monitored.

C. The client has been following up on the recommendations from the medical evaluation.

D. The client has not regularly followed up on his/her medical evaluation recommendations and was redirected to do so.

7. Review Psychoactive Chemicals (7)

A. The client's use of psychoactive chemicals (e.g., nicotine, caffeine, alcohol, street drugs) was reviewed.

B. The client's pattern of psychoactive chemical use was connected to his/her symptoms.

C. The client was supported as he/she acknowledged that his/her psychoactive chemical use is affecting his/her anxiety symptoms.

D. The client was reinforced for decreasing his/her psychoactive chemical use, leading to a decrease in anxiety symptoms.

E. The client denies any connection between his/her psychoactive chemical use and his/her anxiety symptoms and has continued to use psychoactive chemicals, despite encouragement to discontinue this.

8. Recommend Substance Abuse Evaluation and/or Termination (8)

A. It was recommended to the client that he/she terminate the consumption of mood-altering substances that could contribute to anxiety.

B. The client was referred for a substance abuse evaluation to more completely assess his/her substance abuse concerns and how they may trigger anxiety.

C. The client was referred for substance abuse treatment to assist him/her in discontinuing his/her consumption of mood-altering substances.

D. As the client has decreased his/her use of mood-altering substances, he/she has experienced a decrease in anxiety, and this was reviewed.

E. The client has declined any evaluation or treatment related to his/her substance use and was encouraged to seek this out at a later time.

9. Differentiate Anxiety Symptoms (9)

A. The client was assisted in differentiating anxiety symptoms that are a direct effect of his/her severe and persistent mental illness, as opposed to a separate diagnosis of an anxiety disorder.

B. The client was provided with feedback regarding his/her differentiation of symptoms that are related to his/her severe and persistent mental illness, as opposed to a separate diagnosis.

C. The client's specific anxiety disorder, which is freestanding from his/her severe and persistent mental illness, was reviewed.

D. The client has been unsuccessful in identifying ways in which his/her anxiety symptoms are related to his/her mental illness or a separate anxiety disorder.

10. Differentiate Reality versus Hallucinations/Delusions (10)

A. The client was assisted in differentiating between actual life situations and those that appear real but are due to hallucinations or delusions.

B. Positive feedback was provided to the client as he/she identified several situations that have appeared real but are actually due to hallucinations or delusions.

C. Redirection was provided to the client as he/she continues to struggle with reality testing and is uncertain about the reality of his/her hallucinations or delusions.

11. Acknowledge Anxiety Related to Delusional Experiences (11)

A. It was acknowledged that both real and delusional experiences could cause anxiety.

B. The client was provided with support as he/she acknowledged his/her anxieties and worries, which are related to both the real experiences and delusional experiences.

12. Identify Diagnostic Classification (12)

A. The client was assisted in identifying a specific diagnostic classification for his/her anxiety symptoms.

B. Using a description of anxiety symptoms such as that found in Bourne's *The Anxiety and Phobia Workbook,* the client was taken through a detailed review of his/her anxiety symptoms, diagnosis, and treatment needs.

C. The client has failed to clearly understand and classify his/her anxiety symptoms and was given additional feedback in this area.

13. Refer to a Physician (13)

A. The client was referred to a physician for an evaluation for a prescription of psychotropic medications.

B. The client was reinforced for following through on a referral to a physician for an assessment for a prescription of psychotropic medications, but none were prescribed.

C. The client has been prescribed psychotropic medications.

D. The client declined evaluation by a physician for a prescription of psychotropic medications and was redirected to cooperate with this referral.

14. Educate about Psychotropic Medications (14)

A. The client was taught about the indications for and the expected benefits of psychotropic medications.

B. As the client's psychotropic medications were reviewed, he/she displayed an understanding about the indications for and expected benefits of the medications.

C. The client displayed a lack of understanding of the indications for and expected benefits of psychotropic medications and was provided with additional information and feedback regarding his/her medications.

15. Monitor Medications (15)

A. The client was monitored for compliance with his/her psychotropic medication regimen.

B. The client was provided with positive feedback about his/her regular use of psychotropic medications.

C. The client was monitored for the effectiveness and side effects of his/her prescribed medications.

D. Concerns about the client's medication effectiveness and side effects were communicated to the physician.

E. Although the client was monitored for medication side effects, he/she reported no concerns in this area.

16. Review Side Effects of Medications (16)

A. The possible side effects related to the client's medications were reviewed with him/her.

B. The client identified significant side effects, and these were reported to the medical staff.

C. Possible side effects of the client's medications were reviewed, but he/she denied experiencing any side effects.

17. Discuss Anxiety Cycle (17)

A. The client was taught about how anxious fears are maintained by a cycle of unwarranted fear and avoidance that precludes positive, corrective experiences with the feared object or situation.

B. The client was taught about how treatment breaks the anxiety cycle by encouraging positive, corrective experiences.

C. The client was taught information from *Mastery of Your Anxiety and Worry—Therapist Guide* (Craske, Barlow, and O'Leary) regarding the anxiety pattern.

D. The client was reinforced as he/she displayed a better understanding of the anxiety cycle of unwarranted fear and avoidance and how treatment breaks the cycle.

E. The client displayed a poor understanding of the anxiety and was provided with remedial feedback in this area.

18. Discuss Target of Treatment (18)

A. A discussion was held about how treatment targets worry, anxiety symptoms, and avoidance to help the client manage worry effectively.

B. The reduction of overarousal and unnecessary avoidance were emphasized as treatment targets.

C. The client displayed a clear understanding of the target of treatment and was provided with positive feedback in this area.

D. The client struggled to understand the target of treatment and was provided with specific examples in this area.

19. Assign Reading on Anxiety (19)

A. The client was assigned to read psychoeducational chapters of books or treatment manuals on anxiety.

B. The client was assigned information from *Mastery of Your Anxiety and Worry—Client Manual* (Zinbarg, Craske, Barlow, and O'Leary).

C. The client has read the assigned information on anxiety, and key points were reviewed.

D. The client has not read the assigned information on anxiety and was redirected to do so.

20. Teach Relaxation Skills (20)

A. The client was taught relaxation skills.

B. The client was taught progressive muscle relaxation, guided imagery, and slow diaphragmatic breathing.

C. The client was taught how to discriminate better between relaxation and tension.

D. The client was taught how to apply relaxation skills to his/her daily life.

E. The client was taught relaxation skills as described in *Progressive Relaxation Training* (Bernstein and Borkovec).

F. The client was taught relaxation skills as described in *Treating GAD* (Rygh and Sanderson).

G. The client was provided with feedback about his/her use of relaxation skills.

21. Assign Relaxation Homework (21)

A. The client was assigned to do homework exercises in which he/she practices relaxation on a daily basis.

B. The client has regularly used relaxation exercises, and the helpful benefits of these exercises were reviewed.

C. The client has not regularly used relaxation exercises and was provided with corrective feedback in this area.

D. The client has used some relaxation exercises, but does not find these to be helpful; he/she was assisted in brainstorming how to modify these exercises to be more helpful.

22. Assign Reading on Relaxation Calming Strategies (22)

A. The client was assigned to read about progressive muscle relaxation and other calming strategies in relevant books and treatment manuals.

B. The client was directed to read about muscle relaxation and other calming strategies in *Progressive Relaxation Training* (Bernstein and Borkovec).

C. The client was directed to read about muscle relaxation and other calming strategies in *Mastery of Your Anxiety and Worry—Client Guide* (Zinbarg, Craske, Barlow, and O'Leary).

D. The client has read the assigned information on progressive muscle relaxation, and key points were reviewed.

E. The client has not read the assigned information on progressive muscle relaxation and was redirected to do so.

23. Utilize Biofeedback (23)

A. Electromyograph (EMG) biofeedback techniques were used to facilitate the client learning relaxation skills.

B. The client reported that he/she has implemented his/her use of relaxation skills in daily life to reduce levels of muscle tension and the experience of anxiety; the benefits of this technique were reviewed.

C. The client reported that his/her level of anxiety has decreased since relaxation techniques were implemented; he/she was encouraged to continue this technique.

D. The client has not followed through on implementation of relaxation skills to reduce anxiety symptoms; he/she was redirected to do so.

24. Identify Distorted Thoughts (24)

A. The client was assisted in identifying the distorted schemas and related automatic thoughts that mediate anxiety responses.

B. The client was taught the role of distorted thinking in precipitating emotional responses.

C. The client was reinforced as he/she verbalized an understanding of the cognitive beliefs and messages that mediate his/her anxiety responses.

D. The client was assisted in replacing distorted messages with positive, realistic cognitions.

E. The client failed to identify his/her distorted thoughts and cognitions and was provided with tentative examples in this area.

25. Assign Exercises on Self-Talk (25)

A. The client was assigned homework exercises in which he/she identifies fearful self-talk and creates reality-based alternatives.

B. The client's replacement of fearful self-talk with reality-based alternatives was critiqued.

C. The client was reinforced for his/her successes at replacing fearful self-talk with reality-based alternatives.

D. The client was provided with corrective feedback for his/her failures to replace fearful self-talk with reality-based alternatives.

E. The client has not completed his/her assigned homework regarding fearful self-talk and was redirected to do so.

26. Teach Thought Stopping (26)

A. The client was taught thought-stopping techniques that involve thinking of a stop sign and replacing negative thoughts with a pleasant scene.

B. The client was assigned "Making Use of the Thought-Stopping Technique" form the *Adult Psychotherapy Homework Planner,* 2nd ed. (Jongsma).

C. The client's implementation of the thought-stopping technique was monitored and his/her success with this technique was reinforced.

D. The client reported that the thought-stopping technique has been beneficial in reducing his/her preoccupation with anxiety-producing cognitions; he/she was encouraged to continue this technique.

E. The client has failed to use the thought-stopping techniques and his/her attempts to use these techniques were reviewed and problem-solved.

27. Read about Cognitive Restructuring of Fears (27)

A. The client was assigned to read about cognitive restructuring of fears or worries in books or treatment manuals.

B. *Mastery of Your Anxiety and Worry—Client Guide* (Zinbarg, Craske, Barlow, and O'Leary) was assigned to the client to help teach him/her about cognitive restructuring.

C. Key components of cognitive restructuring were reviewed.

D. The client and parents have not done the assigned reading on cognitive restructuring, and they were redirected to do so.

28. Assign Reading on Worry Exposure (28)

A. The client was assigned to read about worry exposure in relevant books or treatment manuals.

B. The client was assigned *Mastery of Your Anxiety and Worry—Client Guide* (Zinbarg, Craske, Barlow, and O'Leary) to learn about worry exposure.

C. Key concepts related to worry exposure were reviewed and processed within the session.

D. The client has not done the reading on worry exposure, and he/she was redirected to do so.

29. Construct Anxiety Stimulus Hierarchy (29)

A. The client was assisted in constructing a hierarchy of anxiety-producing situations associated with two or three spheres of worry.

B. It was difficult for the client to develop a hierarchy of stimulus situations, as the causes of his/her anxiety remain quite vague; he/she was assisted in completing the hierarchy.

C. The client was successful at creating a focused hierarchy of specific stimulus situations that provoke anxiety in a gradually increasing manner; this hierarchy was reviewed.

30. Select Initial Exposures (30)

A. Initial exposures were selected from the hierarchy of anxiety-producing situations, with a bias toward the likelihood of being successful.

B. A plan was developed with the client for managing the symptoms that may occur during the initial exposure.

C. The client was assisted in rehearsing the plan for managing the exposure-related symptoms within his/her imagination.

D. Positive feedback was provided for the client's helpful use of symptom management techniques.

E. The client was redirected for ways to improve his/her symptom management techniques.

31. Assign Homework on Situational Exposures (31)

A. The client was assigned homework exercises to perform worry exposures and record his/her experience.

B. The client was assigned situational exposures homework from *Mastery of Your Anxiety and Worry—Client Guide* (Zinbarg, Craske, Barlow, and O'Leary).

C. The client was assigned situational exposures homework from *Generalized Anxiety Disorder* (Brown, O'Leary, and Barlow).

D. The client's use of worry exposure techniques was reviewed and reinforced.

E. The client has struggled in his/her implementation of worry exposure techniques and was provided with corrective feedback.

F. The client has not attempted to use the worry exposure techniques and was redirected to do so.

32. Assign Imagination Exercises (32)

A. The client was asked to vividly imagine worse-case consequences of worries, holding them in mind until the anxiety associated with them weakens.

B. The client was asked to imagine consequences of his/her worries as described in *Mastery of Your Anxiety and Worry—Therapist Guide* (Craske, Barlow, and O'Leary).

C. The client was supported as he/she has maintained a focus on the worst-case consequences of his/her worry until the anxiety weakened.

D. The client was assisted in generating reality-based alternatives to the worst-case scenarios, and these were processed within the session.

33. Teach Problem-Solving Strategies (33)

A. The client was taught a specific problem-solving strategy.

B. The client was taught problem-solving strategies including specifically defining a problem, generating options for addressing it, implementing a plan, evaluating options, and reevaluating and refining the plan.

C. The client was provided feedback on his/her use of the problem-solving strategies.

34. Assign Problem-Solving Exercise (34)

A. The client was assigned a homework exercise in which he/she problem solves a current problem.

B. The client was assigned a problem to solve as described in *Mastery of Your Anxiety and Worry—Client Guide* (Zinbarg, Craske, Barlow, and O'Leary).

C. The client was assigned a problem to solve as described in *Generalized Anxiety Disorder* (Brown, O'Leary, and Barlow).

D. "Applying Problem-Solving to Interpersonal Conflict" from *Adult Psychotherapy Homework Planner,* 2nd ed. (Jongsma) was assigned to the client.

E. The client was provided with feedback about his/her use of the problem-solving assignment.

35. Differentiate between Lapse and Relapse (35)

A. A discussion was held with the client regarding the distinction between a lapse and a relapse.

B. A lapse was associated with an initial and reversible return of symptoms, fear, or urges to avoid.

C. A relapse was associated with the decision to return to fearful and avoidant patterns.

D. The client was provided with support and encouragement as he/she displayed an understanding of the difference between a lapse and a relapse.

E. The client struggled to understand the difference between a lapse and a relapse and was provided with remedial feedback in this area.

36. Discuss Management of Lapse Risk Situations (36)

A. The client was assisted in identifying future situations or circumstances in which lapses could occur.

B. The session focused on rehearsing the management of future situations or circumstances in which lapses could occur.

C. The client was reinforced for his/her appropriate use of lapse management skills.

D. The client was redirected in regard to his/her poor use of lapse management skills.

37. Encourage Routine Use of Strategies (37)

A. The client was instructed to routinely use the strategies that he/she has learned in therapy (e.g., cognitive restructuring, exposure).

B. The client was urged to find ways to build his/her new strategies into his/her life as much as possible.

C. The client was reinforced as he/she reported ways in which he/she has incorporated coping strategies into his/her life and routine.

D. The client was redirected about ways to incorporate his/her new strategies into his/her routine and life.

38. Apply Secondary Gain (38)

A. The possible secondary gain associated with anxiety symptoms was reviewed.

B. The client identified specific secondary gains that he/she has attained related to anxiety symptoms, such as less involvement in potentially difficult social situations, and these were reviewed.

C. The client denied any pattern of secondary gain related to decreased functioning due to his/her anxiety and was provided with hypothetical examples of the secondary gains.

39. Encourage Daily Routines (39)

A. The client was encouraged to develop a routine daily pattern as a means of reducing stress.

B. The client was assisted in setting a routine daily pattern, including his/her regular waking and resting times, mealtimes, and routinely performing daily chores.

C. The client was reinforced for implementing a regular daily routine, which has increased his/her emotional stability.

D. The client has not maintained his/her regular daily routine and was provided with redirection in this area.

40. Enlist the Client's Support System (40)

A. The help of the client's support system was enlisted in his/her implementation of specific stress reduction techniques.

B. The client's support system was enthusiastic and supportive of his/her stress reduction techniques, and he/she was encouraged to use this support on a regular basis.

C. The client's support system has declined significant involvement in helping him/her to implement specific stress reduction techniques, so alternative means of development of support for stress reduction were developed.

D. The client has declined support from his/her family, friends, and caretakers and was again urged to use this support.

BORDERLINE PERSONALITY

CLIENT PRESENTATION

1. Emotional Reactivity (1)*

A. The client described a history of extreme emotional reactivity when minor stresses occur in his/her life.

B. The client's emotional reactivity is usually quite short lived, as he/she returns to a calm state after demonstrating strong feelings of anger, anxiety, or depression.

C. The client's emotional liability has been reduced, and he/she reported less frequent incidents of emotional reactivity.

2. Chaotic Interpersonal Relationships (2)

A. The client has a pattern of intense, but chaotic, interpersonal relationships as he/she puts high expectations on others and is easily threatened that the relationship might be in jeopardy.

B. The client has had many relationships that have ended because of the intensity and demands that he/she placed on the relationship.

C. The client reported incidents that have occurred recently with friends, whereby he/she continued placing inappropriately intense demands on the relationship.

D. The client has made progress in stabilizing his/her relationship with others by diminishing the degree of demands that he/she places on the relationship and reducing the dependency on it.

3. Identify Disturbance (3)

A. The client has a history of being confused as to who he/she is and what his/her goals are in life.

B. The client has become very intense about questioning his/her identity.

C. The client has become more assured about his/her identity and is less reactive to this issue.

4. Impulsivity (4)

A. The client described a history of engaging in impulsive behaviors that have the potential for producing harmful consequences for himself/herself.

B. The client has engaged in impulsive behaviors that compromise his/her reputation with others.

C. The client has established improved control over impulsivity and considers the consequences of his/her actions more deliberately before engaging in behavior.

5. Suicidal/Self-Mutilating Behavior (5)

A. The client reported a history of multiple suicidal gestures and/or threats.

B. The client has engaged in self-mutilating behavior on several occasions.

C. The client made a commitment to terminate suicidal gestures and threats.

D. The client agreed to stop the pattern of self-mutilating behaviors.

---

* The numbers in parentheses correlate to the number of the Behavioral Definition statement in the companion chapter with the same title in *The Severe and Persistent Mental Illness Treatment Planner,* 2nd ed. (Berghuis and Jongsma) by John Wiley & Sons, 2008.

E. There have been no recent reports of occurrences of suicidal gestures, threats, or self-mutilating behavior.

6. Feelings of Emptiness (6)

A. The client reported a chronic history of feeling empty and bored with life.

B. The client's frequent complaints of feeling bored and that life had no meaning had alienated him/her from others.

C. The client has not complained recently about feeling empty or bored, but appears to be more challenged and at peace with life.

7. Intense Anger Eruptions (7)

A. The client frequently has eruptions of intense and inappropriate anger triggered by seemingly insignificant stressors.

B. The client seems to live in a state of chronic anger and displeasure with others.

C. The client's eruptions of intense and inappropriate anger have diminished in their frequency and intensity.

D. The client reported that there have been no incidents of recent eruptions of anger.

8. Feels Others Are Unfair (8)

A. The client made frequent complaints about the unfair treatment he/she believes that others have given him/her.

B. The client frequently verbalized distrust of others and questioned their motives.

C. The client has demonstrated increased trust of others and has not complained about unfair treatment from them recently.

9. Black-or-White Thinking (9)

A. The client demonstrated a pattern of analyzing issues in simple terms of right or wrong, black or white, trustworthy versus deceitful, without regard for extenuating circumstances before considering the complexity of the situations.

B. The client's black-or-white thinking has caused him/her to be quite judgmental of others.

C. The client finds it difficult to consider the complexity of situations, but prefers to think in simple terms of right versus wrong.

D. The client has shown some progress in allowing for the complexity of some situations and extenuating circumstances, which might contribute to some other people's actions.

10. Abandonment Fears (10)

A. The client described a history of becoming very anxious whenever there is any hint of abandonment present in an established relationship.

B. The client's hypersensitivity to abandonment has caused him/her to place excessive demands of loyalty and proof of commitment on relationships.

C. The client has begun to acknowledge his/her fear of abandonment as being excessive and irrational.

D. Conflicts within a relationship have been reported by the client, but he/she has not automatically assumed that abandonment will be the result.

INTERVENTIONS IMPLEMENTED

1. Assess Behavior, Affect, and Cognitions (1)*

A. The client's experience of distress and disability was assessed to identify targets of therapy.

B. The client's pattern of behaviors (e.g., parasuicidal acts, angry outbursts, overattachment) was assessed to help identify targets for therapy.

C. The client's affect was assessed, including emotional overreactions and painful emptiness, in regard to targets for therapy.

D. The client's cognitions were assessed, including biases such as dichotomous thinking, overgeneralization, and catastrophizing, to assist in identifying targets for therapy.

E. Specific targets for therapy were identified.

2. Explore Childhood Abuse/Abandonment (2)

A. Experiences of childhood physical or emotional abuse, neglect, or abandonment were explored.

B. As the client identified instances of abuse and neglect, the feelings surrounding these experiences were processed.

C. The client's experiences with perceived abandonment were highlighted and related to his/her current fears of this experience occurring in the present.

D. As the client's experience of abuse and abandonment in his/her childhood was processed, he/she denied any emotional impact of these experiences on himself/herself.

E. The client denied any experience of abuse and abandonment in his/her childhood, and he/she was urged to talk about these types of concerns as he/she deems it necessary in the future.

3. Validate Distress and Difficulties (3)

A. The client's experience of distress and subsequent difficulties were validated as understandable, given his/her particular circumstances, thoughts, and feelings.

B. It was reflected to the client that most people would experience the same distress and difficulties, given the same circumstances, thoughts, and feelings.

C. The client was noted to accept the validation about his/her level of distress

4. Orient to Dialectical Behavioral Therapy (DBT) (4)

A. The client was oriented to DBT.

B. The multiple facets of DBT were highlighted, including support, collaboration, challenge, problem solving, and skill building.

C. The biosocial view related to Borderline Personality Disorder was emphasized, including the constitutional and social influences.

D. The concept of dialectics was reviewed with the client.

E. Information from *Cognitive-Behavioral Treatment of Borderline Personality* (Linehan) was reviewed with the client.

---

* The numbers in parentheses correlate to the number of the Therapeutic Intervenion statement in the companion chapter with the same title in *The Severe and Persistent Mental Illness Treatment Planner,* 2nd ed. (Berghuis and Jongsma) by John Wiley & Sons, 2008.

5. Assign Reading on Borderline Personality Disorder (5)

A. The client was asked to read selected sections of books or manuals that reinforce therapeutic interventions.

B. Portions of *Skills Training Manual for Treating Borderline Personality Disorder* (Linehan) were assigned to the client.

C. The client has read assigned information from books or manuals, and key concepts were reinforced.

D. The client has not read assigned portions of books or manuals that reinforce therapeutic interventions and was redirected to do so.

6. Solicit Agreement for DBT (6)

A. An agreement was solicited from the client to work collaboratively within the parameters of the DBT approach.

B. A written agreement was developed with the client to work collaboratively within the parameters of the DBT approach.

C. The client has agreed to work within the DBT approach to overcome the behaviors, emotions, and cognitions that have been identified as causing problems in his/her life.

D. The client was reinforced for his/her commitment to working within the DBT program.

E. The client has not agreed to work within the DBT program and was referred back to "Treatment as Usual."

7. Explore Self-Mutilating Behavior (7)

A. The client's history and nature of self-mutilating behavior were explored thoroughly.

B. The client recalled a pattern of self-mutilating behavior that has dated back several years.

C. The client's self-mutilating behavior was identified as being associated with feelings of depression, fear, and anger, as well as a lack of self-identity.

8. Assess Suicidal Behavior (8)

A. The client's history and current status regarding suicidal gestures were assessed.

B. The secondary gain associated with suicidal gestures was identified.

C. Triggers for suicidal thoughts were identified, and alternative responses to these trigger situations were proposed.

9. Arrange Hospitalization (9)

A. As the client was judged to be harmful of self, arrangements were made for voluntary psychiatric hospitalization.

B. As the client refused a necessary psychiatric hospitalization, the proper steps to involuntary hospitalize the client were initiated.

C. The client has been psychiatrically hospitalized.

D. Ongoing contact with the psychiatric hospital has been maintained in order to coordinate the most helpful treatment while in the hospital.

10. Refer to Emergency Helpline (10)

A. The client was provided with an emergency helpline telephone number that is available 24 hours a day.

B. Positive feedback was provided as the client promised to utilize the emergency helpline telephone number rather than engaging in any self-harm behaviors.

C. The client has not used the emergency helpline telephone system in place of engaging in self-harm behaviors and was reminded about this useful resource.

11. Interpret Self-Mutilating Behavior (11)

A. The client's self-mutilation was interpreted as an expression of the rage and helplessness that could not be expressed as a child victim of emotional abandonment and abuse.

B. The client accepted the interpretation of his/her self-mutilation and more directly expressed his/her feelings of hurt and anger associated with childhood abuse experiences.

C. The client rejected the interpretation of self-mutilating behavior as an expression of rage associated with childhood abandonment or neglect experiences.

D. An expectation that the client will be able to control his/her urge for self-mutilation was expressed.

12. Elicit Nonsuicide Contract (12)

A. A promise was elicited from the client that he/she will initiate contact with the therapist or an emergency helpline if the suicidal urge becomes strong and before any self-injurious behavior is enacted.

B. The client was reinforced as he/she promised to terminate self-mutilation behavior and to contact emergency personnel if urges for such behavior arise.

C. The client has followed through on the nonself-harm contract by contacting emergency service personnel rather than enacting any suicidal gestures or self-mutilating behavior; he/she was reinforced for this healthy use of support.

D. The client's potential for suicide was consistently assessed despite the suicide prevention contract.

13. Resolve Therapy-Interfering Behaviors (13)

A. The client's pattern of therapy-interfering behavior (e.g., missing appointments, noncompliance, abruptly leaving therapy) was consistently monitored.

B. The client was confronted for his/her therapy-interfering behaviors.

C. The clinician took appropriate responsibility for the clinician's own therapy-interfering behaviors.

D. Therapy-interfering behaviors were problem-solved.

14. Refer for Medication Evaluation (14)

A. The client was assessed in regard to the need for psychotropic medication.

B. The client was referred to a physician to be evaluated for psychotropic medications to stabilize his/her mood.

C. The client has cooperated with a referral to a physician and has attended the evaluation for psychotropic medications.

D. The client has refused to attend a physician evaluation for psychotropic medications and was redirected to do so.

15. Monitor Medication Compliance (15)

A. The client's compliance with prescribed medications was monitored, and effectiveness of the medication on his/her level of functioning was noted.

B. The client reported that the medication has been beneficial in stabilizing his/her mood, and he/she was encouraged to continue its use.

C. The client reported that the medication has not been beneficial in stabilizing his/her mood; this was reflected to the prescribing clinician.

D. The client reported side effects of the medication that he/she found intolerable; these side effects were relayed to the physician.

16. Use Strategies to Manage Maladaptive Behaviors, Thoughts, and Feelings (16)

A. Validation, dialectical strategies, and problem-solving strategies were used to help the client manage, reduce, or stabilize maladaptive behaviors, thoughts, and feelings.

B. Therapeutic techniques as described in *Cognitive-Behavioral Treatment of Borderline Personality* (Linehan) were used to help the client manage his/her symptoms.

C. Validation was consistently used to help the client manage, reduce, and stabilize maladaptive behaviors, thoughts, and feelings.

D. Dialectical strategies, such as metaphor or devil's advocacy, were used to help the client manage, reduce, or stabilize maladaptive behaviors, thoughts, and feeling.

E. Problem-solving strategies, such as behavioral analysis, cognitive restructuring, skills training, and exposure, were used to help the client manage, reduce, or stabilize his/her maladaptive behaviors, thoughts, and feelings.

F. It was noted that the client has decreased maladaptive behaviors (e.g., angry outbursts, binge drinking, abusive relationships, high-risk sex, uncontrolled spending), maladaptive thought patterns (e.g., all-or-nothing thinking, catastrophizing, personalizing), and maladaptive feelings (e.g., rage, hopelessness, abandonment).

17. Conduct Skills Training (17)

A. Group skills training was used to teach responses to identified problem behaviors.

B. Individual skills training was used to teach the client responses to identified behavioral problem patterns.

C. The client was taught assertiveness for use in abusive relationships.

D. The client was taught cognitive strategies for identifying and controlling financial, sexual, and other impulsivity.

E. The client has participated in skills training for specific behavioral problems, and the benefit of this treatment was reviewed.

F. The client has not participated in group skills training and was redirected to do so.

18. Teach Skills for Regular Use (18)

A. Behavioral strategies were taught to the client via instruction, modeling, and advising.

B. Role-playing and exposure exercises were used to strengthen the client's use of behavioral strategies.

C. The client was provided with regular homework assignments to help incorporate the behavioral strategies into his/her everyday life.

D. The client was reinforced for his/her regular use and understanding of behavioral strategies.

E. The client has struggled to understand the behavioral strategies and was provided with remedial information in this area.

19. Conduct Trauma Work (19)

A. As the client's adaptive behavior patterns have been evident, work on remembering and accepting the facts of previous trauma was initiated.

B. The client was assisted in using his/her new adaptive behavior patterns and emotional regulation skills to reduce denial and increase insight into the effects of previous trauma.

C. The client was helped to reduce maladaptive emotional and/or behavioral responses to trauma-related stimuli through the regular use of adaptive behavioral patterns and emotional skills.

D. The client was assisted in tolerating the distress of remembering and accepting the facts of previous trauma and in reducing self-blame.

E. The client has been noted to be successful in using his/her adaptive behavioral patterns and emotional regulation skills in managing the effects of previous trauma.

F. The client has become more emotionally disregulated due to the trauma work and was redirected to use behavioral and emotional regulation skills.

20. Explore Schema and Self-Talk (20)

A. The client was assisted in exploring how his/her schema and self-talk mediate his/her trauma-related and other fears.

B. The client's distorted schema and self-talk were reviewed.

C. The client was reinforced for his/her insight into his/her self-talk and schema that support his/her trauma-related and other fears.

D. The client struggled to develop insight into his/her own self-talk and schema and was provided with tentative examples of these concepts.

21. Assign Exercises on Self-Talk (21)

A. The client was assigned homework exercises in which he/she identifies fearful self-talk and creates reality-based alternatives.

B. The client was assigned the homework exercise "Journal and Replace Self-Defeating Thoughts" from the *Adult Psychotherapy Homework Planner,* 2nd ed. (Jongsma).

C. The client was directed to complete the "Daily Record of Dysfunctional Thoughts" from *Cognitive-Behavioral Therapy of Depression* (Beck, Rush, Shaw, and Emery).

D. The client's replacement of fearful self-talk with reality-based alternatives was critiqued.

E. The client was reinforced for his/her successes at replacing fearful self-talk with reality-based alternatives.

22. Reinforce Positive Self-Talk (22)

A. The client was reinforced for implementing positive, realistic self-talk that enhances self-confidence and increases adaptive action.

B. The client noted several instances from his/her daily life that reflected the implementation of positive self-talk, and these successful experiences were reinforced.

23. Develop Hierarchy of Triggers (23)

A. The client was directed to develop a hierarchy of feared and avoided trauma-related stimuli.

B. The client was helped to list many of the feared and avoided trauma-related stimuli.

C. The client was assisted in developing a hierarchy of feared and avoided trauma-related stimuli.

D. The client's journaling was used to assist in developing a hierarchy of feared and avoided trauma-related stimuli.

24. **Direct Imaginal Exposure (24)**

A. Imaginal Exposure was directed by having the client describe a chosen traumatic experience at an increasing, but client-chosen, level of detail.

B. Cognitive restructuring techniques were integrated and repeated until the associated anxiety regarding childhood trauma was reduced and stabilized.

C. The session was recorded and provided to the client to listen to between sessions.

D. "Share the Painful Memory" from the *Adult Psychotherapy Homework Planner,* 2nd ed. (Jongsma) was assigned to help direct the client's imaginal exposure.

E. Techniques from *Posttraumatic Stress Disorder* (Resick and Calhoun) were used to direct the client's imaginal exposure.

F. The client's progress was reviewed, reinforced, and problem solved.

25. **Assign Homework on Exposure (25)**

A. The client was assigned homework exercises to perform exposure to feared stimuli and record his/her experience.

B. The client was directed to listen to the taped exposure session to consolidate his/her skills for exposure to feared stimuli.

C. The client was assigned situational exposure homework from *Posttraumatic Stress Disorder* (Resick and Calhoun).

D. The client's use of exposure techniques was reviewed and reinforced.

E. The client has struggled in his/her implementation of exposure techniques and was provided with corrective feedback.

F. The client has not attempted to use the exposure techniques and was redirected to do so.

26. **Encourage Trust in Own Evaluations (26)**

A. The client was encouraged to value, believe, and trust in his/her evaluations of himself/herself, others, and situations.

B. The client was encouraged to examine situations in a nondefensive manner, independent of others' opinions.

C. The client was encouraged to build self-reliance through trusting his/her own evaluations.

D. The client was reinforced for his/her value, belief, and trust in his/her own evaluations of himself/herself, others, and situations.

E. The client was redirected when he/she tended to devalue, disbelieve and distrust his/her own evaluations.

27. **Encourage Positive Experiences (27)**

A. The client was encouraged to facilitate his/her personal growth by choosing experiences that strengthen self-awareness, personal values, and appreciation of life.

B. The client was encouraged to use spiritual practices and other relative life experiences to help increase his/her positive experiences.

28. Use Multiple Family Group Treatment (28)

A. The client was referred for multiple family group treatment.

B. The client was enrolled in a multiple family group treatment program.

C. The client's family has participated in a multiple family group treatment program, gaining insight into family dynamics and how to cope with the client's symptoms.

D. The family is not enrolled in the multiple family group treatment program, and the reasons for this resistance were reviewed.

CHEMICAL DEPENDENCE

CLIENT PRESENTATION

1. Consistent Abuse of Alcohol (1)*

A. The client described a history of alcohol abuse on a frequent basis, often until intoxicated or passed out.

B. Family members confirmed a pattern of chronic alcohol abuse by the client.

C. The client acknowledged that his/her alcohol use began in adolescence and has continued into adulthood.

D. The client has committed himself/herself to a plan of abstinence from alcohol and participation in a recovery program.

E. The client has maintained total abstinence, which is confirmed by his/her family.

2. Consistent Drug Abuse (1)

A. The client described a history of mood-altering illicit drug abuse on a frequent basis.

B. Family members confirmed a pattern of chronic drug abuse by the client.

C. The client acknowledged that his/her drug abuse began in adolescence and has continued into adulthood.

D. The client has committed himself/herself to a plan of abstinence from mood-altering drugs and participation in a recovery program.

E. The client has maintained total abstinence, which is confirmed by his/her family.

3. Exacerbation of Primary Symptoms (2)

A. The client displayed an increase in his/her primary psychosis symptoms (e.g., hallucinations, delusions, mania) as a result of abuse of mood-altering illicit substances.

B. The client has displayed a compromised reality orientation due to the abuse of mood-altering illicit substances.

C. Due to the client's withdrawal from mood-altering illicit substances, he/she has displayed an increase in primary psychosis symptoms.

D. As the client has terminated his/her use of mood-altering illicit substances, his/her experience of primary psychosis symptoms has decreased significantly.

4. Exacerbation of Secondary Symptoms (2)

A. The client has displayed an exacerbation of secondary psychosis symptoms (e.g., anxiety, unstable affect, disorganization) as a result of abuse of mood-altering illicit substances.

* The numbers in parentheses correlate to the number of the Behavioral Definition statement in the companion chapter with the same title in *The Severe and Persistent Mental Illness Treatment Planner,* 2nd ed. (Berghuis and Jongsma) by John Wiley & Sons, 2008.

B. The client has displayed increased anxiety, unstable affect, and disorganization as a result of withdrawal from mood-altering illicit substances.

C. As the client has terminated his/her use of mood-altering illicit substances, his/her experience of secondary psychosis symptoms has decreased significantly.

5. Inability to Reduce Alcohol/Drug Abuse (3)

A. The client acknowledged that he/she frequently has attempted to terminate or reduce his/her use of mood-altering substances but found that he/she has been unable to follow through.

B. The client acknowledged that in spite of negative consequences and a desire to reduce or terminate the mood-altering substances, he/she has been unable to do so.

C. As the client has participated in a total recovery program, he/she has been able to maintain abstinence from mood-altering drug use.

6. Negative Blood Effects (4)

A. The client's blood work results reflect a pattern of heavy substance use in that his/her liver enzymes are elevated.

B. The client's blood work results indicate that mood-altering drugs have been used.

C. As the client has participated in the recovery program and has been able to maintain abstinence from mood-altering substances, his/her blood work has shown no evidence of ongoing substance abuse.

7. Denial (5)

A. The client presented with denial regarding the negative consequences of his/her substance abuse, in spite of direct feedback from others about its negative impact.

B. The client's denial is beginning to break down as he/she is acknowledging that substance abuse has created problems in his/her life.

C. The client now openly admits to the severe negative consequences brought on by his/her substance abuse.

8. Persistent Alcohol/Drug Abuse Despite Problems (6)

A. The client has continued to abuse alcohol and/or drugs in spite of recurring physical, legal, vocational, social, or relationship problems that were directly caused by the substance use.

B. The client has denied that the many problems in his/her life are directly caused by substance abuse.

C. The client acknowledged that substance abuse has been the cause of multiple problems in his/her life, and he/she verbalized a strong desire to maintain a life free from using all mood-altering substances.

D. As the client has maintained sobriety, some of the direct negative consequences of substance abuse have diminished.

E. The client is now able to face resolution of significant problems in his/her life as he/she has begun to establish sobriety.

9. Diversion of Resources (7)

A. The client displayed a pattern of diverting limited financial or personal resources into obtaining the substance, using the substance, or recovering from the effects of the substance.

B. The client's basic needs have gone unfulfilled due to his/her diverting financial and personal resources into substance use and abuse.

C. As the client has decreased or discontinued his/her substance use, he/she has used financial and personal resources in a more prudent, self-sustaining manner.

10. Medical Warnings (8)

A. The client acknowledged that a physician has warned him/her about the negative consequences of substance abuse.

B. The client has received specific warnings about the interactions of his/her psychotropic medications and illicit substances.

C. The client is suffering from poor health due to his/her substance abuse, but this substance abuse continues in spite of significant negative consequences.

D. The client's physical health has stabilized, and some of the negative consequences have begun to reverse as he/she has maintained a life free of mood-altering substances.

E. The client's psychiatric status has improved as his/her substance abuse has decreased due to the increased potency of his/her psychotropic medication and decreased negative interactions of illicit substances.

11. Increased Tolerance (9)

A. The client described a pattern of increasing tolerance for the mood-altering substance, as he/she needed to use more of it to obtain the desired effect.

B. The client described the steady increase in the amount and frequency of the substance abuse as his/her tolerance for it has increased.

12. Physical Withdrawal (10)

A. The client acknowledged that he/she has experienced physical withdrawal symptoms (e.g., shaking, seizures, nausea, headaches, sweating, insomnia) as he/she withdrew from the substance abuse.

B. The client's physical symptoms of withdrawal have eased as he/she stabilized and maintained abstinence from the mood-altering substance.

C. There is no further evidence of physical withdrawal symptoms associated with chemical dependence.

13. Relapse after Substantial Sobriety (11)

A. The client has relapsed after having been free from substance abuse for several years.

B. The client presented with low self-esteem and feelings of hopelessness and helplessness subsequent to reverting to substance abuse after a substantial period of sobriety.

C. The client is confident that he/she can return to clean and sober living after having relapsed briefly following a period of substantial sobriety.

INTERVENTIONS IMPLEMENTED

1. Remove Substances (1)*

A. After obtaining permission from the client, illicit substances were removed from his/her immediate access and disposed of.

B. The client was assisted with disposing of his/her available illicit mood-altering substances.

C. The client refused to dispose of or give permission for removal of his/her illicit mood-altering substance despite being urged to do so.

2. Refer to an Emergency Room (2)

A. The client was referred to an emergency room for immediate medical assessment and care relative to present substance use and intoxication.

B. Transportation to an emergency room was provided for the client for immediate medical assessment and care.

C. The client required an ambulance to assist him/her in obtaining emergency medical care.

D. The client declined to submit to emergency medical care or assessment relative to his/her present substance use and intoxication.

3. Assess Intoxication (3)

A. The client's current level of intoxication was assessed by subjective means (e.g., reviewing his/her behavior or speech).

B. Based on subjective means, the client is identified as being significantly intoxicated.

C. The client's level of intoxication was reviewed through objective means, such as a Breathalyzer or blood test.

D. Based on objective assessment, the client meets the legal standard for intoxication.

E. Based on the results of both a subjective and objective evaluation, the client is not intoxicated.

4. Refer to Detoxification (4)

A. The client was referred to an acute detoxification unit within a substance abuse treatment program.

B. The client was referred to a hospital-based acute detoxification unit.

C. The client was supported as he/she willingly admitted himself/herself to an acute detoxification unit.

D. The client declined to admit himself/herself to an acute detoxification unit, despite being urged to do so.

* The numbers in parentheses correlate to the number of the Therapeutic Intervention statement in the companion chapter with the same title in *The Severe and Persistent Mental Illness Treatment Planner,* 2nd ed. (Berghuis and Jongsma) by John Wiley & Sons, 2008.

5. Assess Suicide Risk (5)

A. The client was asked to describe the frequency and intensity of his/her suicidal ideation, the details of any suicide plan, the history of any previous suicide attempts, and any family history of depression or suicide.

B. The client was asked to promise to be forthright regarding the current and future strength of his/her suicidal feelings and the ability to control such suicidal urges.

C. The client was monitored on an ongoing basis for his/her suicide potential.

D. The client denied any pattern of suicidal ideation and was assessed to be not at risk for harming himself/herself.

6. Refer to Medical Staff for Immediate Physical Needs (6)

A. An immediate physical examination was arranged for the client, and the medical staff was encouraged to identify rehabilitation programs to aid the client in recovering from chemical dependence.

B. Medical staff examined the client, and specific negative medical effects of chemical dependence were identified.

C. The medical staff has identified specific recommendations to help remediate the immediate effects of the client's chemical dependence.

D. The physician has not identified any physical effects related to the client's chemical dependence.

E. Specific chemical dependence remediation behaviors were reviewed with the client.

7. Encourage Healthy Nutrition (7)

A. The client was encouraged to maintain healthy nutritional practices.

B. Education was provided to the client regarding his/her nutrition needs.

C. The client was provided with positive feedback regarding his/her pattern of healthy nutrition.

D. The client has not been maintaining healthy nutritional practices and was urged to modify this pattern.

8. Refer to a Dietician or Nutritionist (8)

A. The client was referred to a dietician for an assessment regarding basic nutritional knowledge and skills, usual diet, and nutritional deficiencies.

B. The client has met with the dietician, and the results of his/her assessment were reviewed.

C. The client displayed an understanding of his/her nutritional functioning as the assessment was reviewed.

D. The client displayed a lack of understanding about the information contained in the nutritional assessment and was provided with additional feedback in this area.

E. The client has not followed through on his/her referral to a dietician and was redirected to do so.

9. Identify Residential Needs (9)

A. The client was assisted in identifying his/her residential needs that will be most conducive to his/her sobriety and mental health stabilization.

B. The client was provided with feedback as he/she described aspects of his/her current residential needs.

C. The client identified that he/she needs a place to live that will be supportive of his/her abstinence from substance abuse and was praised for his/her understanding.

D. The client was referred to a local crisis residential program.

E. The client was accompanied to a local crisis housing program and advocated for regarding his/her need to be admitted to the program.

F. The client has been admitted to a crisis housing setting.

G. The client refused any involvement in the crisis housing and was redirected to the benefits of this type of service.

10. Facilitate an Agreement with the Landlord or Home Provider (10)

A. An agreement was facilitated between the client and the landlord or home provider regarding expectations for the client to remain in that residential setting.

B. The client's pattern of symptoms and behaviors related to his/her psychiatric status and substance abuse were reviewed and incorporated into the agreement with the landlord or home provider.

C. The client's landlord or home provider was supported for demonstrating an understanding of the client's specific needs within the residential setting.

D. The client continues to be at risk for removal from his/her current residential situation due to his/her exacerbated psychiatric symptoms and substance abuse.

11. Explore Victimization (11)

A. The client was asked about any recent history of having experienced sexual, physical, or other types of victimization.

B. The client identified recent experiences of victimization, and this was reviewed within the session.

C. The client was provided with empathetic support regarding his/her reports of victimization.

D. The client denied any recent experience of sexual, physical, or other types of victimization.

12. Contact Adult Protective Services (12)

A. The local adult protective services agency was contacted regarding abuse that has been occurring to client.

B. Advocacy was provided on behalf of the client regarding the need for intervention by the adult protective services unit due to the client being abused.

C. Adult protective services staff has not followed up on possible abuse, and further advocacy was provided.

13. Provide Information to Legal Authorities (13)

A. After obtaining a proper authorization to release confidential information, information regarding the client's mental illness and its effect on his/her behavior was provided to legal authorities.

B. Legal authorities were provided with feedback regarding the impact of the client's mental illness on his/her behavior, and this assisted in the appropriate adjudication of his/her legal concerns.

C. Legal authorities appear to be disinterested in the client's mental illness issues, and further advocacy was provided in this area.

D. The client refused to provide an authorization to release information, so no information was provided to the police/prosecutor.

14. Urge Personal Responsibility (14)

A. The client was urged to accept personal responsibility for his/her substance abuse and the consequences of his/her erratic behavior.

B. As the client accepted his/her responsibility for his/her substance abuse and erratic behavior, he/she was provided with positive feedback.

C. The client tends to minimize and deny his/her substance abuse and consequent erratic behavior and was given additional feedback in this area.

15. Facilitate Involvement with Legal Needs (15)

A. The client was encouraged to attend legal appointments, court dates, and other legal needs.

B. Transportation to the client's legal appointments, court dates, and other legal needs was provided.

C. The client was accompanied to his/her legal appointments.

D. Despite providing support to help the client keep his/her legal appointments and court dates, he/she continues to be sporadic in his/her attendance.

16. Coordinate Support System Confrontation (16)

A. Family members, friends, and colleagues were coordinated to confront the client about the negative effects that his/her substance abuse has had on their lives and on their relationships with him/her.

B. The client's friends and family were supported in gathering to confront the client about his/her substance abuse and the negative effects it has had on their relationships with the client.

C. The client received positive feedback for his/her ability to accept the confrontation from his/her support system and described an increased determination to discontinue his/her substance use.

D. The client reacted negatively to the confrontation from his/her support system and was urged to review their concerns.

17. Conduct Motivational Interviewing (17)

A. Motivational Interviewing techniques were used to help assess the client's preparation for change.

B. The client was assisted in identifying his/her stage of change regarding his/her substance abuse concerns.

C. It was reflected to the client that he/she is currently building motivation for change.

D. The client was assisted in strengthening his/her commitment to change.

E. The client was noted to be participating actively in treatment.

18. Gather Drug/Alcohol History (18)

A. The client was asked to describe his/her substance abuse in terms of the amount and pattern of use, symptoms of abuse, and negative life consequences that have resulted from chemical dependence.

B. The client was reinforced for openly discussing his/her substance abuse history and giving complete data regarding its nature and extent.

C. The client was confronted for minimizing his/her substance abuse and not giving reliable data regarding the nature and extent of his/her chemical dependence problem.

19. Gather Drug/Alcohol Abuse Information from Support Network (19)

A. Family members, peers, and other treatment staff were requested to provide additional information regarding the client's substance use history.

B. Family members have not given reliable data regarding the nature and extent of the client's chemical dependence problems and were confronted on minimizing the client's substance abuse.

20. Administer Objective Test of Drug/Alcohol Abuse (20)

A. The Alcohol Severity Index was administered to the client.

B. The Michigan Alcohol Screening Test (MAST) was administered to the client.

C. The results of the objective test of drug/alcohol abuse, which indicated a significant substance abuse problem, were processed with the client.

D. The results of the objective test of drug/alcohol abuse indicated that the client's problem with chemical dependence is relatively minor, and this was shared with the client.

21. Refer to a Physician (21)

A. The client was referred to a physician/psychiatrist who is familiar with both mental illness and chemical dependence issues for an evaluation for a prescription of psychotropic medications.

B. The client was reinforced for following through on a referral to a physician for an assessment for a prescription of psychotropic medications, but none were prescribed.

C. The client has been prescribed psychotropic medications.

D. The client declined evaluation by a physician for a prescription of psychotropic medication and was redirected to cooperate with this referral.

22. Monitor Medications (22)

A. The client was monitored for compliance with his/her psychotropic medication regimen.

B. The client was provided with positive feedback about his/her regular use of psychotropic medications.

C. The client was monitored for the effectiveness and side effects of his/her prescribed medications.

D. Concerns about the client's medication effectiveness and side effects were communicated to the physician.

E. Although the client was monitored for medication side effects, he/she reported no concerns in this area.

23. List Reasons Why Substance Abuse Is Attractive (23)

A. Today's clinical contact focused on developing a list of reasons why the client finds substance abuse attractive.

B. The client was assisted in identifying specific reasons why he/she finds substance abuse to be attractive (e.g., self-medication of mental illness symptoms, novelty seeking, euphoria).

C. The client's list of reasons why substance abuse is attractive was processed with the clinician.

D. The client has not developed a list of why substance abuse is attractive for him/her and was redirected to do so.

24. List Negative Impact of Substance Abuse (24)

A. The client was asked to list all of the negative consequences that have resulted from his/her substance abuse.

B. The client's list of the ways substance abuse has had a negative impact was processed, and each negative impact was reinforced with him/her.

C. The client's list of the negative impact of his/her substance abuse was processed, and the shortness of the list was confronted as denial on his/her part.

D. The client has not completed his/her list of the negative impact of his/her substance abuse and was redirected to do so.

25. Assign First Step Paper (25)

A. The client was assigned to complete an Alcoholics Anonymous First Step paper and to share it with a group and the therapist.

B. The client has completed a First Step paper; it was reviewed and noted to reflect that chemical dependence has dominated and controlled his/her life.

C. The client has failed to complete a First Step paper and was redirected to do so.

26. Reinforce Breakdown of Denial (26)

A. The client was reinforced for any statement that reflected acceptance of his/her chemical dependence and acknowledgment of the destructive consequences that it has had on his/her life.

B. The client was noted to have decreased his/her level of denial as evidenced by fewer statements that minimize the amount of his/her alcohol/drug abuse and its negative impact on his/her life.

27. Require More Learning about Chemical Dependence (27)

A. The client was required to learn more about chemical dependence and the recovery process.

B. The client was asked to attend didactic lectures, read, or view films related to chemical dependence and the process of recovery.

C. The client was asked to identify in writing several key points attained from his/her media about chemical dependence.

D. Key points from the media that were noted by the client were processed in individual sessions.

E. The client has become more open in acknowledging and accepting his/her chemical dependence; this openness was noted and reinforced.

F. The client has not sought out recommended media and was redirected to do so.

28. Assign AA/NA Member Contact (28)

A. The client was assigned to meet with an Alcoholics Anonymous/Narcotics Anonymous (AA/NA) member who has been working the 12-step program for several years to find out specifically how the program has helped him/her stay sober.

B. The client has followed through on meeting with the AA/NA member and was encouraged about the role that AA/NA can play in maintaining sobriety.

C. The client met with the AA/NA member but was not encouraged about the role of self-help groups in maintaining sobriety; his/her experience was processed.

D. The client has not followed through on meeting with an AA/NA member and was redirected to do so.

29. Identify Sobriety Expectations (29)

A. The client was requested to write out basic expectations that he/she has regarding sobriety.

B. The client has identified specific expectations that he/she has regarding sobriety (e.g., physical changes, social changes, emotional needs), and these were processed with the clinician.

C. As the client has been assisted in developing a more realistic expectation regarding his/her sobriety, he/she has felt more at ease and willing to work toward sobriety.

D. The client has not identified his/her expectations regarding sobriety and was redirected to do so.

30. Encourage Sobriety Despite Relapses (30)

A. Although the client has relapsed, he/she was refocused on the need for substance abuse recovery and on the need for sobriety.

B. As the client has received continued support for his/her recovery and sobriety despite his/her relapses, he/she has become more confident regarding his/her chances for success.

C. The client lacks confidence in his/her ability to obtain recovery and sobriety due to his/her pattern of relapses; this pessimism was challenged and processed.

31. Plan for Extended Monitoring (31)

A. Due to the chronic nature and high recidivism of mentally ill substance abusers, the client was advised about the need for an extended pattern of monitoring of his/her symptoms.

B. The client was supported for endorsing the need for extended monitoring due to the chronic nature of his/her substance abuse and mental illness symptoms.

C. The client struggled to endorse the need for extended monitoring of his/her symptoms and was provided with additional feedback and information in this area.

32. Assign Good-Bye Letter to Drug (32)

A. The client was assigned to write a good-bye letter to his/her drug of choice as a means of terminating his/her emotional and cognitive involvement with that drug.

B. The client has followed through with writing the good-bye letter to his/her drug of choice, and the contents of it were processed.

C. The client's feelings about writing a good-bye letter to the drug of choice were processed.

D. The client reported that he/she felt some sense of relief at breaking emotional ties with his/her drug of choice; the benefits of this progress were reviewed.

E. The client failed to follow through on the assigned good-bye letter to his/her drug of choice and was redirected to do so.

33. Refer to Alcoholics Anonymous/Narcotics Anonymous (AA/NA) Meetings (33)

A. It was strongly recommended to the client that he/she attend AA/NA meetings on a frequent and regular basis in order to obtain support for his/her sobriety.

B. The client has followed through on consistent attendance at AA/NA meetings and reports that the meetings have been helpful: these benefits were processed.

C. The client has attended AA/NA meetings as requested, but reports that he/she does not find them helpful and is resistive to return to them.

D. The client has not followed through on regular attendance at AA/NA meetings and was redirected to do so.

34. Assess Intellectual, Personality, and Cognitive Functioning (34)

A. The client's intellectual, personality, and cognitive functioning were assessed by means of psychological testing.

B. The client's intellectual, personality, and cognitive functioning were assessed by means of clinical interview.

C. The results of the psychological assessment were given to the client and the factors that may contribute to his/her chemical dependence were highlighted.

35. Review Negative Peer Influence (35)

A. A review of the client's negative peers was performed, and the influence of these people on his/her substance abuse patterns was identified.

B. The client accepted the interpretation that maintaining contact with substance-abusing friends would reduce the probability of successful recovery from his/her chemical dependence.

C. A plan was developed to help the client initiate contact with sober people who could exert a positive influence on his/her own recovery (e.g., sobriety buddies).

D. The client has begun to reach out socially to sober individuals in order to develop a social network that has a more positive influence on his/her recovery; he/she was reinforced for this progress.

E. The client has not attempted to reach out socially to sober individuals in order to develop a social network that has a more positive influence in his/her recovery and was reminded about this important facet of his/her recovery.

36. Plan Social and Recreational Activities (36)

A. A list of social and recreational activities that are free from association with substance abuse was developed.

B. The client was verbally reinforced as he/she agreed to begin involvement in new recreational and social activities that will replace substance abuse-related activities.

C. The client has begun to make changes in his/her social and/or recreational activities and reports feeling good about this change; the benefits of this progress were reviewed.

D. The client was very resistive to any changes in social and recreational activities that have previously been a strong part of his/her life, but was encouraged to begin with small changes in this area.

37. Evaluate Living Situation (37)

A. The client's current living situation was reviewed as to whether it fosters a pattern of chemical dependence.

B. The client was supported as he/she agreed that his/her current living situation does encourage continuing substance abuse.

C. The client could not see any reason why his/her current living situation would have a negative effect on his/her chemical dependence recovery; he/she was provided with tentative examples in this area.

38. Encourage a Change in Living Situation (38)

A. The client was encouraged to develop a plan to find a more positive living situation that will foster his/her chemical dependence recovery.

B. The client was reinforced as he/she found a new living situation that is free from the negative influences that the current living situation brings to his/her chemical dependence recovery.

C. The client is very resistive to moving from his/her current living situation; he/she was assisted in processing this resistance.

39. Identify Sobriety's Positive Family Effects (39)

A. The client was assisted in identifying the positive changes that will occur within family relationships as a result of his/her chemical dependence recovery.

B. The client reported that his/her family is enjoying a reduction in stress and increased cooperation since his/her chemical dependence recovery began; his/her reaction to these changes was processed.

C. The client was unable to identify any positive changes that have or could occur within family relationships as a result of his/her chemical dependence recovery and was provided with tentative examples in this area.

40. Reinforce Making Amends (40)

A. The negative effects that the client's substance abuse has had on family, friends, and work relationships were identified.

B. A plan for making amends to those who have been negatively affected by the client's substance abuse was developed.

C. The client's implementation of his/her plan to make amends to those who have been hurt by his/her substance abuse was reviewed.

D. The client reported feeling good about the fact that he/she has begun to make amends to others who have been hurt by his/her substance abuse; this progress was reinforced.

E. The client has not followed through on making amends to others who have been negatively affected by his/her pattern of substance abuse and was reminded to do so.

41. Obtain Commitment Regarding Making Amends (41)

A. The client was asked to make a verbal commitment to make amends to key individuals.

B. The client was urged to make further amends while working through Steps 8 and 9 of a 12-step program.

C. The client was supported as he/she made a verbal commitment to make initial amends now and to make further amends as he/she works through Steps 8 and 9 (of the 12-step program).

D. The client declined to commit to making amends and was redirected to review the need to make this commitment.

42. Refer for Marital Therapy (42)

A. The couple was referred to a clinician who specializes in Behavioral Marital Therapy.

B. The couple was provided with Behavioral Marital Therapy.

C. The couple was assisted in identifying conflicts that could be addressed using communication, conflict-resolution, and/or problem-solving skills.

D. Techniques described by Holzworth-Monroe and Jacobson in "Behavioral Marital Therapy" in *Handbook of Family Therapy* (Gurman and Knickerson) were used to help the couple develop better communication, conflict-resolution, and problem-solving skills.

43. Teach about Coping Package (43)

A. The client was taught a variety of techniques to help manage urges to use chemical substances.

B. The client was taught calming strategies, such as relaxation and breathing techniques.

C. The client was taught cognitive techniques, such as thought-stopping, positive self-talk, and attention-focusing skills (e.g., distraction from urges, staying focused, behavioral goals of abstinence).

D. The client has used his/her coping package techniques to help reduce his/her urges to use chemical substances; this progress was reinforced.

E. The client has not used the coping package for managing urges to use chemical substances and was redirected to do so.

44. Explore Schema and Self-Talk (44)

A. The client's schema and self-talk that weaken his/her resolve to remain abstinent were explored.

B. The biases that the client entertains regarding his/her schema and self-talk were challenged.

C. The client was assisted in generating more realistic self-talk to correct for his/her biases and build resilience.

D. The client was provided with positive feedback for his/her replacement of self-talk and biases.

E. The client struggled to identify his/her self-talk and biases that weaken his/her resolve to remain abstinent and was provided with tentative examples in this area.

45. Rehearse Replacement of Negative Self-Talk (45)

A. The client was assisted in identifying situations in which his/her negative self-talk occurs.

B. The client was assisted in generating empowering alternatives to his/her negative self-talk.

C. The client was assigned "Negative Thoughts Trigger Negative Feelings" from the *Adult Psychotherapy Homework Planner,* 2nd ed. (Jongsma).

D. The client's success in rehearsing the response to negative self-talk was reviewed and reinforced.

46. Develop Hierarchy of Urge-Producing Cues (46)

A. The client was directed to construct a hierarchy of urge-producing cues to use substances.

B. The client was assisted in developing a hierarchy of urge-producing cues to use substances.

C. The client was helped to identify a variety of cues that prompt his/her use of substances.

47. Practice Response to Urge-Producing Cues (47)

A. The client was assisted in selecting urge-producing cues with which to practice, with a bias toward cues that are likely to result in a successful experience.

B. Behavioral techniques were used to help the client cognitively restructure his/her urge-producing cues.

C. The client's use of cognitive-restructuring strategies was reviewed and processed.

48. Assess Stress-Management Skills (48)

A. The client's current level of skill in managing everyday stressors was assessed.

B. The client was assessed in regard to his/her ability to meet role demands for work, social, and family expectations.

C. Behavioral and cognitive-restructuring techniques were used to help build social and communication skills to manage everyday challenges.

D. The client was provided with positive feedback regarding his/her ability to manage common everyday stressors.

E. The client continues to struggle with common everyday stressors and was provided with remedial feedback in this area.

49. Assign Social and Communication Information (49)

A. The client was assigned to read about social skills.

B. The client was assigned to read about communication skills.

C. The client was assigned to read *Your Perfect Right* (Alberti and Emmons).

D. The client was assigned to read *Conversationally Speaking* (Garner).

E. The client has read the assigned information about social and communication skills and key points were reviewed.

F. The client has not read the assigned information on social and communication skills and was redirected to do so.

50. Differentiate between Lapse and Relapse (50)

A. A discussion was held with the client regarding the distinction between a lapse and a relapse.

B. A lapse was associated with an initial and reversible return of symptoms or urges to use substances.

C. A relapse was associated with the decision to return to regular use of substances.

D. The client was provided with support and encouragement as he/she displayed an understanding of the difference between a lapse and a relapse.

E. The client struggled to understand the difference between a lapse and a relapse and was provided with remedial feedback in this area.

51. Discuss Management of Lapse Risk Situations (51)

A. The client was assisted in identifying future situations or circumstances in which lapses could occur.

B. The session focused on rehearsing the management of future situations or circumstances in which lapses could occur.

C. The client was asked to identify how family and peer conflict contribute to his/her stress levels.

D. The client was reinforced for his/her appropriate use of lapse management skills.

E. The client was redirected in regard to his/her poor use of lapse management skills.

52. Identify Relapse Triggers (52)

A. The client was assisted in developing a list of potential relapse signs and triggers that could lead him/her back to substance abuse.

B. The client was requested to identify specific primary psychotic symptoms that affect his/her desire for substances.

C. The client was supported for identifying specific primary psychotic symptoms and how these increase his/her desire for substances.

D. The client was assisted in developing a specific strategy for constructively responding to his/her substance abuse relapse triggers.

E. The client was reinforced for his/her successful implementation of the coping strategies for the substance abuse relapse triggers.

F. A review was conducted regarding the client's pattern of relapse subsequent to failing to use constructive coping strategies in a trigger situation.

53. Encourage Routine Use of Strategies (53)

A. The client was instructed to routinely use the strategies that he/she has learned in therapy (e.g., cognitive restructuring exposure).

B. The client was urged to find ways to build his/her new strategies into his/her life as much as possible.

C. The client was reinforced as he/she reported ways in which he/she has incorporated coping strategies into his/her life and routine.

D. The client was redirected about ways to incorporate his/her new strategies into his/her routine and life.

54. Refer to Supported Employment (54)

A. The client was referred to a supported employment program to assist him/her in developing independent job skills.

B. The client was reinforced for his/her involvement in the supported employment program that has assisted him/her in skill building regarding employment needs.

C. The client has not actively participated in the supported employment program and was redirected to do so.

55. Coach Regarding Employment Issues (55)

A. The client was coached regarding his/her preparation for employment, searching for a job, and maintaining employment.

B. The client was assisted in role-playing and rehearsing specific techniques necessary for obtaining and maintaining employment.

C. The client was provided with positive feedback regarding his/her increased understanding of issues related to obtaining and maintaining employment.

D. The client continues to have a poor understanding of basic concepts related to obtaining and maintaining employment and was provided with additional feedback in this area.

56. Solicit Family Support (56)

A. The client was directed to solicit support from family members for his/her sobriety.

B. The client was reinforced for developing specific support from his/her family members for his/her sober lifestyle.

C. The client's family members have been reluctant to support his/her sober lifestyle due to his/her mental illness and substance abuse pattern, and this was processed within the session.

D. The client described that his/her family has been reluctant to support his/her sober lifestyle due to their own substance abuse concerns, and this was processed within the session.

E. The client has not solicited family support for his/her sober lifestyle and was provided with additional encouragement and redirection in this area.

57. Coordinate Meeting with a 12-Step Recovery Program Sponsor (57)

A. A meeting was set up between the client and a sponsor from a 12-step program to find out specifically how the program has helped the sponsor stay sober.

B. The client's sponsor was provided with additional information regarding mental illness issues to assist in his/her relationship with the client.

C. The client was reinforced for following through with the planned meeting with the 12-step program sponsor, and for reporting that he/she felt encouraged about the role of a 12-step program in maintaining his/her sobriety.

D. The client kept the planned meeting with a 12-step recovery program sponsor but was not encouraged about the role of self-help groups in maintaining sobriety; this meeting was processed.

E. The client has not followed through on meeting with a 12-step recovery program sponsor and was redirected to do so.

58. Refer Family to a Support Group (58)

A. The client's family was referred to a community-based support group for loved ones of chronically mentally ill substance abusers.

B. Family members were reinforced for becoming involved in a community-based support group for the loved ones of chronically mentally ill substance abusers and for reporting that this has been helpful in dealing with the stress that occurs due to the client's substance abuse and mental illness symptoms.

C. Family members have not been involved in a community-based support group and were redirected to do so.

59. Encourage Consistent Attendance at Recovery Meetings (59)

A. The client was strongly encouraged to consistently attend 12-step recovery program meetings three or more times per week in order to obtain support for his/her sobriety.

B. The client was reinforced for following through with consistent attendance to 12-step recovery program meetings, and he/she reports that the meetings have been helpful.

C. The client has not followed through on regular attendance to 12-step recovery program meetings and was redirected to do so.

D. The client has attended 12-step recovery meetings as requested, but he/she reports that he/she does not find them helpful and is resistive to return to them; this resistance was processed.

60. Develop Aftercare Plan (60)

A. The client was assisted in developing an aftercare plan that will support the maintenance of long-term sobriety.

B. The client has listed several components to an aftercare plan that will support his/her sobriety, such as family activities, counseling, self-help support groups, and sponsors; feedback about his/her list was provided.

C. The client has not followed through on developing an aftercare plan and was redirected to do so.

61. Coordinate Contact with Recovering Mentally Ill Individual (61)

A. Contact between the client and another mentally ill individual who is further along in his/her substance abuse recovery was coordinated in order to help the client process how others have achieved sobriety.

B. The client has followed up on his/her contact with another mentally ill individual who is further along in substance abuse recovery, and this contact was processed within the session.

C. The client has not followed up on contact with another mentally ill individual in recovery and was redirected to do so.

DEPRESSION

CLIENT PRESENTATION

1. Changes in Appetite (1)*

A. The client reported that he/she has had a significant decrease in his/her appetite.

B. The client reported that he/she has had a significant increase in his/her appetite.

C. The client's change in appetite has resulted in significant weight changes associated with the depression.

D. As the depression has begun to lift, the client's appetite has returned to normal.

E. The client reported that his/her appetite is at normal levels.

2. Depressed Affect (2)

A. The client reported that he/she feels deeply sad and has periods of tearfulness on an almost daily basis.

B. The client's depressed affect was clearly evident within the session as tears were shed on more than one occasion.

C. The client reported that he/she has begun to feel less sad and can experience periods of joy.

D. The client appeared to be happier within the session, and there was no evidence of tearfulness.

E. The client reported no experience of depressed affect.

3. Lack of Activity Enjoyment (3)

A. The client reported a diminished interest in or enjoyment of activities that he/she previously found pleasurable.

B. The client has begun to involve himself/herself with activities that he/she previously found pleasurable.

C. The client has returned to an active interest in and enjoyment of activities.

4. Sleeplessness/Hypersomnia (4)

A. The client reported periods of inability to sleep and other periods of sleeping for many hours without the desire to get out of bed.

B. The client's problem with sleep disturbance has diminished as the depression has lifted.

C. Medication has improved the client's problems with sleep disturbance.

D. The client reported a normal sleep routine resulting in his/her feeling rested.

5. Decreased Energy Level (5)

A. The client reported that he/she feels a very low level of energy compared with normal times in his/her life.

B. It was evident within the session that the client has low levels of energy as demonstrated by slowness of walking, minimal movement, lack of animation, and slow responses.

---

* The numbers in parentheses correlate to the number of the Behavior Definition statement in the companion chapter with the same title in *The Severe and Persistent Mental Illness Treatment Planner*, 2nd ed. (Berghuis and Jongsma) by John Wiley & Sons, 2008.

C. The client's energy level has increased as the depression has lifted.

D. It was evident within the session that the client is demonstrating normal levels of energy.

6. Psychomotor Agitation (6)

A. The client demonstrated psychomotor agitation within the session.

B. The client reported that with the onset of the depression, he/she has felt unable to relax or sit quietly.

C. The client reported a significant decrease in psychomotor agitation and an increase in the ability to sit more quietly.

D. It was evident within the session that the client has become more relaxed and less agitated.

7. Psychomotor Retardation (6)

A. The client demonstrated evidence of psychomotor retardation within the session.

B. The client moved and responded very slowly, showing a lack of energy and motivation.

C. As the depression has lifted, the client has responded more quickly and his/her psychomotor retardation has diminished.

8. Social Withdrawal (7)

A. The client has withdrawn from social relationships that were important to him/her.

B. As the client's depression has deepened, he/she has increasingly isolated himself/herself.

C. The client has begun to reach out to social contacts as the depression has begun to lift.

D. The client has resumed normal social interactions.

9. Feelings of Hopelessness and Worthlessness (8)

A. The client has reported feelings of hopelessness and worthlessness that began as the depression deepened.

B. The client's feelings of hopelessness and worthlessness have diminished as the depression begins to lift.

C. The client expressed hope for the future and affirmation of his/her own self-worth.

10. Inappropriate Guilt (8)

A. The client described feelings of pervasive, irrational guilt.

B. Although the client verbalized an understanding that his/her guilt is irrational, it continues to plague him/her.

C. The depth of irrational guilt has lifted as the depression has subsided.

D. The client no longer experiences feelings of irrational guilt.

11. Hallucinations or Delusions (9)

A. The client has experienced mood-related hallucinations or delusions, indicating that the depression has a psychotic component.

B. The client's thought disorder has begun to diminish as the depression has been treated.

C. The client reported no longer experiencing any thought disorder symptoms.

12. Losses Leading to Unresolved Grief (10)

A. The client has experienced losses related to his/her severe and persistent mental illness symptoms.

B. The client has been unable to resolve the grief that he/she experiences regarding his/her losses due to mental illness symptoms.

C. The client's feelings of grief have turned to major depression as energy has diminished and sadness and hopelessness dominate his/her life.

D. The client has begun to resolve the feelings of grief that are associated with the loss in his/her life.

E. The client has verbalized feelings of hopefulness regarding the future and acceptance of the losses of the past.

13. Suicidal Ideation (11)

A. The client expressed that he/she is experiencing suicidal thoughts but has not taken any action on these thoughts.

B. The client reported strong suicidal thoughts that have resulted in suicidal gestures or attempts.

C. The client reported that suicidal urges have diminished as the depression has lifted.

D. The client denied any suicidal thoughts or gestures and is more hopeful about the future.

14. Low Self-Esteem (12)

A. The client stated that he/she has a very negative perception of himself/herself.

B. The client's low self-esteem was evident within the session as he/she made many self-disparaging remarks and maintained very little eye contact.

C. The client's self-esteem has increased as he/she begins to affirm his/her self-worth.

D. The client verbalized positive feelings toward himself/herself.

INTERVENTIONS IMPLEMENTED

1. Assess Mood Episodes (1)*

A. An assessment was conducted on the client's current and past mood episodes, including the features, frequency, intensity, and duration of the mood episodes.

B. The *Inventory to Diagnose Depression* (Zimmerman, Coryell, Corenthal, and Wilson) was used to assess the client's current and past mood episodes.

C. The results of the mood episode assessment reflected severe mood concerns and this was presented to the client.

D. The results of the mood episode assessment reflected moderate mood concerns, and this was presented to the client.

E. The results of the mood episode assessment reflected mild mood concerns, and this was presented to the client.

2. Display Symptoms Graphically (2)

A. A graphic time line display was used to help the client chart his/her pattern of depression symptoms.

---

* The numbers in parentheses correlate to the number of the Therapeutic Intervention statement in the companion chapter with the same title in *The Severe and Persistent Mental Illness Treatment Planner*, 2nd ed. (Berghuis and Jongsma) by John Wiley & Sons, 2008.

B. The client's precursors, triggers, and pattern of depression symptoms were reviewed on a time line to explore how he/she experiences and is affected by depression.

C. The client displayed a greater understanding of his/her pattern of depression problems and was given support and feedback in this area.

D. The client struggled to understand his/her pattern of depression symptoms and was redirected in this area.

3. Obtain Feedback Regarding Depression Pattern (3)

A. The client's family, friends, and caregivers were asked about the client's pattern of depression symptoms.

B. The client's family was asked about the family history of depression.

C. Family, friends, and caregivers identified a pattern of depression for the client and within the family, and this was reviewed.

4. Log Current Level of Functioning (4)

A. The client, family, or caretaker was provided with sleeping, eating, and activity logs in which to document the client's current level of functioning.

B. Daily logs related to the client's sleeping, eating, and activity levels have been filled out regularly, and the aggregate results were reviewed, indicating a pattern of depression.

C. The client's symptom logs were reviewed, but do not indicate a pattern of depression symptoms.

D. Symptom logs have not been filled out regularly, and this assignment was reinforced as a helpful way to monitor the client's symptoms.

5. Encourage Expression of Depression Feelings (5)

A. The client was encouraged to identify and share his/her feelings of depression in order to clarify them and gain insight into the causes.

B. The client was provided with support and empathy as he/she described his/her feelings of depression.

C. As the client has expressed his/her pattern of depression feelings, he/she has been assisted in gaining insight into the causes for his/her depression.

D. The client was unable to clearly identify his/her depression feelings and was provided with additional feedback in this area.

6. Identify Losses Due to Severe and Persistent Mental Illness Symptoms (6)

A. Inquiries were made about specific losses that the client might have experienced due to his/her severe and persistent mental illness symptoms.

B. Empathy was provided as the client identified concerns related to loss of independence, income, freedom, dignity, or relationships due to his/her pattern of severe and persistent mental illness symptoms.

C. The client was provided with feedback about how his/her losses due to severe and persistent mental illness symptoms may contribute to secondary symptoms related to depression.

D. The client denied any specific losses due to his/her severe and persistent mental illness symptoms, and this was accepted.

7. Administer Psychological Tests for Depression (7)

A. Psychological testing was arranged to objectively assess the client's depression and suicide risk.

B. The Beck Depression Inventory—2 was used to assess the client's depression and suicide risk.

C. The Beck Hopelessness Scale was used to assess the client's depression and suicide risk.

D. The results of the testing indicated severe concerns related to the client's depression and suicide risk, and this was reflected to the client.

E. The results of the testing indicated moderate concerns related to the client's depression and suicide risk, and this was reflected to the client.

F. The results of the testing indicated mild concerns related to the client's depression and suicide risk, and this was reflected to the client.

8. Review Use of Stimulants and Depressants (8)

A. The client's acknowledged use of stimulants (e.g., nicotine, caffeine, street drugs) was reviewed.

B. The client's acknowledged use of depressants (e.g., barbiturates, alcohol) was reviewed.

C. The client was provided with feedback about his/her use of stimulants and depressants and the relationship to his/her symptoms.

D. The client denied any use of stimulants or depressants and was warned about the effect of such mood-altering substances on his/her pattern of symptoms.

9. Evaluate Substance Abuse (9)

A. The client was evaluated for his/her use of substances, the severity of his/her substance abuse, and treatment needs/options.

B. The client was referred to a clinician knowledgeable in both substance abuse and severe and persistent mental illness treatment in order to assess accurately his/her substance abuse concerns and treatment needs.

C. The client was compliant with the substance abuse evaluation, and the results of the evaluation were discussed with him/her.

D. The client did not participate in the substance abuse evaluation and was encouraged to do so.

10. Review Sleep Hygiene (10)

A. Basic steps to sleep hygiene (e.g., decreasing stimulants in the evening; having a quiet, comfortable place to sleep; spending time winding down) were reviewed.

B. The client's sleep hygiene pattern was reviewed, and he/she was reinforced for positive use of sleep induction techniques.

C. As the client has developed more structure to his/her sleep hygiene pattern, he/she has experienced a better pattern of sleep, and this was reviewed.

D. The client has not used the sleep hygiene techniques, continues to have poor sleep, and was given additional feedback in this area.

E. Behavior strategies to reinforce a structured sleep routine were introduced.

11. Refer for Sleep Study (11)

A. The client was referred to a sleep disorder specialist for an evaluation of his/her sleeping patterns.

B. The client has participated in an evaluation of his/her sleep pattern, and was found to have a specific sleep disorder.

C. The client has participated in a sleep disorder evaluation, but no specific sleep disorder was identified.

D. The client has been assisted in implementing steps to ameliorate his/her sleep disorder concerns.

12. Refer to a Supervised Environment (12)

A. Because the client was judged to be uncontrollably harmful to himself/herself, arrangements were made for psychiatric hospitalization.

B. The client was referred to a crisis residential facility due to concerns about his/her inability to manage himself/herself within a less restrictive setting.

C. The client was supported for cooperating voluntarily with admission to a more supervised environment.

D. The client refused to voluntarily admit himself/herself to a more supervised environment, and therefore civil commitment procedures were initiated.

13. Develop a Suicide Prevention Plan (13)

A. A suicide prevention plan was developed with the client focusing on how he/she will be monitored and to whom he/she should turn if suicidal ideation increases.

B. The client was given positive feedback for adhering to his/her structured suicide prevention plan.

C. The client has not adhered to the structured suicide prevention plan and was redirected to do so.

14. Refer for Medication Evaluation (14)

A. The client was referred to a physician for an evaluation for a prescription of psychotropic medications.

B. The client has followed through on a referral to a physician and has been assessed for a prescription of psychotropic medications, but none were prescribed.

C. The client has been prescribed psychotropic medications.

D. The client declined an evaluation by a physician for a prescription of psychotropic medications and was redirected to do so.

15. Educate about Psychotropic Medications (15)

A. The client was taught about the indications for and the expected benefits of psychotropic medications.

B. As the client's psychotropic medications were reviewed, he/she displayed an understanding about the indications for and expected benefits of the medications.

C. The client displayed a lack of understanding of the indications for and expected benefits of psychotropic medications and was provided with additional information and feedback regarding his/her medications.

16. Monitor Medications (16)

A. The client was monitored for compliance with his/her psychotropic medication regimen.

B. The client was provided with positive feedback about his/her regular use of psychotropic medications.

C. The client was monitored for the effectiveness and side effects of his/her prescribed medications.

D. Concerns about the client's medication effectiveness and side effects were communicated to the physician.

E. Although the client was monitored for medication side effects, he/she reported no concerns in this area.

17. Monitor Symptom Increase Due to an Antidepressant (17)

A. The client's pattern of severe and persistent mental illness symptoms was monitored due to the possibility of these being exacerbated by the introduction of an antidepressant medication.

B. The client's severe and persistent mental illness symptoms appear to have increased subsequent to the introduction of an antidepressant, and this information was reflected to the prescribing physician.

C. Medication adjustments have been implemented in order to decrease the negative effects of the antidepressant medication on the client's severe and persistent mental illness symptoms.

D. No exacerbation of severe and persistent mental illness symptoms has been identified subsequent to the introduction of antidepressants.

18. Discuss Depression Development, Maintenance, and Changes (18)

A. Factors that were related to the development and maintenance of the client's depression were discussed.

B. The focus was placed on how treatment will target specific factors that develop and maintain the client's depression.

C. The client has been able to disclose factors that develop and maintain his/her depression and is accepting of the ways in which treatment will target these factors for change.

D. The client has been uncertain about the factors that develop and maintain his/her depression and was provided with remedial feedback in this area.

19. Identify Depressogenic Schemata (19)

A. The client was assisted in developing an awareness of his/her automatic thoughts that reflect depressogenic schemata.

B. The client was assisted in developing an awareness of his/her distorted cognitive messages that reinforce hopelessness and helplessness.

C. The client was helped to identify several cognitive messages that occur on a regular basis and feed feelings of depression.

D. The client recalled several instances of engaging in negative self-talk that precipitated feelings of helplessness, hopelessness, and depression; these were processed.

20. Assign Dysfunctional-Thinking Journal (20)

A. The client was requested to keep a daily journal that lists each situation associated with depressed feelings and the dysfunctional thinking that triggered the depression.

B. The client was assigned to use the "Daily Record of Dysfunctional Thoughts," as described in *Cognitive Therapy of Depression* (Beck, Rush, Shaw, and Emery).

C. The client was directed to complete the "Negative Thoughts Trigger Negative Feelings" assignment from the *Adult Psychotherapy Homework Planner,* 2nd ed. (Jongsma).

D. The Socratic method was used to challenge the client's dysfunctional thoughts and to replace them with positive, reality-based thoughts.

E. The client was reinforced for instances of successful replacement of negative thoughts with more realistic positive thinking.

F. The client has not kept his/her record of automatic thoughts and was redirected to do so.

21. Conduct Behavioral Experiments (21)

A. The client was encouraged to do "behavioral experiments" in which depressive automatic thoughts are treated as hypotheses/predictions and are tested against reality-based alternative hypothesis.

B. The client's automatic depressive thoughts were tested against the client's past, present, and/or future experiences.

C. The client was assisted in processing the outcome of his/her behavioral experiences.

D. The client was encouraged by his/her experience of the more reality-based hypothesis/ predictions; this progress was reinforced.

E. The client continues to focus on depressive automatic thoughts and was redirected toward the behavioral evidence of the more reality-based alternative hypotheses.

22. Reinforce Positive Self-Talk (22)

A. The client was reinforced for any successful replacement of distorted negative thinking with positive, reality-based cognitive messages.

B. It was noted that the client has been engaging in positive,, reality-based thinking that has enhanced his/her self-confidence and increased adaptive action.

C. The client was assigned to complete the "Positive Self-Talk" assignment from the *Adult Psychotherapy Homework Planner,* 2nd ed. (Jongsma).

23. Teach Behavioral Coping Strategies (23)

A. The client was taught behavioral coping strategies such as physical exercise, increased social involvement, sharing of feelings, and increased assertiveness as ways to reduce feelings of depression.

B. The client has implemented behavioral coping strategies to reduce feelings of depression and was reinforced for doing so.

C. The client reported that the utilization of behavioral coping strategies has been successful at reducing feelings of depression; the benefits of this progress were reviewed.

D. The client was assisted in identifying several instances in which behavioral coping strategies were helpful in reducing depressive feelings.

E. The client has not used behavioral coping strategies and was redirected to use this important resource.

24. Engage in Behavioral Activation (24)

A. The client was engaged in "behavioral activation" by scheduling activities that have a high likelihood for pleasure and mastery.

B. The client was directed to complete tasks from the "Identify and Schedule Pleasant Events" assignment from the *Adult Psychotherapy Homework Planner,* 2nd ed. (Jongsma).

C. Rehearsal, role-playing, role reversal, and other techniques were used to engage the client in behavioral activation.

D. The client was reinforced for his/her successes in scheduling activities that have a high likelihood for pleasure and mastery.

E. The client has not engaged in pleasurable activities and was redirected to do so.

25. Employ Self-Reliance Training (25)

A. Self-reliance training was used to help the client assume increased responsibility for routine activities (e.g., cleaning, cooking, shopping).

B. The client was urged to take responsibility for routine activities in order to overcome depression symptoms.

C. The client was reinforced for his/her increased self-reliance.

D. The client has not assumed increased responsibility for routine activities and his/her struggles in this area were redirected.

26. Assess the Interpersonal Inventory (26)

A. The client was asked to develop an "interpersonal inventory" of important past and present relationships.

B. The client's interpersonal inventory was assessed for potentially depressive themes (e.g., grief, interpersonal disputes, role transitions, interpersonal deficits).

C. The client's interpersonal inventory was found to have significant depressive themes, and this was reflected to the client.

D. The client's interpersonal inventory was found to have minimal depressive themes, and this was reflected to the client.

27. Explore Unresolved Grief (27)

A. The client's history of losses that have triggered feelings of grief were explored.

B. The client was assisted in identifying losses that have contributed to feelings of grief that have not been resolved.

C. The client's unresolved feelings of grief are noted to be contributing to current feelings of depression and were provided a special focus.

28. Teach Assertiveness (28)

A. The client was referred to an assertiveness training group that will educate and facilitate assertiveness skills.

B. Role-playing, modeling, and behavioral rehearsal were used to train the client in assertiveness skills.

C. The client has demonstrated a clearer understanding of the difference between assertiveness, passivity, and aggressiveness; he/she was urged to use these skills.

D. The client displayed a poor understanding of assertiveness skills and was provided with remedial training in this area.

29. Teach Conflict Resolution Skills (29)

A. The client was taught conflict resolution skills such as practicing empathy, active listening, respectful communication, assertiveness, and compromise.

B. Using role-playing, modeling, and behavioral rehearsal, the client was taught implementation of conflict resolution skills.

C. The client reported implementation of conflict resolution skills in his/her daily life and was reinforced for this utilization.

D. The client reported that resolving interpersonal conflicts has contributed to a lifting of his/her depression; the benefits of this progress were emphasized.

E. The client has not used the conflict-resolution skills that he/she has been taught and was provided with specific examples of when to use these skills.

30. Help Resolve Interpersonal Problems (30)

A. The client was assisted in resolving interpersonal problems through the use of reassurance and support.

B. The "Applying Problem-Solving to Interpersonal Conflict" assignment from the *Adult Psychotherapy Homework Planner,* 2nd ed. (Jongsma) was used to help resolve interpersonal problems.

C. The client was helped to clarify cognitive and affective triggers that ignite conflicts.

D. The client was taught active problem-solving techniques to help him/her resolve interpersonal problems.

E. It was reflected to the client that he/she has significantly reduced his/her interpersonal problems.

F. The client continues to have significant interpersonal problems, and he/she was provided with remedial assistance in this area.

31. Address Interpersonal Conflict through Conjoint Sessions (31)

A. A conjoint session was held to assist the client in resolving interpersonal conflicts with his/her partner.

B. The client reported that the conjoint sessions have been helpful in resolving interpersonal conflicts with his/her partner, and this has contributed to a lifting of his/her depression.

C. It was reflected that ongoing conflicts with a partner have fostered feelings of depression and hopelessness.

32. Teach Decision-Making Strategy (32)

A. The client was taught specific decision-making strategies.

B. The client was encouraged to identify one problem at a time, break the decision down into relevant parts, examine the pros and cons of relevant choices, and develop a decision based on that procedure.

C. The client was reinforced for his/her successful use of decision-making skills.

D. The client gave specific examples of his/her use of decision-making strategies.

E. The client has not used appropriate decision-making strategies and was redirected to do so.

33. Discourage Major Decisions While Depressed (33)

A. The client was discouraged from making major life decisions until after his/her mood disorder improves.

B. The client acknowledges the need to improve his/her mood before making major life decisions and was commended for this restraint.

C. The client continues to attempt to make major life changes despite the presence of his/her mood disorder and was provided with additional feedback in this area.

34. Reinforce Physical Exercise (34)

A. A plan for routine physical exercise was developed with the client, and a rational for including this in his/her daily routine was made.

B. The client and therapist agreed to make a commitment toward implementing daily exercise as a depression reduction technique.

C. The client has performed routine daily exercise, and he/she reports that it has been beneficial; these benefits were reinforced.

D. The client has not followed through on maintaining a routine of physical exercise and was redirected to do so.

35. Recommend Exercising Your Way to Better Mental Health (35)

A. The client was encouraged to read *Exercising Your Way to Better Mental Health* (Leith) to introduce him/her to the concept of combating stress, depression, and anxiety with exercise.

B. The client has followed through with reading the recommended book on exercise and mental health and reported that it was beneficial; key points were reviewed.

C. The client has implemented a regular exercise regimen as a depression reduction technique and reported successful results; he/she was verbally reinforced for this progress.

D. The client has not followed through with reading the recommended material on the effect of exercise on mental health and was encouraged to do so.

36. Build Relapse Prevention Skills (36)

A. The client was assisted in building relapse prevention skills through the identification of early warning signs of relapse.

B. The client was directed to consistently review skills learned during therapy.

C. The client was assisted in developing an ongoing plan for managing his/her routine challenges.

37. Connect Repressed Emotions with Depression (37)

A. The client was taught about the possible connection between previously unexpressed feelings and his/her current state of depression.

B. As the client has been assisted in gaining insight into his/her suppressed feelings from the past, his/her current feelings of depression have diminished.

C. The client verbalized an understanding of the relationship between his/her current depressed mood and the repression of anger, hurt, and sadness, and this was processed.

D. The client was unable to connect his/her repressed feelings and his/her current state of depression and was provided with additional feedback in this area.

38. Teach Expression of Repressed Emotions (38)

A. The client was taught about healthy ways in which he/she can express his/her repressed emotions.

B. To help the client express repressed emotions, specific techniques were modeled.

C. Physical techniques for expressing emotions (e.g., beating a pillow) were reviewed.

D. Verbal and written expressions of emotions (e.g., writing a letter) were reviewed.

E. Specific rituals for expressing repressed emotions were reviewed (e.g., writing the emotion down, then tearing it up, and tossing it into the wind).

F. The client was reinforced for his/her use of healthy techniques to express his/her repressed emotions and reports decreased feelings of depression.

G. The client continues to struggle with depressed feelings despite having been assisted in expressing his/her repressed emotions.

39. Refer to an Activity Therapist (39)

A. The client was referred to an activity therapist for recommendations regarding physical fitness activities that are available in the community.

B. The client was referred to community physical fitness resources (e.g., health clubs and other recreational programs).

C. The client has been actively participating in community physical fitness programs and was reinforced for this.

D. The client has declined involvement in community physical fitness programs and was redirected to do so.

40. Educate the Family (40)

A. The client's family was educated about his/her mental illness concerns.

B. The client's family was referred to *What to Do When Someone You Love Is Depressed: A Practical and Helpful Guide* by Golant and Golant.

C. Family members were praised for displaying an increased understanding of the client's mental illness concerns.

41. Teach Support Changes (41)

A. The family members were taught about how to support the changes the client has made through treatment.

B. Specific examples were listed from the family members regarding the ways in which the client's changes may affect the family functioning.

C. Family members were reinforced for their positive support of the client's changes within treatment.

D. Family members have sought a return to the previous status quo and have not supported the client through his/her treatment; this pattern was reflected to the family members.

42. Educate about Maintenance Treatment (42)

A. The client was educated about the ongoing need for maintenance treatment (e.g., following up on appointments, continuing to take medications, or attending support groups) despite the lack of identifiable symptoms.

B. The client acknowledged his/her need for maintenance treatment despite the lack of identifiable symptoms and was reinforced for this understanding.

C. The client continues to use maintenance treatment despite the lack of identifiable symptoms and was provided with positive feedback in this area.

D. The client has not used maintenance treatment and was redirected to do so.

43. Identify Symptom Indicators of Depression (43)

A. The client was requested to identify a list of symptom triggers and indicators of his/her depression deepening.

B. The client has developed a list of symptom triggers and indicators, and this was reviewed.

C. The client was urged to share information about symptom indicators with his/her support network to assist them in monitoring his/her symptoms.

D. The client has not developed a list of symptom triggers or indicators and was redirected in this area.

EMPLOYMENT PROBLEMS

CLIENT PRESENTATION

1. Chronic Unemployment (1)*

A. The client described a history of unemployment and underemployment.

B. Although the client has attempted to work on a regular basis, he/she has been unable to sustain regular periods of employment.

C. The client has little motivation to maintain regular patterns of work.

D. Although the client has been working on a regular basis, his/her employment is in a setting that is less than his/her capability.

E. As treatment has progressed, the client has been more regularly involved in work activity.

2. History of Job Loss (2)

A. The client reported that he/she has often been terminated from his/her occupational setting due to interpersonal conflicts or an inability to control his/her primary psychosis symptoms.

B. The client described that he/she has been fired due to psychotic symptoms.

C. The client reported that his/her current job is at risk due to his/her severe mental illness symptoms.

D. As the client's severe and persistent mental illness symptoms have stabilized, he/she has been able to be more regular in employment.

3. Decreased Desire for Employment (3)

A. The client reported a low pattern of motivation to seek employment.

B. The client reported a lack of desire to maintain his/her current employment position.

C. The client's low energy level has placed his/her current work setting in jeopardy.

D. As the client has stabilized his/her mood, he/she reports an increased desire to actively seek and maintain employment.

4. Lack of Training (4)

A. The client's lack of training has contributed to his/her failure to obtain employment.

B. The client has not received formal or on-the-job training to assist in securing employment.

C. As the client has developed specific training and job skills, he/she has been able to obtain and maintain employment.

5. Failure to Achieve Expected Success (5)

A. The client reports a pattern of failure to achieve or maintain expected levels of occupational involvement, duration, and success.

B. The client described his/her pattern of employment as functioning below the age-appropriate level of occupational involvement, duration, and success.

---

* The numbers in parentheses correlate to the number of the Behavioral Definition statement in the companion chapter with the same title in *The Severe and Persistent Mental Illness Treatment Planner,* 2nd ed. (Berghuis and Jongsma) by John Wiley & Sons, 2008.

C. As the client's severe and persistent mental illness symptoms have stabilized, he/she has reported an increase in his/her level of occupational involvement, duration, and success.

6. Conflicts Due to Paranoia (6)

A. The client described his/her pattern of conflict with authority figures due to unfounded suspiciousness or paranoia.

B. The client described that he/she has often rebelled against authority figures due to his/her unfounded suspiciousness or paranoia.

C. As the client's pattern of suspiciousness and paranoia have been reduced, he/she reports decreased conflicts with authority figures.

D. The client does not experience conflicts with authority figures due to any suspiciousness or paranoia.

7. Psychiatric Destabilization Due to Job Loss (7)

A. The client described feelings of anxiety, depression, or other psychiatric destabilization secondary to being fired or laid off.

B. The client describes fears, feelings of worthlessness, and bizarre thoughts as a reaction to the stress of being fired or laid off.

C. As treatment has progressed, the client reports increased psychiatric stability despite employment problems.

D. The client's employment problems have stabilized with a commensurate stabilization in his/her psychiatric functioning.

8. Fears Returning to Work (8)

A. The client is fearful, due to his/her history of employment problems and failures, about returning to the workplace.

B. The client's fears of returning to the workplace have exacerbated his/her employment problems.

C. The client was able to identify and verbalize his/her fears about returning to the workplace.

D. As the client has worked through his/her fears about returning to the workplace, he/she has shown more interest in employment.

9. Emotional Reaction to Job Placement (9)

A. The client identified specific negative emotions that he/she experiences due to the nature of his/her job placement.

B. The client described that his/her anxiety symptoms have increased due to the menial or repetitive nature of his/her job placement.

C. The client identified depressed thoughts and feelings due to the nature of his/her job placement.

D. As the client has worked through his/her feelings of depression and anxiety, he/she has become more emotionally stable.

E. The client reports that he/she is content in his/her job placement.

10. Symptom Exacerbation Due to Increased Expectations (10)

A. The client described that he/she has been anxious due to his/her increased job expectations.

B. The client has experienced an increase in his/her primary mental illness symptoms due to his/her anxiety related to job tasks and expectations.

C. As the client has adjusted to his/her increased job expectations, he/she has experienced a decrease in his/her primary psychosis symptoms.

INTERVENTIONS IMPLEMENTED

1. Outline Employment History (1)*

A. The client was asked to prepare a chronological outline of his/her previous employment.

B. The client was assisted in preparing a chronological outline of his/her previous employment.

C. The client's employment history was reviewed.

D. Specific incidents of the client's employment success and failure were identified and processed within the session.

E. The client has not prepared a chronological outline of his/her previous employment and was redirected to do so.

2. Identify Successful and Unsuccessful Employment Experiences (2)

A. The client was asked to describe his/her previous successful employment situations.

B. The client was asked to describe his/her negative job experiences.

C. Attentive listening and encouragement were used to support the client as he/she reviewed his/her previous successful and unsuccessful employment situations.

D. The client was unable to identify any previous successful employment situations and was given feedback in this area.

3. Relate Symptom Pattern to Employment Difficulties (3)

A. The client was requested to identify situations in which the primary symptoms of his/her mental illness have negatively affected his/her job performance.

B. The client was asked to identify situations in which his/her primary symptoms of mental illness have affected his/her social interactions at work.

C. The client's job performance and social interaction difficulties were processed within the clinical contact.

D. The client was unable to identify ways in which his/her primary symptoms have affected his/her job performance or social interaction and was given additional feedback in this area.

4. Educate about Mental Illness (4)

A. The client was educated about the expected or common symptoms of his/her mental illness that may negatively impact his/her employment.

B. As his/her symptoms of mental illness were discussed, the client displayed an understanding of how these symptoms may affect his/her level of employment.

C. The client struggled to identify how symptoms of his/her mental illness may negatively impact his/her employment and was given additional feedback in this area.

5. Identify and Evaluate Reasons against Employment (5)

A. The client was assisted in identifying possible reasons for not obtaining employment.

* The numbers in parentheses correlate to the number of the Therapeutic Intervention statement in the companion chapter with the same title in *The Severe and Persistent Mental Illness Treatment Planner,* 2nd ed. (Berghuis and Johnsma) by John Wiley & Sons, 2008.

B. The client identified specific reasons why he/she is hesitant to obtain employment (e.g., his/her loss of disability payments or fear of increased responsibility or expectations), and this was accepted as an important factor.

C. The client's reasons for not wishing to obtain employment were evaluated, reviewed, and processed.

D. The client has been unable to identify any reasons why he/she would not desire to gain employment and was challenged to pursue employment.

E. As the client has worked through his/her reasons for not wishing to obtain or maintain employment, he/she was assisted in acknowledging his/her tendency to sabotage his/her employment.

F. As the client has processed his/her reasons for not obtaining or maintaining employment, he/she has rejected them and is noted to have an increased commitment to obtaining and maintaining employment.

6. Identify Positive Reasons for Employment (6)

A. The client was asked to identify positive reasons for obtaining or maintaining employment.

B. The client was assisted in developing positive reasons for obtaining or maintaining employment

C. As the client has developed his/her positive reasons for obtaining or maintaining employment, he/she has been provided with feedback and support.

D. The client has struggled to identify positive reasons for obtaining or maintaining employment and was given additional support in this area.

7. Arrange Psychiatric Evaluation (7)

A. The client was referred to a physician for an evaluation for a prescription of psychotropic medications.

B. The client has followed through on a referral to a physician and has been assessed for a prescription of psychotropic medications, but none were prescribed.

C. The client has been prescribed psychotropic medications.

D. The client declined evaluation by a physician for a prescription of psychotropic medication and was redirected to do so.

8. Encourage Consistent Use of Medications (8)

A. The client was encouraged to take his/her medications on a consistent basis.

B. The client was provided with positive reinforcement for his/her regular use of psychiatric medications.

C. The client has been erratic with his/her use of psychiatric medications and was provided with feedback in this area.

9. Coordinate Privacy at Work Site (9)

A. The availability of a secure, private area where the client can keep and take his/her medications was coordinated at his/her work site.

B. The client's employer has provided a secure, private area where the client can store and take his/her medications, and the benefits of this accommodation were reviewed.

C. The client has been able to regularly take his/her medications in a secure, private area at his/her work site, and the benefits of this were reviewed within the session.

D. The client has not taken advantage of using a secure, private area to keep and take his/her medications and has continued to be erratic with the use of his/her medications. The effects of this were reviewed within the clinical contact.

10. Monitor Medications (10)

A. The client was monitored for compliance with his/her psychotropic medication regimen.

B. The client was provided with positive feedback about his/her regular use of psychotropic medications.

C. The client was monitored for the effectiveness and side effects of his/her prescribed medications.

D. Concerns about the client's medication effectiveness and side effects were communicated to the physician.

E. Although the client was monitored for medication side effects, he/she reported no concerns in this area.

11. Educate about Psychotropic Medications (11)

A. The client was taught about the indications for and the expected benefits of psychotropic medications.

B. As the client's psychotropic medications were reviewed, he/she displayed an understanding about the indications for and expected benefits of the medications.

C. The client displayed a lack of understanding of the indications for and expected benefits of psychotropic medications and was provided with additional information regarding his/her medications.

12. Educate Regarding Medication Effect on Employment (12)

A. The client was educated about the expected positive effect of his/her psychiatric medications on his/her employment functioning.

B. The client identified that his/her functioning in the employment situation has significantly improved as he/she has been more stable on his/her medication, and this was processed within the session.

C. The client continues to struggle with his/her employment setting despite his/her improved functioning subsequent to the use of psychiatric medications, and this was reviewed.

13. Encourage Employment as Central to Recovery (13)

A. The client was advised about how employment is a central goal in the recovery process.

B. The personal, social, financial, and other relevant benefits of employment were discussed with the client.

C. The client was reinforced in his/her motivation to obtain employment as a central goal in recovery.

D. The client has not developed employment as a central goal for recovery, and was redirected to do so.

14. Refer to Supported Employment (14)

A. The client was referred to a supported employment program.

B. The client has engaged in the support employment program and the benefits of this program were reviewed.

C. The client has not utilized the supported employment program and was redirected to do so.

15. Identify Target Social Behaviors (15)

A. The client was asked to identify three social behaviors that will promote better interpersonal functioning in the work situation.

B. The client was assisted in identifying three social behaviors that will promote his/her better interpersonal functioning in the work situation.

C. The client was reinforced for making a commitment to work on specific social behaviors (e.g., eye contact, dress, and politeness) to promote better interpersonal functioning in the work situation.

D. The client has failed to identify his/her needs regarding increased social behaviors and was provided with additional feedback in this area.

16. Identify Setting for New Social Behaviors (16)

A. The client was assisted in identifying employment situations in which his/her new prosocial behaviors could be used.

B. The client was given positive feedback regarding the situations in which he/she has been using his/her new, prosocial behaviors in the work setting.

17. Practice Target Social Behaviors (17)

A. Behavioral rehearsal, role playing, and role reversal were used to help the client practice targeted interpersonal behaviors.

B. The client was praised for displaying a good understanding of how to use his/her targeted interpersonal behaviors.

C. The client was urged to implement his/her targeted interpersonal behaviors in real-life settings.

D. The client has continued to struggle with his/her targeted interpersonal behaviors and was given additional practice in this area.

18. Teach Assertiveness (18)

A. The client was taught assertiveness skills.

B. The client was referred to written material regarding how to implement assertiveness.

C. The client was referred to *The Assertiveness Workbook* by Pfeiffer or *Assert Yourself* by Lindenfield to learn more about assertiveness skills.

D. Role modeling, role playing, modeling, and behavioral rehearsal were used to train the client in assertiveness skills.

E. The client has demonstrated a clearer understanding of the difference between assertiveness, passivity, and aggressiveness and was commended for this success.

19. Refer to an Assertiveness-Training Workshop (19)

A. The client was referred to an assertiveness-training workshop to assist in his/her education regarding assertiveness skills.

B. The client was reinforced for attending lectures, completing assignments, and cooperating with role-playing situations to help learn more about his/her assertiveness through the training workshop.

C. The client failed to demonstrate an understanding of assertiveness and was provided with additional feedback in this area.

20. Identify Marketable Skills (20)

A. The client was asked to identify marketable skills for which he/she has displayed mastery and could form a basis for employment search.

B. The client was provided with feedback about his/her marketable skills.

C. As the client's marketable skills have been reviewed, he/she has become more positive about his/her ability to obtain employment.

21. Refer to a Skill Program (21)

A. The client was referred for employment skill assessment and training (e.g., community education, technical center training, vocational rehabilitation, or occupational therapy).

B. The client has attended an employment skill assessment and training program, and his/her new vocational skills were reviewed.

C. The client has been sporadic in his/her attendance at the employment skill assessment and training program and was urged to be more regular.

D. The client has declined to be involved in the employment skill assessment and training program and was given additional encouragement in this area.

22. Monitor Progress in Educational/Rehabilitation Program (22)

A. The client's ongoing attendance, functioning, and progress in the educational or employment rehabilitation program was monitored.

B. The client was accompanied to the employment training program to assist in increasing his/her functioning within the program.

C. The client was provided feedback about his/her attendance, functioning, and progress in the employment educational or rehabilitation program.

23. Identify Occupational Interests (23)

A. Interest testing was administered to identify specific types of occupations in which the client has interest.

B. The client has participated in interest testing, and occupations in which he/she has shown interest were reviewed.

C. The client's interest testing has been completed, and he/she has been given feedback in this area.

D. The client refused to cooperate with the interest testing and was urged to do so.

24. Review Testing to Identify Occupational Placement (24)

A. The client's interest testing was reviewed with him/her to help brainstorm specific jobs in which he/she would be interested.

B. The client has been able to identify a variety of jobs in which he/she has an interest, and this was noted to be consistent with his/her interest testing.

C. The client has struggled to identify occupational interests that are consistent with his/her interest testing.

25. Develop a Resume (25)

A. The client was assisted in developing his/her resume.

B. Resources from *101 Quick Tips for a Dynamite Resume* by Fein or *Resumes for the First Time Job Hunter* by VGM Career Horizons editors were used to assist the client in developing his/her resume.

C. The client has completed his/her resume and was given helpful feedback.

D. The client has not completed his/her resume and was redirected to do so.

26. Obtain Letters of Reference (26)

A. The client was requested to identify family, friends, teachers, former employers, or other clinicians from whom letters of reference for employment may be requested.

B. The client was assigned to procure letters of reference from family, friends, teachers, former employers, or other clinicians.

C. The client has obtained his/her letters of reference, and these were reviewed.

D. The client has not obtained his/her letters of reference and was redirected to do so.

27. Review Classified Ads (27)

A. The local classified advertisements for job placements were reviewed with the client.

B. Feedback was shared with the client about specific job advertisements.

C. The client identified specific jobs for which he/she would like to apply and was given feedback about these selections.

D. The client has neglected to identify jobs from the classified advertisements for which he/she would like to apply and was redirected to do so.

28. Assign Interviewing Techniques Material (28)

A. The client was assigned to read material related to interviewing techniques.

B. The client was assigned to read from selections from *What Color Is Your Parachute?* by Bowles or *10 Minute Guide to Job Interviews* by Morgan.

C. The client has read specific material on job interview techniques, and this was processed.

D. The client has not reviewed the information regarding job interview techniques and was redirected to do so.

29. Practice Job Interviews (29)

A. Role-playing, behavioral rehearsal, and role reversal were used to help increase the client's confidence and skill in the interview process.

B. As the client practiced his/her interview techniques, he/she was provided with feedback and support.

30. Assist in Planning and Coordinating Interview Appointment (30)

A. The client was assisted in planning his/her interview appointment.

B. As the client developed specific plans for his/her interview appointment, he/she was monitored and provided feedback to make sure that he/she had covered all areas.

C. The client has developed a comprehensive plan for his/her interview appointment and was provided with positive feedback in this area.

D. Transportation to the client's interview was coordinated for him/her.

E. The client indicated that he/she had transportation to the job interview but was reminded about other resources as a backup plan.

F. The client was assisted in identifying public modes of transportation.

G. The client has not developed a comprehensive plan for his/her interview appointment and was redirected in this area.

31. Process Interview/Decide about Job (31)

A. Subsequent to the interview, the client's overall interview experience was processed, identifying positive and negative aspects of his/her performance.

B. The client has been offered a job position, and he/she was assisted in making decisions about whether to accept the job offer.

C. The client has made a decision about accepting the job offered to him/her and was provided with feedback and support in this area.

32. Secure Reliable Transportation (32)

A. The client was assisted in planning for reliable transportation to and from work.

B. The client secured reliable transportation to and from work, and he/she was reinforced for planning ahead in this manner.

C. The client has not developed reliable options for transportation to and from work, and was redirected to do so.

33. Arrange for a Job Coach (33)

A. It was arranged for a job coach to meet regularly with the client in the job setting to review job needs, skills, and problem areas.

B. The client was supported for cooperating with the job coach, who has assisted in helping the client coordinate all needs, skills, and problem resolution to maintain his/her position.

C. The client has been stable in his/her job setting, and the services of the job coach have been discontinued.

34. Educate the Employer (34)

A. After obtaining the proper authorization for release of information, the client's mental illness symptoms were reviewed with his/her employer.

B. The employer was supported for verbalizing a better understanding of the client's needs within the employment setting.

C. The employer reacted negatively to the information regarding the client's mental illness, and this was reviewed with the client.

35. Educate Fellow Employees (35)

A. After obtaining the proper authorization to release confidential information, specific information was provided to the client's fellow employees regarding his/her mental illness concerns.

B. Sensitivity training regarding the client's mental illness and his/her needs were provided to his/her fellow employees.

C. The client reports increased support in the workplace due to his/her fellow employees being aware of his/her mental illness concerns, and this was discussed.

D. The client reported that his/her fellow employees have reacted negatively to the disclosure about his/her mental illness, and this was processed within the session.

36. Develop Crisis Intervention Plan with Employer (36)

A. The client assisted in developing an agreed-upon intervention plan with his/her employer related to symptom exacerbation.

B. The client and his/her employer have utilized the crisis plan and were provided with feedback about how useful this has been.

C. The client and his/her employer have not used the agreed upon intervention plan and were redirected to do so.

37. Provide Feedback (37)

A. The client was visited at the job site and provided with feedback about his/her hygiene, dress, behavior, and technical skills.

B. The client has improved his/her hygiene, dress, behavior, and technical skills as a result of the feedback provided for him/her.

C. The client continues to struggle with basic hygiene, dress, behavior, and technical skills and was provided with additional feedback in this area.

38. Review Rules and Etiquette (38)

A. A review of the workplace rules for the client was completed.

B. The client was informed regarding basic etiquette expectations within the workplace.

C. The client reports his/her employment functioning has increased as he/she regularly adheres to workplace rules and etiquette, and this success was reflected back to him/her.

D. The client continues to not comply with basic workplace rules and etiquette and was provided with additional feedback in this area.

39. Meet with the Employer (39)

A. A meeting was held with the employer to review the client's functioning and needs.

B. Specific issues related to the client's functioning and needs within the employment setting were identified, and specific techniques to ameliorate these needs were developed.

C. As the employer has indicated ongoing satisfaction with the client's functioning, the frequency of the meetings with the employer has been reduced.

D. The client is no longer in need of outside coordination or review of his/her employment functioning.

FAMILY CONFLICTS

CLIENT PRESENTATION

1. Estranged Relationships (1)*

A. The client described an atmosphere of frequent conflict with parents and siblings.

B. Family members have little contact with the client and are not seen as a positive influence or source of support.

C. The client has taken the initiative to increase the closeness he/she experiences with family members.

D. The client indicated that he/she feels more a part of a family unit and is supported by his/her family members.

2. Abuse toward Family (2)

A. A series of incidents have occurred in which the client was abusive toward family members.

B. The client tends to project the blame for his/her aggressive or abusive behaviors onto other people.

C. The client has begun to take steps to control his/her abusive behavior.

D. The client has recently demonstrated good self-control and not engaged in any abusive or aggressive behaviors toward family members.

3. Manipulation/Intimidation (2)

A. The client described a pattern of incidents in which he/she has been manipulative or attempted to intimidate family members.

B. Family members reported that the client has displayed a pattern of threatening behavior to manipulate or intimidate them, without becoming physically abusive.

C. The client has recently become more cooperative and respectful, rather than being manipulative or intimidating.

D. The client has been supportive and respectful toward family members on a consistent basis.

4. Overcontrol by Family (3)

A. The client displayed a pattern of lower-than-expected functioning in a variety of areas due to overcontrol of his/her basic needs and decisions by the family.

B. The client described a pattern of his/her family members making basic choices for him/her despite his/her ability to take care of these basic needs.

C. The client has begun to take control of some of his/her own basic needs.

D. The client has become more independent and displayed the ability to care for many of his/her needs despite his/her mental illness concerns.

---

* The numbers in parentheses correlate to the number of the Behavioral Definition statement in the companion chapter with the same title in *The Severe and Persistent Mental Illness Treatment Planner,* 2nd ed. (Berghuis and Jongsma) by John Wiley & Sons, 2008.

5. Family Denial/Rejection (4)

A. Family members have often demonstrated rejection toward the client due to his/her mental illness.

B. The family members have often denied the client's diagnosis of mental illness.

C. The client described family conflicts due to his/her family's difficulty accepting him/her and his/her diagnosis.

D. The client reported that he/she has begun to feel more accepted by family members despite his/her mental illness concerns.

E. The client described a consistent pattern of his/her family members accepting him/her despite his/her mental illness.

6. Lack of Prodromal Knowledge (5)

A. Family members displayed a consistent pattern of ignorance about the client's chronic mental illness symptoms and indicators of decompensation.

B. Family members have often been slow to assist the decompensating client due to their lack of knowledge about his/her chronic mental illness symptoms and indicators of decompensation.

C. Family members have begun to learn about the client's mental illness symptoms and indicators of decompensation.

D. Family members have been more supportive as they have learned about the client's pattern of symptoms and indicators of decompensation.

7. Lack of Treatment Knowledge (6)

A. Family members displayed a poor understanding of the treatment options available to the client.

B. Family members have not accessed helpful treatment for the client due to their lack of knowledge or understanding of treatment options.

C. Family members have inadvertently thwarted treatment due to their lack of understanding of the treatment options available to the client.

D. As family members have become knowledgeable about treatment options, they have been more supportive of the client's treatment.

8. Embarrassment (7)

A. Family members described a feeling of embarrassment and a tendency to hide the client because of his/her erratic behaviors related to his/her severe mental illness symptoms.

B. The client feels rejected when his/her family members display embarrassment and a tendency to hide him/her because of his/her mental illness symptoms.

C. Family members have begun to support the client and accept his/her pattern of symptoms.

D. The client reports that he/she feels more accepted and has experienced decreased family conflicts due to his/her family members being more open about his/her symptoms and needs.

INTERVENTIONS IMPLEMENTED

1. Explore Family Relationships (1)*

A. The client was asked to describe his/her experiences in family relationships.

B. The client was probed as to the nature, frequency, and intensity of the family conflict.

C. Causes for conflict within family relationships were explored.

D. The client outlined the nature of the family conflicts and his/her perspective on the causes for them, and these data were processed.

2. Describe Specific Family Interactions (2)

A. The client was requested to provide examples of positive family experiences.

B. The client's identification of positive family experiences was reviewed and processed.

C. The client was requested to provide examples of negative family experiences.

D. The client's description of negative family experiences was reviewed and processed.

E. The client struggled to identify examples of positive and negative family experiences, and was urged to develop this information more fully.

3. Create a Family Genogram (3)

A. The client's description of family members, patterns of interaction, rules, and secrets was translated into a graphical genogram.

B. A family session was conducted in which a genogram was developed that was complete, denoting family members, patterns of interaction, rules, and secrets.

C. The dysfunctional communication patterns between nuclear and extended family members were highlighted.

D. Family members were supported as they acknowledged the lack of healthy communication that permeates the extended family.

E. The client displayed increased understanding of his/her family's pattern of unhealthy communication and was encouraged for this progress.

F. The client failed to develop insight into family interactions and was given tentative interpretations of these patterns.

4. Describe Problematic Relationships (4)

A. The client was requested to list and describe his/her problematic relationships.

B. The client's description of his/her problematic relationships was processed.

C. The client has failed to develop a comprehensive list of his/her problematic relationships and was redirected to do so.

5. Clarify Impact on Relationships (5)

A. The client's specific behaviors that contribute to positive relationships and interactions were highlighted and clarified.

B. Specific behaviors in which the client engages that have a negative impact on relationships were highlighted and clarified.

* The numbers in parentheses correlate to the number of the Therapeutic Intervention statement in the companion chapter with the same title in *The Severe and Persistent Mental Illness Treatment Planner,* 2nd ed. (Berghuis and Jongsma) by John Wiley & Sons, 2008.

C. The client was given positive feedback as he/she displayed insight into the positive and negative effects that his/her behavior has on relationships.

D. The client failed to connect his/her behavior with the positive or negative impact on relationships and was given additional feedback in this area.

6. Identify Past Positive Interactions (6)

A. Solution-focused techniques were used to assist the client in identifying how he/she has facilitated positive social interaction in the past.

B. The client identified specific situations in which he/she has been able to facilitate some positive social interactions in the past, and these were processed.

C. Solution-focused techniques were used to help the client generate a list of additional situations in which he/she could use his/her positive social skills.

D. The client struggled to identify positive interactions from the past and was provided with additional feedback and support in this area.

7. Facilitate Family Emotional Expression (7)

A. Family members were assisted in identifying and expressing emotions regarding the client's mental illness.

B. Family members were supported as they expressed their emotions regarding the client's mental illness concerns.

C. Family members expressed multiple emotions regarding the client's mental illness, which were processed within the session.

D. Family members have been reluctant to express emotions relating to the client's mental illness concerns and were encouraged to do so when they felt more comfortable with it.

8. Use Magical Question (8)

A. A magical question (i.e., "What would happen in your family if the client did not have any mental illness symptoms?") was used to help the family members identify the impact of the mental illness symptoms on the family.

B. Family members identified specific ways in which the client's mental illness symptoms have impacted the family, and these were reviewed and clarified.

C. Family members displayed a greater understanding of the impact on the family relative to the client's mental illness symptoms and were reinforced for this increased understanding.

9. Use Multiple Family Group Treatment (9)

A. The client was referred for multiple family group treatment.

B. The client was enrolled in a multiple family group treatment program.

C. The client's family has participated in a multiple family group treatment program, gaining insight into family dynamics and how to cope with the client's symptoms.

D. The family is not enrolled in the multiple family group treatment program, and the reasons for this resistance were reviewed.

10. Conduct Family-Focused Treatment (10)

A. The client and significant others were included in the family-focused treatment model.

B. Family-focused treatment was used with the client and significant others as indicated in *Bipolar Disorder: A Family Approach* (Miklowitz and Goldstein).

C. As family members were not available to participate in therapy, the family-focused treatment model was adapted to individual therapy.

11. Refer to a Lending Library (11)

A. The client and his/her family were referred to a lending library within the agency to access books or tapes on the topic of severe mental illness.

B. The client and his/her family were referred to the community library resources to access books or tapes on severe mental illness.

C. The client and his/her family's increased understanding of severe mental illness symptoms through the use of the educational materials was reviewed and noted.

D. The client and his/her family have not sought out available reading materials and were redirected to do so.

12. Teach Family Members about Severe and Persistent Mental Illness (12)

A. The client's family members were referred to a didactic session on the topic of severe and persistent mental illness.

B. The client's family members were provided with didactic information about the topic of severe and persistent mental illness.

C. The client's family members were reinforced for displaying new knowledge about his/her mental illness symptoms.

D. The client's family members have not attended didactic sessions on psychosis and were redirected to do so.

13. Educate about Mood Episodes (13)

A. A variety of modalities were used to teach the family about signs and symptoms of the client's mood episodes.

B. The phasic relapsing nature of the client's mood episodes was emphasized.

C. The client's mood episode concerns were normalized.

D. The client's mood episodes were destigmatized.

14. Teach Stress Diathesis Model (14)

A. The client was taught a stress diathesis model of Bipolar Disorder.

B. The biological predisposition to mood episodes was emphasized.

C. The client was taught about how stress can make him/her more vulnerable to mood episodes.

D. The manageability of mood episodes was emphasized.

E. The client was reinforced for his/her clear understanding of the stress diathesis model of Bipolar Disorder.

F. The client struggled to display a clear understanding of the stress diathesis model of Bipolar Disorder and was provided with additional remedial information in this area.

15. Provide Rational for Treatment (15)

A. The client was provided with the rationale for treatment involving ongoing medication and psychosocial treatment.

B. The focus of treatment was emphasized, including recognizing, managing, and reducing biological and psychological vulnerabilities that could precipitate relapse.

C. A discussion was held about the rationale for treatment.

D. The client was reinforced for his/her understanding of the appropriate rational for treatment.

E. The client was redirected when he/she displayed a poor understanding of the rationale for treatment.

16. Identify Relapse Triggers (16)

A. Sources of the client's stress and triggers of potential relapse were identified.

B. Negative events, cognitive interpretations, aversive communication, poor sleep hygiene, and medication noncompliance were investigated as potential stressors or triggers of potential relapse.

C. Cognitive-behavioral techniques were used to address the sources of stress and triggers for potential relapse.

17. Enhance Engagement in Medication Use (17)

A. Motivational interviewing approaches were used to help enhance the client's level of engagement in his/her medication use and compliance to the medication regimen.

B. Modeling, role-playing, and behavioral rehearsal were used to help the client use problem-solving skills to work through several current conflicts.

C. The client was taught about the risk for relapse when medication is discontinued.

D. Commitment was obtained to continuous prescription adherence.

E. As a result of motivational interviewing approaches for medication compliance, the subject's use of medication has significantly improved.

F. The client continues to be medication noncompliant despite use of motivational interviewing approaches; the client was refocused onto this task.

18. Assess Prescription Noncompliance Factors (18)

A. Factors that have precipitated the client's prescription noncompliance were assessed.

B. The client was checked for specific thoughts, feelings, and stressors that might contribute to his/her prescription noncompliance.

C. A plan was developed for recognizing and addressing the factors that have precipitated the client's prescription noncompliance.

19. Educate about Lab Work (19)

A. The client was educated about the need to stay compliant with necessary lab work involved in regulating his/her medication levels.

B. The client was encouraged to stay compliant with necessary lab work.

C. The client was reinforced for his/her compliance to completing necessary lab work to help regulate his/her medication levels.

D. The client has not been regular in his/her compliance to lab work for regulating his/her medication levels and was redirected to do so.

20. Assess Potential Crises (20)

A. The client was assisted in assessing potential crises, including his/her most likely route to decompensation.

B. The client was assisted in problem solving how to manage his/her potential crises.

C. Family members were engaged in discussing the client's likely potential crises and how to manage them.

D. Family members have been assisted in developing a comprehensive plan for managing the client's potential crises.

E. The family members are not in agreement on how to manage the client's potential crises and were provided with additional coordination in this area.

21. Develop Relapse Drill (21)

A. The client and family were assisted in drawing up a relapse drill, detailing roles and responsibilities.

B. Family members were asked to take responsibility for specific roles (e.g., who will call a meeting of the family to problem solve potential relapse; who will call physician, schedule a serum level, or contact emergency services, if needed).

C. Obstacles to providing family support to the client's potential relapse were reviewed and problem solved.

D. The family was asked to make a commitment to adherence to the relapse response plan.

E. The family was reinforced for their commitment to the adherence to the relapse response plan.

F. The family has not developed a clear commitment to the relapse prevention plan and was redirected in this area.

22. Assess and Educate about Aversive Communication (22)

A. The family was assessed for the role of aversive communication in family distress and in the risk for the client's manic relapse.

B. The family was educated about the role of aversive communication (e.g., highly expressed emotion) in developing greater family stress and in increasing the client's risk for manic relapse.

C. The family displayed a clear understanding of the effects of aversive communication, and this was reinforced.

D. The family was provided with remedial feedback, as they did not display a clear understanding of the risk for relapse due to aversive communication.

23. Teach Communication Skills (23)

A. Behavioral techniques were used to teach communication skills.

B. Communication skills such as offering positive feedback, active listening, making positive requests for behavioral change, and giving negative feedback in an honest, respectful manner were taught to the client and family.

C. Behavioral techniques were used to teach the family healthy communication skills.

D. Education, modeling, role-playing, corrective feedback, and positive reinforcement were used to teach communication skills.

24. Assign Communication Skills Homework (24)

A. The client and family were assigned homework exercises to use and record newly learned communication skills.

B. Family members have used newly learned communication skills, and the results were processed within the session.

C. Family members have not used the newly learned communication skills and were redirected to do so.

25. Increase Sensitivity to Effects of Behavior (25)

A. Role-playing, role reversal, and behavioral rehearsal were used to increase the client's sensitivity to the negative effects of his/her impulsive behavior.

B. The client was reinforced for his/her increased sensitivity to the negative effects of his/her impulsive behavior on others.

26. Confront Mania and Enforce Rules (26)

A. Unhealthy, impulsive, or manic behaviors that occur during contacts with the clinician were identified and confronted.

B. Clear rules and roles in the relationship were identified and enforced with immediate, short-term consequences for breaking such boundaries.

C. The client's unhealthy, impulsive, or manic behaviors have diminished in response to limit setting within the session.

27. Address Problem Solving (27)

A. The client was asked to identify conflicts that can be addressed through problem-solving techniques.

B. The family members were asked to give input about conflicts that could be addressed with problem-solving techniques.

C. The client and family arrived at a list of conflicts that could be addressed with problem-solving techniques.

28. Teach Problem-Solving Skills (28)

A. Behavioral techniques such as education, modeling, role-playing, corrective feedback, and positive reinforcement were used to teach the client and family problem-solving skills.

B. Specific problem-solving skills were taught to the family, including defining the problem constructively and specifically, brainstorming options, evaluating options, choosing options, implementing a plan, evaluating results, and reevaluating the plan.

C. Family members were asked to use the problem-solving skills on specific situations.

D. The family was reinforced for positive use of problem-solving skills.

E. The family was redirected for failures to properly use problem-solving skills.

29. Assign Problem-Solving Homework (29)

A. The client and family were assigned to use newly learned problem-solving skills and record their use.

B. The client and family were assigned "Applying Problem-Solving to Interpersonal Conflict" in the *Adult Psychotherapy Homework Planner,* 2nd ed. (Jongsma).

C. The results of the family members' use of problem-solving skills were reviewed within the session.

30. Assess Family Support Network (30)

A. The family was assessed for the extent to which it has a support network.

B. The family was encouraged to use extended family, neighbors, church friends, social relationships, and other portions of their support network to provide diversion, emotional support, and/or respite care for the client.

C. The family has limited support to assist in diversion, emotional support, or respite care for the client and was encouraged to develop more supports.

31. Refer the Family to Respite Services (31)

A. The family was referred to a community-based respite care service.

B. Respite services have assisted in providing supervision or taking responsibility for the client on a short-term basis.

C. The family was supported for using respite services and reporting less stress and strain on the family.

D. The family has not used respite services and was encouraged to do so.

32. Acknowledge Family Frustration Regarding Services (32)

A. The family was facilitated in expressing their frustration and anger regarding not having received services that they desired in the past.

B. The family's experience of not having received services that they desired in the past was acknowledged.

C. The family reported feeling validated about having experienced past service difficulties and are being redirected to current available services.

D. The family's frustration and anger regarding past service failures has caused decreased desire to attempt current services, and they were encouraged to attempt these resources again.

33. Refer Family Members to Support Group (33)

A. The client's family members were referred to a support group for families of the mentally ill.

B. The client's family members have used the support group for families of the mentally ill, and their positive experience was reviewed.

C. The client's family members have attended a support group for families of the mentally ill but did not find this a helpful experience; this was reviewed in order to help problem solve obstacles to gaining benefits from this resource.

D. The client's family members have not attended the support group for families of the mentally ill and were redirected to do so.

34. Schedule Maintenance Sessions (34)

A. The client was scheduled for a maintenance session between one and three months after therapy ends.

B. The client was advised to contact the therapist if he/she needs to be seen prior to the maintenance session.

C. The client's maintenance session was held, and he/she was reinforced for his/her successful implementation of therapy techniques.

D. The client's maintenance session was held, and he/she was coordinated for further treatment, as his/her progress has not been sustained.

35. Identify Social Activities (35)

A. The client was assisted in identifying mutually satisfying social activities for himself/herself and his/her family.

B. The client was supported for identifying mutually satisfying social activities for himself/herself and his/her family.

C. The client and his/her family have participated in mutually satisfying social activities, and this was reviewed and supported.

D. The client has not identified helpful social activities and was redirected to do so.

36. Refer to an Activity or Recreational Therapist (36)

A. The client was referred to an activity or recreational therapist for assistance in developing leisure skills or activities to share with family members.

B. The client has met with the activity or recreational therapist and is developing leisure skills to share with family members.

C. The client was reinforced for developing more leisure skills and reporting better relationships with family members.

D. The client has not followed through on the referral to an activity or recreational therapist and was redirected to do so.

37. Identify Family Patterns That Limit the Client's Functioning (37)

A. Family roles and behavioral patterns that have developed as a result of the family's reaction to the client's mental illness were identified.

B. An analysis of family roles and behavioral patterns focused on how the client's independent functioning has been limited and dependence has been encouraged.

C. The client was reinforced for displaying insight into his/her family's reaction to his/her mental illness symptoms and how this affects his/her functioning.

D. The client's family members were supported for displaying insight into their reaction to his/her severe and persistent mental illness symptoms and how this affects his/her functioning.

E. The client and his/her family members did not display any insight into their family patterns of behavior, so they were given feedback in this area.

38. Encourage Independence (38)

A. The client was encouraged to make all possible choices and demonstrate maximum independence in daily events.

B. The client's family members were encouraged to allow him/her to make all possible choices and demonstrate maximum independence in daily events.

C. The client's growing pattern of independence and ability to make his/her own choices were reviewed within the session.

D. The client was given positive feedback for his/her increase in independence.

E. The client reported that he/she has not focused on making his/her own choices and maximizing independence, and this resistance was reviewed.

39. Review Backup Caregiver/Advocate (39)

A. The options available for backup to the primary caregiver/advocate were reviewed.

B. A specific plan was developed for the client's care and advocacy should the primary caregiver/advocate be unable to care for the client.

C. The client and his/her family have developed a comprehensive plan in the event that the primary caregiver/advocate is unable to care for the client, and they received positive feedback for this.

D. The client and his/her family reported minimal resources for his/her care and advocacy should the primary caregiver be unable to care for him/her, and they were referred to community resources.

40. Encourage Sibling Involvement (40)

A. The client's siblings were encouraged to be regularly involved in his/her treatment and social contacts.

B. The client reported increased involvement with his/her siblings, and this was reviewed and supported.

C. The client's siblings have developed a more involved relationship with him/her, and this development was reinforced.

D. The client's siblings continue to avoid involvement with him/her, and this pattern was reviewed and confronted.

41. Encourage Religious Involvement (41)

A. Family members were encouraged to continue regular involvement of the client in church or other religious practices.

B. Family members have worked to include the client in the family's regular religious practices and were provided with reinforcement for this.

C. Family members continue to exclude the client from the family's religious activities and were encouraged to involve him/her in this area.

42. Monitor Religiously Themed Symptoms/Issues (42)

A. The potency of the client's religious interest was assessed.

B. The client was assisted in differentiating between religiously oriented mental illness symptoms and legitimate spiritual issues.

C. The client was reinforced for displaying a clear understanding of legitimate spiritual issues versus his/her religiously oriented mental illness symptoms, and this was noted to be helpful in his/her involvement in family religious practices.

D. The client displayed confusion regarding his/her religiously oriented mental illness symptoms and legitimate spiritual issues and was provided with additional feedback in this area.

43. Provide Symptom Information to Religious Leaders (43)

A. A release of information was obtained to allow information to be provided to the clergy or other church leaders regarding assistance that the client may need in accessing spiritual practices and programs.

B. Specific information was provided to the clergy and other church leaders regarding the client's special needs related to spiritual practices and programs.

C. Church leaders were supported for responding positively to information about the client's specific needs related to spiritual practices and programs.

D. The client reported ongoing difficulty engaging in family-oriented spiritual practices and was provided with additional feedback in this area.

44. Resolve Family Self-Blame (44)

A. Family members were assisted in identifying feelings of responsibility and self-blame for the client's mental illness.

B. Family members were provided with information regarding the etiology of the client's severe and persistent mental illness.

C. Family members were assisted in resolving any unrealistic feelings of responsibility and self-blame regarding the client's mental illness.

FINANCIAL NEEDS

CLIENT PRESENTATION

1. Low Income (1)*

A. The client described a history of low income due to the effects of psychotic and other severe mental illness symptoms.

B. The client is on a limited, state-supported income.

C. The client reported that his/her psychosis and other severe mental illness symptoms have resulted in a significant loss of income.

D. As the client has stabilized, he/she reports increased financial stability.

2. Chronic Homelessness (2)

A. The client described a pattern of chronic homelessness.

B. The client described that he/she often uses supported transitional living services (e.g., homeless shelters or adult foster care placements).

C. The client described a pattern of financial difficulty, which has contributed to his/her homelessness.

D. As treatment has progressed, the client has become more financially stable and is able to sustain his/her living situation.

3. Unemployment (3)

A. The client has become unemployed and has no source of income.

B. The client described a consistent pattern of unemployment or underemployment and is not capable of providing sufficient funds to meet his/her basic needs.

C. The client has developed a plan to obtain emergency financial relief through community services.

D. The client has developed a plan to seek employment.

E. The client has become employed again, and income has been restored.

4. Impulsive Spending (4)

A. The client described a pattern of his/her impulsive spending that does not consider the eventual financial consequences of such actions.

B. The client was in defensive denial regarding his/her pattern of impulsive spending.

C. The client acknowledged his/her impulsive spending and has begun to develop a plan to help cope with this problem.

D. The client identified that his/her impulsive spending often occurs in relation to psychotic or manic episodes.

E. The client has established a pattern of delaying any purchase until the financial consequences of the purchase can be planned for and met.

---

* The numbers in parentheses correlate to the number of the Behavioral Definition statement in the companion chapter with the same title in *The Severe and Persistent Mental Illness Treatment Planner,* 2nd ed. (Berghuis and Jongsma) by John Wiley & Sons, 2008.

5. Failure to Budget (5)

A. The client described a long-term lack of discipline and money management that has led to a failure to budget for basic financial responsibilities.

B. The client described that his/her financial information is poorly organized, which results in unpaid bills and greater financial liability.

C. The client has never established a budget with spending guidelines and savings goals that would allow for prompt payment of bills.

D. The client has developed a budget and has begun to live within it, making timely payments of bills.

6. Lack of Entitlements (6)

A. The client described a history of not applying for or accessing monetary entitlements or other available welfare benefits.

B. The client displayed a lack of knowledge of the available monetary entitlements or other available welfare benefits.

C. The client has been reluctant to access monetary entitlements or other welfare benefits due to his/her perceived stigma regarding these resources.

D. The client has applied for and accessed monetary entitlements or other available welfare benefits.

7. Illegal Activity (7)

A. The client described a pattern of illegal activity used to meet his/her financial needs.

B. The client described legal concerns due to his/her illegal activity.

C. As the client has become more financially stable, he/she has discontinued his/her illegal activity.

8. Bad Credit (8)

A. The client described his/her poor credit history.

B. The client has attempted to qualify for credit but has been turned down.

C. The client described a pattern of unpaid bills and outstanding debts, which have negatively affected his/her credit history.

D. As the client has become more financially secure, he/she has taken responsibility for his/her bad debts and is improving his/her credit.

INTERVENTIONS IMPLEMENTED

1. Request Financial History (1)*

A. The client was requested to relate his/her history or pattern of financial problems.

B. The client was assisted in developing an understanding of his/her pattern of financial problems.

---

* The numbers in parentheses correlate to the number of the Therapeutic Intervention statement in the companion chapter with the same title in *The Severe and Persistent Mental Illness Treatment Planner,* 2nd ed. (Berghuis and Jongsma) by John Wiley & Sons, 2008.

C. The client displayed an increased understanding of his/her syndrome of financial difficulties and how they relate to his/her severe and persistent mental illness symptoms; he/she was provided with positive feedback about this insight.

D. The client has little understanding of his/her pattern of financial problems and was provided with additional feedback in this area.

2. Provide Support and Decrease Blame (2)

A. The client was provided with support and empathy regarding his/her financial difficulties.

B. An emphasis was placed on decreasing the client's sense of guilt and blame for his/her financial difficulties.

C. The client reports, due to the increased support, diminished feelings of guilt or being overwhelmed by his/her financial difficulties.

D. The client reported ongoing feelings of guilt for his/her financial problems and was provided with additional feedback in this area.

3. Identify Beneficial Financial Practices (3)

A. The client was requested to identify at least two financial practices that he/she uses that are beneficial or that add stability.

B. The client identified specific financial practices that are helpful (e.g., saving, budgeting, and comparison shopping) and was provided with positive feedback for these.

C. The client could not identify any positive financial practices and was provided with prompts to assist in identifying beneficial financial practices.

4. Identify Negative Financial Practices (4)

A. The client was asked to identify at least two financial practices that have led to his/her financial difficulty.

B. The client was assisted in identifying specific patterns of financial behavior that have led to financial difficulty (e.g., unstable work history, impulsive spending, failure to pay on commitments).

C. The client could not identify his/her pattern of negative financial practices and was provided with specific examples in this area.

5. Process Financial Patterns (5)

A. The client's financial successes and failures were processed, focusing on patterns, triggers, and consequences of successes and failures.

B. The client received positive feedback for his/her identification of patterns, triggers, and consequences of his/her financial decisions.

C. The client found it difficult to identify patterns, triggers, and consequences of his/her financial successes and failures and was given additional feedback about these areas.

6. List Current Financial Obligations (6)

A. The client was directed to write out a list of all current financial obligations.

B. The client's list of current financial obligations was reviewed for accuracy and completeness.

C. The client has not written out a complete list of all current financial obligations and was redirected to do so.

7. Review Financial Obligations (7)

A. The client's list of financial obligations was compared with normally expected obligations (e.g., those listed on the budgeting worksheet in *Personal Budget Planner: A Guide for Financial Success* by Gelb).

B. The client's list of financial obligations appears to be complete when compared with normally expected obligations, and this was processed with him/her.

C. The client has omitted many typical financial obligations and was provided with feedback in this area.

8. Educate about Mental Illness (8)

A. The client was educated about the expected or common symptoms of his/her mental illness that may negatively impact his/her financial functioning.

B. As his/her symptoms of mental illness were discussed, the client displayed an understanding of how these symptoms may affect his/her financial stability.

C. The client did not understand how symptoms of his/her mental illness may negatively impact basic financial functioning and was given additional feedback in this area.

9. Relate Symptom Pattern to Financial Difficulties (9)

A. The client was requested to identify situations in which the primary symptoms of his/her mental illness have negatively affected his/her financial stability.

B. The client's financial difficulties related to mental illness symptoms were processed.

C. The client was unable to identify ways in which his/her primary symptoms have affected his/her financial functioning and was given additional feedback in this area.

10. Suggest a Payee (10)

A. It was suggested to the client that he/she use a payee to receive public aid funds on his/her behalf.

B. The client was directed to consider allowing someone else to exercise general control over his/her finances.

C. The client agreed with the suggestion to obtain a payee and allow outside control over his/her finances in order to decrease his/her erratic, impulsive spending; the effects of this decision were processed.

D. The client declined using a payee or allowing other control over his/her finances and was provided with additional encouragement in this area.

11. Coordinate a Payee (11)

A. The client was assisted in initiating the procedures for obtaining a payee for benefits.

B. The client was given instructions about what steps to take to obtain a payee.

C. A payee was obtained for administration of the client's benefits.

12. Coordinate a Cosigner (12)

A. The client was assisted in requiring a cosigner to be necessary for all bank withdrawal transactions.

B. The client was reinforced for obtaining a cosigner to be necessary for all bank withdrawal transactions, which has helped to limit his/her erratic, impulsive spending.

C. The client refused to allow a cosigner to be required for any bank withdrawal transactions; additional encouragement was given to him/her to reconsider.

13. Pursue Involuntary Legal Control (13)

A. Involuntary legal control over the client's finances was pursued through the guardianship process.

B. Involuntary legal control over the client's finances was obtained through the guardianship process.

C. Although involuntary legal control has been sought, the legal process did not allow for outside control of the client's finances.

14. Refer to a Physician (14)

A. The client was referred to a physician for an evaluation for a prescription of psychotropic medications.

B. The client was reinforced for following through on a referral to a physician for an assessment for a prescription of psychotropic medications, but none were prescribed.

C. The client has been prescribed psychotropic medications.

D. The client declined evaluation by a physician for a prescription of psychotropic medications and was redirected to cooperate with this referral.

E. The client's medications were coordinated.

15. Educate about Psychotropic Medications (15)

A. The client was taught about the indications for and the expected benefits of psychotropic medications.

B. As the client's psychotropic medications were reviewed, he/she displayed an understanding about the indications for and expected benefits of the medications.

C. The client displayed a lack of understanding of the indications for and expected benefits of psychotropic medications and was provided with additional information and feedback regarding his/her medications.

16. Monitor Medications (16)

A. The client was monitored for compliance with his/her psychotropic medication regimen.

B. The client was provided with positive feedback about his/her regular use of psychotropic medications.

C. The client was monitored for the effectiveness and side effects of his/her prescribed medications.

D. Concerns about the client's medication effectiveness and side effects were communicated to the physician.

E. Although the client was monitored for medication side effects, he/she reported no concerns in this area.

17. Coordinate Adult Foster Care Placement (17)

A. The client was placed in an adult foster care placement to create a stable residence that is not dependent on financial management skills.

B. The client was supported for accepting adult foster care placement, which has helped him/her to obtain a stable residence regardless of his/her personal financial management.

C. The client has declined involvement in the adult foster care placement and is continuing to have an unstable living situation due to his/her financial mismanagement; additional encouragement to reconsider this decision was given.

18. Coordinate Placement within the Support System (18)

A. The client was assisted in coordinating placement with family or friends to create a stable residence that is not dependent on financial management skills.

B. The client was supported for accepting placement with family or friends, which has helped him/her to obtain a stable residence regardless of his/her personal financial management.

C. The client has declined placement with family or friends and is continuing to have an unstable living situation due to his/her financial mismanagement; he/she was urged to reconsider this decision.

19. Provide Support for Independent Living Situation (19)

A. The client was assisted in developing an independent or semi-independent living situation.

B. The client received guidance for obtaining financial assistance related to developing an independent or semi-independent living situation.

C. The client has been able to successfully develop, after obtaining assistance on the financial aspects, an independent or semi-independent living situation; he/she was given support for this step.

D. The client has not created a more independent living situation and was provided with additional direction in this area.

20. Review Financial Needs and Management (20)

A. The client's financial needs and money management practices were reviewed.

B. The client was supported as he/she reviewed his/her financial needs and management practices.

C. The client refused to provide data regarding how he/she manages his/her money and was urged to do so.

21. File for Benefits (21)

A. The client was assisted in obtaining, completing, and filing forms for Social Security Disability benefits or other public aid.

B. The client has completed all necessary documentation for filing for Social Security Disability benefits or other public aid, and this material was reviewed.

C. The client's application for Social Security Disability benefits and other public aid was incomplete, and he/she received assistance in completing these applications.

22. Coordinate Transportation (22)

A. Transportation was coordinated for the client to all necessary appointments related to obtaining financial assistance benefits.

B. The client was praised for attending all necessary appointments related to obtaining benefits.

23. Assign Social Security Readings (23)

A. The client was assigned to read information about maximizing his/her Social Security benefits.

B. The client was assigned to read specific portions in *How to Get Every Penny You're Entitled to from Social Security* by Bosley and Gurwitz.

C. The client has read important information regarding how to obtain benefits from Social Security, and this information was processed.

D. The client has not done appropriate reading from Social Security information and was redirected to do so.

24. Provide Agency as an Address (24)

A. The client was directed to use the agency address as a mail drop for his/her benefit checks.

B. The client has regularly obtained his/her government check by having it sent to the agency address, which has stabilized his/her financial concerns; this procedure was supported.

C. The client refused to allow the agency to receive his/her mailed benefit checks; additional urging to reconsider this decision was given.

25. Provide Financial Assistance Lists (25)

A. The client received a list of available and relevant financial assistance resources.

B. The client was advised about financial assistance resources in his/her area (e.g., home heating assistance, scholarships, or housing funds).

C. The client has accessed relevant financial assistance resources, which has helped to stabilize his/her financial concerns, and this assistance was reviewed.

26. Help with Assistance Programs (26)

A. The client was assisted in coordinating appointments and filling out forms to obtain assistance from area programs.

B. The client has accessed area assistance programs, and the benefits of these programs were reviewed.

C. The client has not attempted to obtain assistance from area programs and was provided with additional direction to do so.

27. Coordinate Health Insurance Application (27)

A. The client was assisted in making his/her application for the appropriate public health insurance program.

B. The client has successfully obtained health insurance, and the benefits of this were reviewed with him/her.

C. The client has failed to complete the necessary documentation for applicable public insurance and was provided with additional assistance in this area.

28. Educate about Budgeting Skills (28)

A. The client was educated about basic budgeting procedures.

B. Specific budget information, contained in *Personal Budget Planner: A Guide for Financial Success* by Gelb, was reviewed.

C. The client was supported for displaying a mastery of the basic budgeting skills that he/she has been taught.

D. The client has failed to master basic budgeting skills and was provided with additional information and guidance in this area.

29. Develop a Budget (29)

A. The client was requested to develop a basic budget, including income, necessary expenses, additional spending, and savings plans.

B. The client has developed a basic budget, and this material was reviewed.

C. The client was given positive feedback for his/her comprehensive, realistic budget.

D. The client has not developed a basic budget and was redirected to do so.

30. Refer to Budgeting Classes (30)

A. The client was referred to a community education class related to managing personal finances.

B. The client has attended the community education class related to managing personal finances, and the concepts learned were reviewed.

C. The client has not obtained any benefit from his/her community education class on personal finances, but was encouraged to continue.

D. The client has not attended the community education class regarding personal finances and was redirected to do so.

31. Develop Long-Term Financial Plans (31)

A. The client was requested to identify his/her realistic, long-term financial plans.

B. The client was provided with feedback regarding his/her long-term financial plans.

C. The client has not developed a long-term financial plan and was redirected to do so.

32. Teach Banking Procedures (32)

A. The client was taught about typical banking procedures.

B. The client received positive feedback as he/she displayed mastery of how to complete basic banking procedures.

C. The client displayed a poor understanding of typical banking procedures and was provided with additional training in this area.

33. Tour a Bank (33)

A. A tour of a bank was arranged for the client.

B. The client was supported for participating in the bank tour, with a focus on becoming more comfortable with the procedures and security measures expected within the bank.

C. As the client has become more comfortable with the procedures and security measures within the bank, he/she has been able to more appropriately use the bank; this process was reviewed.

D. The client did not attend the bank tour, and this resistance was processed.

34. Practice Banking Procedures (34)

A. The client was assisted in practicing typical banking procedures within the session (e.g., check writing or check cashing) using imitation supplies or forms.

B. The client was reinforced for displaying the skills necessary to do basic banking procedures.

C. The client continues to display a poor understanding of basic banking procedures and was provided with additional education in this area.

35. Obtain Proper Identification (35)

A. The client was assisted in obtaining proper identification necessary for banking functions.

B. The client was assisted in obtaining a state identification card.

C. The client was reinforced for completing necessary banking functions after obtaining proper identification.

GRIEF AND LOSS

CLIENT PRESENTATION

1. Death of Significant Other (1)*

A. The client presented as visibly upset and distressed over the recent loss of his/her significant other.

B. The client displayed symptoms of depression, confusion, and feelings of insecurity regarding the future.

C. The client reported severe emotional reactions and uncertainty due to his/her grief and loss.

D. The client revealed that feelings of being alone and hopeless have been overwhelming for him/her since the death of his/her significant other.

E. The client has started to talk about the loss of his/her significant other and has begun to accept consolation, support, and encouragement from others.

F. The client has resolved the debilitating grief over the death of his/her significant other.

2. Preoccupation with Loss (2)

A. The client's thoughts have been dominated by the loss experienced, and he/she has not been able to maintain normal concentration on other tasks.

B. The client reported a reduction in his/her preoccupation with the experience of loss and slightly improved concentration.

C. The client's concentration has improved significantly, and his/her thoughts are no longer dominated by the loss he/she has experienced.

3. Exacerbation of Mental Illness Symptoms (2)

A. The client's recent loss has caused an emotional upheaval, which has caused an exacerbation of his/her mental illness symptoms.

B. The client has not regularly maintained his/her medications or monitored his/her prodromals due to his/her preoccupation by the loss, which has resulted in an exacerbation of his/her primary mental illness symptoms.

C. The client has regressed due to his/her recent loss.

D. As the client has worked through his/her feelings related to the loss, his/her primary mental illness symptoms have decreased.

4. Depression Symptoms (3)

A. The client described a lack of appetite, sad affect, low energy, and a disturbance of his/her sleep, as well as other depression signs that have occurred since the experience of the loss.

B. The client has experienced thoughts of suicide, crying, or depressed mood since the experience of the loss.

---

* The numbers in parentheses correlate to the number of the Behavioral Definition statement in the companion chapter with the same title in *The Severe and Persistent Mental Illness Treatment Planner,* 2nd ed. (Berghuis and Jongsma) by John Wiley & Sons, 2008.

C. The client's depression symptoms have diminished as he/she has begun to resolve the feelings of grief.

D. The client's depression symptoms have lifted.

5. Hopelessness/Worthlessness (4)

A. The client verbalized feelings of hopelessness and worthlessness subsequent to his/her experience of the loss of the significant other.

B. The client verbalized an unreasonable pattern of feeling hopeless and worthless as he/she struggles to meet the needs previously met by the lost significant other.

C. The client reports that his/her feelings of hopelessness and worthlessness have diminished.

D. The client reports a pattern of feeling hopeful and worthwhile despite the loss.

6. Inappropriate Guilt (4)

A. The client expressed feelings of guilt about having acted in some way to cause the death of his/her significant other.

B. The client has continued to hold onto the unreasonable belief that he/she behaved in some manner that either caused the death of the significant other or failed to prevent it from occurring.

C. The client has started to work through his/her feelings of guilt about the death of the significant other.

D. The client verbalized that he/she is not responsible for the death of the significant other.

E. The client has successfully worked through his/her feelings of guilt and no longer blames himself/herself for the death of the significant other.

7. Fear of Abandonment (4)

A. The client reported that he/she fears being abandoned by all significant others due to his/her experience of multiple losses.

B. The client reported being confused about what the future of his/her life would be like due to his/her traumatic loss.

C. The client is beginning to talk about his/her future and reports a decreased fear of abandonment as he/she struggles to resolve the experience of loss.

D. The client has begun to return to a more normal, hopeful outlook on his/her life, and he/she does not fear being abandoned by others who care for him/her.

8. Grief Avoidance (5)

A. The client has shown a pattern of avoidance of talking about the loss except on a very superficial level.

B. The client's feelings of grief are coming more to the surface as he/she faces the loss issue more directly.

C. The client is able to talk about the loss more directly without being overwhelmed by feelings of grief.

9. Loss Due to the Effects of Mental Illness (6)

A. The client described a pattern of loss of ability, status, relationships, and competence due to his/her incapacitating effects of psychosis and other severe mental illness symptoms.

B. The client described his/her pattern of grief-related emotions due to the personal losses he/she has experienced subsequent to his/her severe mental illness symptoms.

C. As the client has stabilized, he/she has regained some abilities, status, and competence and reports less of a sense of loss.

D. The client has become more at ease with the incapacitating effects of his/her severe mental illness symptoms.

10. Low Self-Esteem (7)

A. The client stated that he/she has a very negative perception of himself/herself.

B. The client's low self-esteem was evident within the session as he/she made many self-disparaging remarks and maintained very little eye contact.

C. The client related his/her low self-esteem to his/her history of losses.

D. The client's self-esteem has increased as he/she is beginning to find reasons to affirm his/her self-worth.

E. The client verbalized positive feelings toward himself/herself.

11. Childhood Trauma (8)

A. The client reported that he/she had a history of childhood traumas that includes abuse.

B. The client reported that painful memories of his/her abusive childhood experiences are intrusive and unsettling.

C. The client reported that nightmares and other disturbing thoughts related to childhood abuse have interfered with his/her sleep.

D. The client reported that his/her emotional reactions associated with the childhood abusive experiences have been resolved.

E. The client was able to discuss his/her childhood abusive experience without being overwhelmed with negative emotions.

12. Abusive Parent Figures (8)

A. The client described his/her parents as rigid, perfectionist, and hypercritical, resulting in consistent feelings of inadequacy.

B. The client reported that his/her parents were threatening and demeaning, resulting in feelings of low self-esteem.

C. The client reported that his/her parents were hyperreligious, resulting in rigid, high expectations of behavior and harsh discipline.

D. The client described an emotionally repressive atmosphere at home during his/her childhood as a result of his/her parents' lack of nurturance, encouragement, and positive reinforcement.

E. The client is able to affirm himself/herself now, in spite of a history of parental rejection.

13. Dissociative Phenomena (9)

A. The client described a pattern of dissociative experiences.

B. The client displayed periods of lost time, depersonalization, and other dissociative phenomena.

C. The client's dissociative experiences have diminished in frequency and intensity.

D. The client no longer experiences dissociative phenomena.

14. Paranoia (9)

A. The client's speech and thought patterns displayed paranoid ideation.

B. The client is distrustful and reactive subsequent to his/her experience of significant losses.

C. The client's paranoid thoughts and speech have become less frequent.

D. The client no longer gives evidence of paranoia.

15. Spiritual Conflicts (10)

A. The client described confusing and conflicting thoughts and feelings regarding his/her spiritual understanding of the losses he/she has experienced.

B. The client described that he/she is angry with God for the losses that he/she has experienced.

C. The client has begun to work through his/her spiritual conflicts.

D. The client has become more settled regarding his/her spiritual conflicts and made his/her peace with God.

16. Loss of Support Network (11)

A. The client expressed grief over having lost important portions of his/her support network due to his/her psychotic or other severe mental illness symptoms.

B. The client's support network members have identified their inability to continue supporting him/her due to the effects of his/her severe mental illness symptoms.

C. As the client has stabilized, his/her support network has become more available to him/her, and his/her grief has resolved.

INTERVENTIONS IMPLEMENTED

1. Provide Emotional Support (1)*

A. Active and empathic listening, consistent eye contact, unconditional positive regard, and warm acceptance were used to help provide direct emotional support to the client.

B. The client was supported as he/she began to express feelings more freely as rapport and trust levels increased.

C. The client has continued to experience difficulties being open and direct in his/her expression of painful feelings and was encouraged to discuss these as he/she feels safe to do so.

2. Assess Suicidal Intent (2)

A. The client was asked to describe the frequency and intensity of his/her suicidal ideation, the details of any existing suicidal plan, the history of any previous suicide attempts, and any family history of depression or suicide.

B. The client was encouraged to be forthright regarding the current strengths of his/her suicidal feelings and his/her ability to control such suicidal urges.

C. The client was provided with positive feedback and support as he/she described his/her thoughts and feelings regarding suicide.

D. The client was assessed to have a low potential for suicide and was advised that suicide monitoring will continue.

E. The client was assessed to have a high potential for suicide and was referred for a more intensive level of supervision.

---

* The numbers in parentheses correlate to the number of the Therapeutic Intervention statement in the companion chapter with the same title in *The Severe and Persistent Mental Illness Treatment Planner,* 2nd ed. (Berghuis and Jongsma) by John Wiley & Sons, 2008.

3. Arrange for Hospitalization/Crisis Residential Placement (3)

A. The client was judged to be uncontrollably harmful to himself/herself and psychiatrically unstable; therefore, arrangements were made for psychiatric hospitalization.

B. The client was judged to be at risk for harm to himself/herself; therefore, arrangements were made for a crisis residential admission.

C. The client was reinforced for cooperating voluntarily with admission to a more intensive level of treatment.

D. The client refused to cooperate voluntarily with admission to a psychiatric facility, and therefore commitment procedures were indicated.

4. List Relationship Losses (4)

A. The client was asked to elaborate on the circumstances, feelings, and effects of the loss or losses in his/her life.

B. The client was supported as he/she identified the losses that have been experienced in his/her life and shared the feelings of pain and grief associated with these losses.

C. The client talked about the losses experienced, but the feelings associated with these losses were not shared; continued efforts to explore these feelings were implemented.

5. Resolve Relationship Problems (5)

A. The client was assisted in resolving specific relationship problems.

B. The client was provided with specific examples of how to resolve relationship problems.

C. The client was provided with feedback as he/she explained his/her attempts at resolving his/her relationship problems.

D. As the client has resolved relationship problems, he/she has improved his/her overall functioning and was provided with positive feedback in this area.

6. Explore Losses Due to Mental Illness (6)

A. The client was asked to describe his/her experience of job losses and other losses related to his/her mental illness symptoms.

B. The client was provided with feedback and support as he/she described the losses that he/she has experienced due to the loss of occupational and other functional abilities.

C. The client avoided providing meaningful feedback about the losses that he/she has experienced related to mental illness concerns and was given further encouragement to focus on these losses.

7. Resolve Occupational Problems (7)

A. The client was assisted in resolving specific occupational problems.

B. The client was provided with specific examples of how to resolve occupational problems.

C. The client was provided with feedback as he/she explained his/her attempts at resolving his/her occupational problems.

D. As the client has resolved occupational problems, he/she has improved his/her overall functioning and was provided with positive feedback in this area.

8. Vent Emotions (8)

A. The client was assisted in identifying, clarifying, and expressing feelings associated with his/her losses.

B. The client was praised as he/she has become more open in expressing feelings of grief.

C. The client minimizes and denies feelings of grief associated with the loss and was encouraged to be more open about these feelings.

9. Refer to a Physician (9)

A. The client was referred to a physician for an evaluation for a prescription of psychotropic medications.

B. The client was reinforced for following through on a referral to a physician for an assessment for a prescription of psychotropic medications, but none were prescribed.

C. The client has been prescribed psychotropic medications.

D. The client declined an evaluation by a physician for a prescription of psychotropic medications and was redirected to cooperate with this referral.

10. Educate about Psychotropic Medications (10)

A. The client was taught about the indications for and the expected benefits of psychotropic medications.

B. As the client's psychotropic medications were reviewed, he/she displayed an understanding about the indications for and expected benefits of the medications.

C. The client displayed a lack of understanding of the indications for and expected benefits of psychotropic medications and was provided with additional information and feedback regarding his/her medications.

11. Monitor Medications (11)

A. The client was monitored for compliance with his/her psychotropic medication regimen.

B. The client was provided with positive feedback about his/her regular use of psychotropic medications.

C. The client was monitored for the effectiveness and side effects of his/her prescribed medications.

D. Concerns about the client's medication effectiveness and side effects were communicated to the physician.

E. Although the client was monitored for medication side effects, he/she reported no concerns in this area.

12. Reinforce Medication Compliance (12)

A. The client was urged to continue his/her strict compliance with his/her prescription medications.

B. The client was assessed for refusal to take his/her psychotropic medications as prescribed.

C. The client was reinforced for his/her regular use and strict compliance with medication prescriptions.

D. The client has not regularly used his/her prescription medications in the manner in which it was ordered and was redirected to comply with these directions.

13. Assign Grief Books (13)

A. Several books on the grieving process were recommended to the client.

B. The client was assigned specific readings from *The Grief Recovery Handbook: The Action Program for Moving Beyond Death* (James and Friedman).

C. The client has read the material on the grieving process, and content from that material was processed.

D. The client was reinforced for showing an increased understanding of the steps of the grieving process as a result of reading the recommended grief material.

E. The client has not followed through on reading any of the grief material and was encouraged to do so.

14. Teach Grief Stages (14)

A. The client was educated regarding the stages of the grieving process.

B. The client verbalized an increased understanding of the steps of the grieving process and identified the stages that he/she has experienced personally, and this was processed.

C. The client could not apply the grief stages to his/her own experience and was provided with additional support and feedback in this area.

15. Educate about Mental Illness (15)

A. The client was educated about the expected or common symptoms of his/her mental illness that may contribute to his/her grief and loss issues.

B. As the client's symptoms of mental illness were discussed, he/she displayed an understanding of how these symptoms may affect his/her grief process.

C. The client did not understand how symptoms of his/her mental illness may negatively impact his/her grief process and was given additional feedback in this area.

16. Apply Knowledge of Mental Illness to Symptoms (16)

A. The client's specific symptoms were reviewed.

B. The client's pattern of mental illness symptoms was reviewed relative to the impact that his/her symptoms have had on his/her pattern of personal losses.

C. The client was provided with positive feedback as he/she displayed insight into his/her pattern of mental illness symptoms and his/her symptoms' impact on his/her losses.

D. The client continued to struggle with his/her understanding of how his/her symptoms have contributed to grief and loss issues and was provided with additional feedback in this area.

17. Refer to a Support Group (17)

A. The client was referred to a support group for individuals with severe and persistent mental illness.

B. The client has attended the support group for individuals with severe and persistent mental illness, and the benefits of this support group were reviewed.

C. The client reported that he/she has not experienced any positive benefit from the use of a support group but was encouraged to continue attending.

D. The client has not used the support group for individuals with severe and persistent mental illness and was redirected to do so.

18. Teach about Defense Mechanisms (18)

A. The client was taught about the common tendency for people to use defense mechanisms.

B. The client was provided with specific examples of the use of defense mechanisms regarding mental illness concerns (e.g., some people deny problems rather than face the reality of a chronic mental illness).

C. The client's description of his/her own pattern of defense mechanisms was processed within the session.

D. The client denied any pattern of defense mechanisms, and this was processed as a defense mechanism itself.

19. Identify Defense Mechanisms (19)

A. The client was assisted in identifying ways in which he/she uses defense mechanisms to delay or avoid facing grief and loss issues.

B. The client accepted his/her pattern of defense mechanisms to delay or avoid facing grief and loss issues, and this was processed within the session.

C. The client denied any use of defense mechanisms and was urged to apply this more appropriately to himself/herself.

20. Assign Reading on Grieving Mental Illness (20)

A. The client was assigned to read material on the process of grief associated with accepting his/her mental illness.

B. The client was referred to sections of *Grieving Mental Illness: A Guide for Patients and Their Caregivers* by Lafond.

C. The client has read the material on grief and mental illness issues, and the content on that material was processed.

D. The client has shown an increase in understanding of his/her losses related to his/her mental illness, and this was reviewed.

E. The client has not followed through on the reading material related to grief associated with mental illness and was encouraged to do so.

21. List the Effects of Mental Illness (21)

A. The client was requested to develop a list of ways in which his/her mental illness symptoms have affected him/her.

B. The client has developed a list of the effects of his/her mental illness on his/her life, and these were processed.

C. The client was assisted in clarifying and identifying those feelings of grief associated with the effect of mental illness, and he/she began to resolve them.

D. The client has not followed through on listing ways in which his/her mental illness symptoms have affected him/her and was redirected to do so.

22. Review Basic Emotions (22)

A. The client was assisted in reviewing a list of basic emotions.

B. The client was helped to identify the social, verbal, and body language cues used to identify basic emotions.

C. As the client has developed an increased understanding of basic emotions, he/she was assisted in applying this to his/her own pattern of feelings.

D. The client was reinforced for improving his/her pattern of functioning as he/she has begun to express his/her emotions.

23. Review Emotion Identification (23)

A. The client was assisted in identifying ways in which he/she labels specific emotions that he/she has experienced.

B. As the client has identified his/her pattern of emotions and how he/she identifies and labels them, he/she was provided with positive feedback in this area.

C. The client was not able to identify how to label specific emotions and was provided with remedial information in this area.

24. Clarify Unidentified Emotional States (24)

A. The client was probed for emotional states that he/she has previously been unable to identify.

B. The client was assisted in uncovering previously unidentified emotional states that have contributed to his/her pattern of symptoms.

25. Assign a Grief Journal/Tape (25)

A. It was recommended that the client keep a daily grief journal to be shared in future sessions.

B. The client has limited writing skills; therefore, he/she was assigned to record grief feelings on an audiotape to be shared in future sessions.

C. The client has kept a grief journal/tape on a daily basis and verbalized the feelings of grief that he/she has experienced, and these were reviewed.

D. The client was provided with positive feedback for using a grief journal to help clarify and identify feelings of grief, and he/she is beginning to resolve them.

26. Journal/Tape Acceptance of Feelings (26)

A. It was recommended to the client that he/she keep a daily journal of his/her feelings of acceptance of the losses.

B. It was recommended to the client that he/she use an audiotape to describe his/her feelings of acceptance of his/her losses.

C. The client's record of his/her feelings of acceptance of losses was shared with the clinician.

D. As the client has kept a record of his/her feelings of acceptance of his/her losses, he/she has begun to resolve his/her grief issues, and he/she was encouraged for this progress.

27. Assign Forgiveness Readings (27)

A. The client was assigned to read information on the process of forgiveness.

B. The client was referred to read portions of *Forgive and Forget: Healing the Hurts We Don't Deserve* by Smedes.

C. Portions of the written material on forgiveness were reviewed to help the client overcome his/her feelings of resentment.

D. The client has failed to read any of the recommended grief material and was redirected to do so.

28. Encourage Mourning Events (28)

A. The client was encouraged to use typical mourning events (e.g., visit the grave site of a deceased relative or write a good-bye letter to someone who is deceased).

B. The client has followed through on implementing the grieving ritual, and his/her experience was processed.

C. The client's involvement in an appropriate grieving ritual was coordinated.

D. The client has not followed through on development of a grieving ritual and was encouraged to do so.

29. Develop a Meaningful Release (29)

A. The client was assisted in developing and safely carrying out a meaningful ritual for letting go of the loss.

B. The client was provided with specific examples of meaningful personal rituals for letting go of the loss (e.g., tying a journal entry, letter, or picture to a helium balloon and letting it go).

C. The client has selected his/her own personalized, meaningful ritual for letting go of the loss and was assisted in completing this.

D. The client has not developed his/her own meaningful ritual for letting go of the loss and was provided with additional encouragement in this area.

30. Develop Meaningful Activities (30)

A. The client was assisted in developing meaningful activities that assist in resolving grief issues (e.g., volunteering to help in a support group that focuses on his/her loss issue).

B. The client has identified his/her own meaningful activities to assist in resolving grief issues and was assisted in implementing these activities.

C. The client's experience of involvement in meaningful activities to assist in resolving grief issues was processed.

D. The client has not instituted the use of meaningful activities to assist in resolving grief issues and was redirected to do so.

31. Encourage Increased Activities (31)

A. The client was encouraged to increase his/her involvement in social activities, hobbies, or volunteer placements.

B. The client's increased involvement in social activities, hobbies, or volunteer placements was coordinated.

C. As the client has increased his/her involvement in social activities, hobbies, or volunteer placements, he/she has reported increased emotional stability, and this progress was processed.

D. The client has not become more involved in social activities, hobbies, or volunteer placements and was encouraged to do so.

32. Explore or Refer Spiritual Issues (32)

A. The client's spiritual struggles were explored.

B. The client was referred to an appropriate clergy person to allow for further discussion of the client's spiritual struggles.

C. The client was reinforced for resolving his/her spiritual struggles and demonstrating an increased pattern of functioning.

D. The client has not focused on his/her spiritual struggles and was redirected to do so.

33. Suggest Faith Readings (33)

A. The client was urged to read spiritual material suitable to his/her faith.

B. The client was urged to read *How Could It Be All Right When Everything Is All Wrong?* by Smedes.

C. The client was urged to read *When Bad Things Happen to Good People* by Kushner.

D. The client has read material appropriate to his/her faith, and pertinent issues were reviewed.

E. The client has not read faith-related material and was encouraged to do so.

34. Coordinate a Family Session (34)

A. A family therapy session was conducted with all members of the family expressing their experience related to the history of losses.

B. Each family member was supported as he/she expressed his/her feelings of grief and related how he/she is coping with the losses.

C. Family members displayed an increased understanding of the client's history of losses and were encouraged to provide additional support to him/her.

D. Family members were confronted regarding not being supportive of the client despite their increased understanding of his/her history.

35. Facilitate Support from Others (35)

A. The client was assisted in identifying other people who are struggling with similar issues.

B. The client was directed to develop supportive relationships with people outside his/her family who are dealing with grief and loss.

C. The client has developed mutually supportive relationships with people outside of his/her family, and the benefits of these relationships were reviewed.

D. The client has failed to develop better relationships with people outside of his/her family that are struggling with similar loss issues, and such a relationship was facilitated for the client.

HEALTH ISSUES

CLIENT PRESENTATION

1. Serious Medical Condition (1)*

A. The client presented with serious medical problems.

B. The client's medical problems cause serious impact on his/her daily living.

C. The client's severe and persistent mental illness symptoms are exacerbated by his/her medical problems.

D. The client's medical condition has improved.

2. Receiving Treatment (2)

A. The client has pursued treatment for his/her medical condition.

B. The client has refused treatment for his/her medical condition.

C. The client has not sought treatment for his/her medical condition because of a lack of insurance and financial resources.

D. The client's physical health concerns have improved due to his/her medical treatment.

3. HIV-Positive (3)

A. The client has tested positive for the human immunodeficiency virus (HIV).

B. The client has been HIV-positive for an extended period of time but has had no serious deterioration in his/her condition.

C. The client is obtaining consistent medical care for his/her HIV status.

D. The client has refused medical care for his/her HIV-positive status and tends to be in denial about the seriousness of the situation.

4. AIDS (3)

A. The client's HIV-positive status has resulted in the development of acquired immune deficiency syndrome (AIDS).

B. The client's medical condition resulting from AIDS has deteriorated, and his/her severe and persistent mental illness symptoms have increased.

C. Although the client has serious AIDS complications, he/she remains at peace and is getting good medical care.

5. Poor Understanding of Medical Issues (4)

A. The client displayed a poor understanding of his/her medical needs.

B. The client is uncertain about his/her available treatment options and medical services for his/her medical concerns.

C. As the client has obtained more specific information related to his/her medical needs, he/she has stabilized his/her medical condition.

---

* The numbers in parentheses correlate to the number of the Behavioral Definition statement in the companion chapter with the same title in *The Severe and Persistent Mental Illness Treatment Planner,* 2nd ed. (Berghuis and Jongsma) by John Wiley & Sons, 2008.

6. Barriers to Treatment (5)

A. The client described difficulties with gaining access to medical facilities or health care providers.

B. Health care providers have discriminated against the client due to his/her severe and persistent mental illness symptoms.

C. The client has failed to make his/her medical needs known due to the effects of his/her severe and persistent mental illness symptoms.

D. As the client has gained better access to medical facilities and health care providers, his/her overall level of functioning has increased.

7. Failure to Access Medical Treatment (6)

A. The client has failed to access appropriate medical treatment due to his/her severe and persistent mental illness symptoms.

B. The client's health status has suffered due to his/her failure to access appropriate medical treatment.

C. As the client's severe and persistent mental illness symptoms have been stabilized, his/her medical treatment has been more easily accessed.

D. The client's medical status has improved due to his/her accessing appropriate medical treatment.

8. Poor Health Habits (7)

A. The client displayed poor oral hygiene.

B. The client bathes infrequently and has significant body odor on a consistent basis.

C. The client lives in unsanitary living conditions.

D. The client displayed poor health habits due to his/her pattern of severe and persistent mental illness symptoms.

E. As the client has stabilized his/her severe and persistent mental illness symptoms, he/she has displayed better health habits.

9. Financial Limitations (8)

A. The client has failed to access or follow through with medical treatment due to financial limitations.

B. The client has obtained financial resources to assist with his/her medical treatment.

C. The client's medical problems have improved due to economically available medical treatment.

10. Chemical Dependence Complications (9)

A. The client has developed medical complications because of his/her chronic chemical dependence history.

B. The client has accepted that he/she has deteriorated medically because of his/her chemical dependence pattern and has terminated substance abuse.

C. The client is in denial about the negative medical effects of his/her substance abuse and continues his/her self-destructive pattern.

D. The client's medical condition has improved subsequent to termination of substance abuse.

INTERVENTIONS IMPLEMENTED

1. Refer to a Physician (1)*

A. The client was referred to a physician for a complete physical to evaluate his/her medical condition.

B. The essential arrangements were made for the client to obtain necessary medical testing.

C. The client followed through with a referral to a physician for a medical evaluation and was reinforced for obtaining proper health care.

D. The client was supported for following through with the recommended medical testing, and the results were processed.

E. The client has failed to follow through on the recommendation to obtain a medical evaluation and was redirected to do so.

2. Consult with a Physician (2)

A. The client's physician has been contacted in order to review his/her orders with the client.

B. The client was encouraged to follow the treatment orders as described by his/her physician during a consultation contact.

C. The client signed a release of information allowing the clinician to obtain medical information from the physician for the purposes of treatment coordination and follow-through monitoring.

3. Provide Medical Information for Making Treatment Decisions (3)

A. The client was provided with appropriate literature and references to material that would increase his/her understanding of his/her medical condition.

B. The client was encouraged to contact medical resources to obtain more information regarding his/her medical condition.

C. The client was assisted in making decisions about his/her current medical treatment needs.

D. Arrangements were made for the client to obtain the necessary medical services.

E. The client was supported for obtaining appropriate medical treatment.

F. The client has declined to seek further information regarding his/her medical condition, its treatment, and the prognosis and was redirected to do so.

4. Acknowledge Denial/Avoidance while Reinforcing Acceptance (4)

A. The client's denial of the seriousness of his/her medical condition was acknowledged as a common emotional response.

B. The client's denial of the seriousness of his/her medical condition was confronted, and he/she was reinforced for showing any acceptance of the medical condition.

C. The client accepted the confrontation regarding the seriousness of his/her medical condition and verbalized increased acceptance of the need for medical intervention.

D. The client was reinforced for showing acceptance of the reality of his/her medical problems.

E. The client was supported for his/her realistic statements regarding his/her medical condition.

---

* The numbers in parentheses correlate to the number of the Therapeutic Intervention statement in the companion chapter with the same title in *The Severe and Persistent Mental Illness Treatment Planner,* 2nd ed. (Berghuis and Jongsma) by John Wiley & Sons, 2008.

F. The client continues to be in denial regarding the seriousness of his/her medical condition and was given additional feedback in this area.

G. The client continues to struggle with the reality of his/her medical problems and was provided with additional feedback in this area.

5. Inform/Encourage Support from Family and Friends (5)

A. A proper authorization to release information was obtained in order to provide family and friends with information regarding the client's medical needs.

B. In a conjoint session, family members, friends, or other important individuals in the client's life were provided with specific information regarding his/her medical needs.

C. Family, friends, and other important individuals in the client's life have been more supportive of him/her subsequent to learning about his/her medical needs, and this was processed.

D. The client's family, friends, and support network received encouragement regarding their emotional support and positive reinforcement for his/her adherence to medical treatment.

E. The client's experience of emotional support from his/her family and friends was processed.

F. Despite additional information regarding the client's medical needs, family, friends, and others have not been supportive of his/her medical needs, and he/she was given emotional support in this area.

6. Educate about Nutrition (6)

A. The client was educated about healthy food choices.

B. The client was educated about the effect of a healthy diet on long-term medical well-being.

C. The client was supported for his/her increased understanding of his/her nutritional choices.

D. The client was reinforced for healthy nutritional choices that have assisted in stabilizing his/her medical well-being.

E. The client continues to make poor nutritional choices, and he/she was redirected in this area.

7. Facilitate Access to a Grocery Store (7)

A. The client was assisted in attaining regular access to a full-service grocery store to help meet his/her nutritional needs.

B. The client was accompanied to the grocery store to help increase his/her comfort level.

C. The client reported feeling more comfortable in accessing the services of a grocery store, and the benefits of this were reviewed.

D. The client continues to struggle with obtaining appropriate supplies for his/her nutritional well-being due to limited access and comfort with the grocery store and was assisted in problem-solving this situation.

8. Educate about Healthy Foods (8)

A. The client was educated about his/her food shopping choices.

B. The client was taught how to compare healthy foods with unhealthy foods.

C. The client was provided with positive reinforcement for making healthier food choices.

D. The client continues to make unhealthy choices regarding his/her foods and was given remedial information in this area.

9. Refer to a Dietician (9)

A. The client was referred to a dietician who will explain proper nutrition that will enhance his/her medical recovery.

B. The client was reinforced for accepting the dietician referral and attending an appointment.

C. The client has verbalized an increased knowledge about how proper nutrition can have a positive impact on his/her medical condition, and he/she was provided with encouragement in this area.

D. The client has refused to follow through on the referral to a dietician and was encouraged to do so.

10. Assess for and Refer for Substance Abuse (10)

A. The client was assessed for substance abuse that may exacerbate his/her medical problems.

B. The client was referred for a substance abuse evaluation.

C. The client was identified as having a concomitant substance abuse problem and was referred for treatment.

D. The client was referred to a 12-step recovery program (e.g., Alcoholics Anonymous or Narcotics Anonymous).

E. The client has been admitted to a substance abuse treatment program and was supported for this follow-through.

F. Upon review, the client does not display evidence of a substance abuse problem, which was reflected to him/her.

G. The client has refused the referral to a substance abuse treatment program, and this refusal was processed.

11. Educate about Substance Abuse Effects (11)

A. The client was educated about the short-term effects of substance abuse.

B. The client was educated about the long-term effects of substance abuse.

C. The client was provided with positive feedback about his/her understanding about the long- and short-term effects of substance abuse.

12. Assess Personal Hygiene Needs (12)

A. The client was asked to prepare an inventory of positive and negative functioning regarding his/her personal hygiene needs.

B. The client prepared his/her inventory of positive and negative functioning regarding his/her personal hygiene needs, and this was reviewed within the session.

C. The client was given positive feedback regarding his/her accurate inventory of positive and negative functioning regarding his/her personal hygiene needs.

D. The client prepared his/her inventory of positive and negative functioning regarding his/her personal hygiene needs but needed additional feedback to develop an accurate assessment.

E. The client has not prepared an inventory of positive and negative functioning regarding his/her personal hygiene needs and was redirected to do so.

13. Refer to a Psychoeducational Group (13)

A. The client was referred to a psychoeducational group focused on teaching personal hygiene skills.

B. The client learned, through the psychoeducational group, to give and receive feedback about personal hygiene skill implementation.

C. The client has attended a psychoeducational group and received feedback about personal hygiene skill implementation, which was processed within the session.

D. The client was verbally reinforced for using the group feedback about personal hygiene skill implementation.

E. The client has not attended the psychoeducational group for personal hygiene skill implementation and was redirected to do so.

14. Institute a Checklist Regarding Personal Hygiene Needs (14)

A. The client was assisted in developing a self-monitoring program for performing his/her personal hygiene needs.

B. The client was provided with positive feedback and encouragement regarding his/her use of a self-monitoring program for performing his/her personal hygiene needs.

C. The client has not implemented or used a self-monitoring program for performing personal hygiene needs and was encouraged to do so.

15. Teach about Exercise (15)

A. The client was taught about the benefits of the regular use of exercise.

B. The client was provided with information about the health benefits that are related to exercise.

C. The client was provided with positive feedback as he/she displayed an understanding of his/her need for exercise.

D. The client denies any need for exercise, and this was processed within the session.

16. Refer to an Activity Therapist (16)

A. The client was referred to an activity therapist for recommendations regarding physical fitness activities that are available in the community.

B. The client was referred to community physical fitness resources (e.g., health clubs and other recreational programs).

C. The client has been actively participating in community physical fitness programs and was reinforced for this.

D. The client has declined involvement in community physical fitness programs and was redirected to do so.

17. Refer to an Exercise Group (17)

A. The client was referred to a community-sponsored exercise group (e.g., aerobics or a walking club).

B. An agency-sponsored exercise group has been developed and offered to the client.

C. The client has participated in the exercise group, and his/her increased health functioning was noted.

D. The client's membership at a local health club or YMCA/YWCA was facilitated.

E. The client has joined a local health club or YMCA/YWCA fitness program and was reinforced for doing so.

F. The client has declined involvement in the exercise opportunities and was redirected to do so.

18. Coordinate Ongoing Medical Care (18)

A. The client was referred to a general physician for routine and ongoing medical evaluation and care.

B. The client's access to a general physician for routine and ongoing medical evaluation and care was coordinated.

C. The client's regular access to routine medical care was reviewed.

D. The client continues to struggle with access to basic health care services and was provided with additional assistance in this area.

19. Plan a Psychiatric Hospitalization (19)

A. A psychiatric hospitalization has been planned on an intermittent basis to complete all needed medical services in a structured, safe, familiar setting.

B. The client's medical services were coordinated to coincide with his/her planned psychiatric hospitalization.

C. The client has received the necessary medical services during his/her psychiatric hospitalization.

D. The client has declined the planned, intermittent psychiatric hospitalization to complete his/her medical needs.

20. Facilitate Attendance at Health Care Appointments (20)

A. The client's attendance at his/her medical, dental, and other health care appointments was monitored.

B. The client was provided with transportation to medical, dental, and other health care appointments.

C. The client was accompanied to his/her doctor's appointments.

D. The scheduling receptionist at the client's health care facility was requested to contact the clinician regarding appointment changes scheduling so that the clinician can guarantee the client's attendance.

E. The clinician was actively involved in maintaining the client's attendance at his/her health care appointments.

F. The client has maintained regular attendance at his/her health care appointments and was provided with positive reinforcement for this.

G. The client continues to be sporadic in his/her attendance at health care appointments and was redirected to be more consistent.

21. Educate Providers Regarding Mental Illness Symptoms (21)

A. An authorization to release information was obtained in order to share information with the client's other health care providers.

B. The client's other health care providers were educated regarding his/her needs relative to his/her mental illness symptoms.

C. The client's health care providers have displayed an increased understanding about his/her needs relative to his/her mental illness symptoms and were thanked for their increased cooperation.

D. The client declined to allow the sharing of information with other health care providers and was urged to reconsider this.

22. Coordinate Regular Dental Care (22)

A. The client was referred to a dentist to determine his/her dental treatment needs.

B. Specific dental treatment needs were identified, and ongoing care was coordinated.

C. No specific dental treatment needs were identified, but a routine follow-up appointment was made.

D. The client has not followed through on the referral for dental services and was redirected to do so.

23. Increase Dental Care (23)

A. The client was trained in the proper use of brushing teeth and flossing.

B. The client was encouraged to use regular brushing and flossing practices.

C. The client was reinforced for his/her regular use of brushing and flossing.

D. The client has not regularly used brushing and flossing and was provided with redirection to do so.

24. Coordinate Hearing/Vision Evaluations (24)

A. A hearing evaluation was coordinated for the client.

B. A vision evaluation was coordinated for the client.

C. The client has attended his/her appropriate evaluations, and the results of these appointments were reviewed.

D. The client has been assisted in following up on recommendations from the hearing and vision evaluations.

E. The client has not participated in hearing and vision evaluations and was redirected to do so.

25. Assist the Client in Filing for Benefits (25)

A. The client was assisted in making his/her application for the appropriate public health insurance program and other entitlements.

B. The client has successfully obtained health insurance or other benefits, and the positive effects of this were reviewed with him/her.

C. The client has failed to complete the necessary documentation for applicable benefits and was provided with additional assistance in this area.

26. Refer to Low-Cost Health Care Providers (26)

A. The client was provided with a list of health care providers who accept public insurance or provide services at a reduced cost or at no cost.

B. The client has used the agency list of available health care providers to obtain appropriate medical care, and the results of these services were discussed.

C. The client has not used the list of health care providers available to him/her and was redirected to do so.

27. Maintain a Stable Residence (27)

A. The client was assisted in developing a more stable residence.

B. The client was provided with assistance to help maintain his/her current residence.

C. As the client has been able to remain in a stable residence, his/her severe and persistent mental illness symptoms have lessened.

D. The client continues to have an unstable residence and was provided with additional suggestions to improve this situation.

28. Refer to a Personal Safety Class (28)

A. The client was referred to a personal safety class, focusing on self-defense and precautions for safety.

B. The client has participated in personal safety classes, and key points from this class were reviewed.

C. The client has not used personal safety classes and was redirected to do so.

29. Access Client in Own Environment (29)

A. Health care services were delivered to the client in his/her own environment.

B. The client was provided with services through his/her homeless shelter.

C. The client was provided with health care services through a mobile health care van.

D. The client continues to avoid using health care services, despite these services being provided where he/she is accessible, and this was reflected to him/her.

30. Refer to a Physician or Psychiatrist for Physical Evaluation (30)

A. The client was referred to a physician who is knowledgeable about the client's medical condition for an evaluation for a prescription of psychotropic medications.

B. The client's psychiatric evaluator was urged to also provide a complete physical evaluation for the client.

C. The client was provided with a physical examination in conjunction with his/her psychiatric evaluation.

D. The client was reinforced for following through on a referral to a physician for an assessment for a prescription of psychotropic medications, but none were prescribed.

E. The client has been prescribed psychotropic medications.

F. The client's physical examination was used to compliment his/her psychiatric evaluation.

G. The client declined evaluation by a physician for a prescription of psychotropic medications and was redirected to cooperate with this referral.

31. Educate about Psychotropic Medications (31)

A. The client was taught about the indications for and the expected benefits of psychotropic medications.

B. The client was monitored for compliance with, effectiveness of, and the side effects of his/her psychotropic medication regimen.

C. The client was provided with positive feedback about his/her regular use of psychotropic medications.

D. The possible side effects of the client's medications were reviewed with him/her.

E. Medical staff were specifically consulted regarding the confounding effects of polypharmacy.

F. Possible side effects of the client's medication were reviewed, but he/she denied experiencing any side effects.

32. Educate about Sexually Transmitted Diseases (STDs) (32)

A. The client was provided with education regarding precautions to take to avoid HIV infection and other STDs.

B. The client was provided with information specific to his/her gender, sexual orientation, and mental illness pattern to help shape his/her perspective of his/her own HIV risk.

C. The client was reinforced for displaying an understanding of the risk of HIV and other STDs.

D. The client has not displayed an understanding of his/her HIV/STD risk and was provided with additional information in this area.

33. Obtain Condoms or Clean Needles (33)

A. The client was referred to programs that will supply free condoms and/or needles to help reduce the risk of HIV infection and other STDs.

B. The client has reduced his/her risk for HIV and other health concerns through the use of condoms and clean needles, and this was reviewed with him/her.

C. The client continues to be at high risk for HIV and other health concerns due to his/her health behaviors and was strongly redirected to take precautions.

34. Use Peer Education (34)

A. The client was assisted through a peer education model in learning more about HIV and other STD concerns.

B. The client was reinforced for an increased understanding of STDs through the use of the peer education model.

C. The client has begun to educate others using the peer education model regarding HIV and other STDs and was supported for this.

D. The client refused involvement in the peer education model and was urged to seek out involvement in this area.

35. Include Partner in STD Education (35)

A. The client's partner was included in education about HIV and other STDs.

B. With proper authorization to release confidential information, the client and his/her partner were assisted in discussing HIV and other STD issues.

C. The client's partner has declined any involvement in discussion about HIV or other STDs and was reminded of this option.

36. Observe and Support Caregivers (36)

A. The client's caregivers were observed for signs of frustration that may reduce their ability to interact effectively with him/her.

B. The client's caregivers were provided with opportunities to express their feelings of frustration relative to providing care for him/her.

C. As the client's caregivers have been assisted in venting their frustrations with providing care for the severely and persistently mentally ill client, his/her care has improved.

D. The client's caregivers were confronted if they became demeaning toward him/her while venting.

E. The client's caregivers denied any pattern of frustration or difficulty in providing care for him/her and were invited to access the clinical support should they feel more stressed by his/her pattern of symptoms.

37. Refer Caregivers to a Support Group (37)

A. The client's caregivers were referred to a support group for those who are affected by another's mental illness.

B. The client's caregivers were supported for attending the support group for caregivers of the mentally ill and reporting positive experiences.

C. The client's caregivers have attended the support group but do not believe that it has been helpful for them, and this negative perception was processed.

D. The client's caregivers have not attended the support group and were redirected to do so.

38. Teach Stress Reduction to Caregivers (38)

A. The client's caregivers were taught stress reduction techniques (e.g., muscle relaxation, abdominal breathing, and safe-place imagery).

B. The client's caregivers have used stress reduction techniques, and the benefits of this were discussed.

C. The client's caregivers have not used stress reduction techniques and were redirected to do so.

39. Refer to a Respite Program (39)

A. The client was referred to a respite program to provide his/her caregivers with a brief rest from the demands of caring for a mentally ill patient.

B. As the client has used the respite program, caregivers report decreased stress subsequent to the brief reprieve, and this was noted.

C. The respite program has not been used, even though caregivers report an ongoing pattern of significant stress; therefore, they were provided with additional encouragement.

HOMELESSNESS

CLIENT PRESENTATION

1. Living on the Streets (1)*

A. The client described a history of living on the street on a short-term, sporadic basis.

B. The client has adopted a lifestyle of living on the streets on a long-term basis.

C. The client has moved into a residence.

2. No Permanent Address (2)

A. The client described chronic periods in which he/she has not maintained a permanent address.

B. The client has moved around to a variety of residences within his/her support network.

C. The client has not been able to access services or entitlements due to his/her failure to maintain a permanent address.

D. The client has maintained a permanent address.

3. Extensive Use of Homeless Programs (3)

A. The client has often used shelters for the homeless.

B. The client has used transitional housing or other supportive living placements.

C. As the client has stabilized his/her severe and persistent mental illness symptoms, he/she has established a more permanent residence.

4. Failure to Make Payments (4)

A. The client described a pattern of a failure to make rent, mortgage, or utility payments, leading to a loss of residence.

B. The client presented his/her bill invoices, which indicated that he/she has failed to make payments necessary to maintain a residence and is at risk of losing his/her residence.

C. The client has been more regular in making his/her bill payments, leading to a more stable pattern of residence.

5. Behavioral Problems Due to Mental Illness (5)

A. The client is at risk of eviction from his/her residence due to behavioral problems related to his/her severe mental illness symptoms.

B. The client described a pattern of eviction from his/her residence due to his/her psychotic or other severe mental illness symptoms.

C. As the client's psychotic or other severe mental illness symptoms have been better controlled, his/her risk of eviction has ended.

6. Lack of Basic Skills (6)

A. The client described a lack of knowledge regarding the basic skills that are needed to maintain a residence (e.g., cleaning, small repairs, budgeting).

---

* The numbers in parentheses correlate to the number of the Behavioral Definition statement in the companion chapter with the same title in *The Severe and Persistent Mental Illness Treatment Planner,* 2nd ed. (Berghuis and Jongsma) by John Wiley & Sons, 2008.

B. The client has been taught about basic skills needed to maintain a residence but does not apply these on a regular basis.

C. The client has used his/her knowledge regarding the basic skills to maintain a residence, and this has helped create a more stable living situation.

INTERVENTIONS IMPLEMENTED

1. Refer to a Homeless Shelter (1)*

A. The client was referred to a local shelter for the homeless.

B. The client was provided with information about how to access a local homeless shelter.

C. The client has used a local homeless shelter and was provided with reinforcement for doing so.

D. The client has declined to use a local homeless shelter and was redirected to use this service.

2. Coordinate Crisis Residential Funds (2)

A. The client was placed in a crisis residential program.

B. Funds for the crisis residential program were coordinated (e.g., motel voucher or transitional program placement).

C. The client was provided with positive reinforcement for his/her use of the crisis residential placement.

D. The client has declined the use of a crisis residential placement and was redirected in this area.

3. Facilitate Placement within Support Network (3)

A. The placement of the client at the home of a family member, friend, or peer was facilitated.

B. Family members, friends, or peers have volunteered to take the client into their home, and he/she was encouraged to use this resource.

C. The client reported greater satisfaction due to living with a family member, friend, or peer, and this was processed.

D. The client has declined offers of placement in the home of a family member, friend, or peer and was redirected in this area.

4. Inquire about History of Homelessness (4)

A. The client was requested to describe his/her history of successful and problematic residential situations.

B. The client was directed to prepare a time line of living in a residence, periods of homelessness, and use of transitional housing.

C. Factors contributing to the client's lifestyle of sporadic homelessness were processed.

D. Empathy and active listening were used as the client reviewed his/her history of successful and problematic residential situations.

E. The client was supported as he/she gave a complete account of his/her history of homelessness.

---

* The numbers in parentheses correlate to the number of the Therapeutic Intervention statement in the companion chapter with the same title in *The Severe and Persistent Mental Illness Treatment Planner,* 2nd ed. (Berghuis and Jongsma) by John Wiley & Sons, 2008.

5. Express Emotions (5)

A. The client was encouraged to share his/her feelings regarding his/her pattern of homelessness (e.g., fear, sadness, loss).

B. The client has shared his/her feelings and has been assisted in identifying causes for the emotions.

C. Emotions such as frustration, discouragement, and embarrassment were acknowledged as natural emotions related to the client's experience of homelessness.

D. The distorted cognitive messages that contribute to the client's emotional response were identified and processed.

E. The client was provided with support and understanding regarding his/her emotional concerns relative to his/her homeless situation.

F. The client was supported as he/she presented with a sad affect and tearfulness when describing his/her feelings.

G. The client described increased acceptance of his/her emotions regarding homelessness, and this was processed within the session.

6. Explore Fears Regarding Seeking a Permanent Residence (6)

A. Possible fears associated with seeking a permanent residence were explored, including the fear of rejection, embarrassment, or failure.

B. The client was provided with support and empathy as he/she described his/her fears related to seeking a permanent residence.

C. The client tended to avoid and deny any expression of negative emotions related to seeking a permanent residence and was encouraged to share these when he/she is able to do so.

7. Provide Feedback Regarding Paranoia (7)

A. The client was provided with realistic feedback regarding his/her paranoia or other irrational delusions.

B. The client accepted the more realistic feedback provided regarding his/her paranoia or other irrational delusions and was reinforced for becoming more reality focused.

C. The client denied the realistic feedback provided regarding his/her paranoia or other irrational delusions and was encouraged to seek a reality check for his/her perceptions.

8. Encourage Maintaining Relationships When Becoming Independent (8)

A. The client was encouraged to maintain important relationships at the homeless shelter when he/she moves to a more independent status.

B. The client has moved into a more independent status and was encouraged to continue his/her important relationships at the homeless shelter regardless of his/her more independent status.

C. The client was reinforced for maintaining important relationships that have helped to ease the emotional stress of a more independent living situation.

D. The client has not maintained important relationships at the homeless shelter, and this was reviewed.

9. Describe Barriers to Maintaining Housing (9)

A. The client was asked to describe specific barriers to maintaining his/her housing.

B. The client was provided with feedback regarding his/her specific barriers to maintaining his/her housing.

C. The client was assisted in resolving specific barriers to housing.

D. The client struggled to identify his/her barriers to maintaining his/her long-term housing and was provided with tentative ideas in this area.

10. Educate about Residential Supports and Services (10)

A. The client was educated about the available options regarding the continuum of supports and services that are available to assist with his/her residential status.

B. The client was assisted in developing a list of pros and cons for each of the housing options available to him/her.

C. The supports and services that are available to assist the client with his/her residential status seem to be well understood, and he/she was provided with positive feedback about this knowledge.

D. The client was provided with a structure for making his/her own decision regarding housing.

E. The client was provided with support for his/her decisions regarding his/her housing.

F. The client continued to display a poor understanding about the continuum of supports and services that are available to help with his/her residential status, and he/she was given additional, remedial information in this area.

11. Apply for Housing Programs (11)

A. The client was assisted in beginning the application process for desired housing programs.

B. The client was provided with directions and given feedback regarding completing the application process for a desired housing program.

C. The client was accompanied to begin the application process for a desired housing program.

D. The client has refused to complete the application process for housing, and his/her resistance was processed.

12. Refer to a Physician (12)

A. The client was referred to a physician for an evaluation for a prescription of psychotropic medications.

B. The client was reinforced for following through on a referral to a physician for an assessment for a prescription of psychotropic medications, but none were prescribed.

C. The client has been prescribed psychotropic medications.

D. The client declined evaluation by a physician for a prescription of psychotropic medications and was redirected to cooperate with this referral.

13. Educate about and Monitor Psychotropic Medications (13)

A. The client was taught about the indications for and the expected benefits of psychotropic medications.

B. As the client's psychotropic medications were reviewed, he/she displayed an understanding about the indications for and expected benefits of the medications.

C. The client displayed a lack of understanding of the indications for and expected benefits of psychotropic medications and was provided with additional information and feedback regarding his/her medications.

D. The client was monitored for compliance with his/her psychotropic medication regimen.

E. The client was provided with positive feedback about his/her regular use of psychotropic medications.

F. The client was monitored for the effectiveness and side effects of his/her prescribed medications.

G. Concerns about the client's medication effectiveness and side effects were communicated to the physician.

14. Review Side Effects of Medications (14)

A. The possible side effects of the client's medications were reviewed with him/her.

B. The client identified significant medication side effects, and these were reported to the medical staff.

C. Possible side effects of the client's medication were reviewed, but he/she denied experiencing any side effects.

15. Store Medications (15)

A. The homeless client's medications were stored in a safe, easily accessible facility.

B. The client was assisted in making certain that his/her storage site for his/her medications was safe and easily accessible.

C. The client was reinforced for more regular use of his/her medications that have been stored safely.

D. The client has not used the safe, easily accessible storage facility for his/her medications and was redirected to do so.

16. Provide Smaller, Immediate Supplies of Medication (16)

A. The client was provided with smaller supplies of medications, as he/she has no site available to store them.

B. The client was reinforced for using smaller, immediate supplies of medications, which has contributed to his/her consistent use of them.

C. The client does not regularly come to obtain his/her smaller, immediate supplies of medications and was redirected to do so.

17. Rent a Secure Storage Space (17)

A. A secure storage space was rented for the client (e.g., locker or mailbox) in which he/she may store necessary medications.

B. The client was reinforced for regularly using a secure storage space to store his/her necessary medications.

C. The client does not use the secure storage space and was redirected to do so.

18. Assess for Safety (18)

A. The client was assessed for his/her level of safety to himself/herself and to others regarding his/her readiness for independent living.

B. The client was provided with feedback regarding his/her level of safety relative to his/her readiness for independent living.

C. The client was provided with remedial assistance to assist in making him/her safer regarding his/her independent housing options.

D. The client refused to accept that his/her safety was in jeopardy and was confronted with additional concerns.

19. Refer for an Intellectual Assessment (19)

A. The client was referred for an assessment of cognitive abilities and deficits.

B. The client received objective psychological testing to assess his/her cognitive strengths and weaknesses.

C. The client cooperated with the psychological testing, and feedback about the results was given to him/her.

D. The psychological testing confirmed the presence of specific cognitive abilities and deficits.

E. The client was not compliant with taking the psychological evaluation and was encouraged to participate completely.

20. Coordinate a Physical Evaluation (20)

A. The client was referred for a complete physical evaluation by a medical professional that is knowledgeable in both physical health and mental illness concerns.

B. The client has completed his/her physical evaluation, and the results of this evaluation were processed.

C. The client has not submitted to a physical evaluation and was redirected to do so.

21. Obtain Financial Entitlements and Subsidies (21)

A. The client was assisted in obtaining, completing, and filing forms for Social Security Disability benefits or other public aid.

B. The client has completed all necessary documentation for filing for Social Security Disability benefits or other public aid, and this material was reviewed.

C. The client's application for Social Security Disability benefits and other public aid was incomplete, and he/she received assistance in completing these applications.

D. The client was assisted in applying for subsidies for housing that are available for mentally ill individuals.

E. The client has appropriately applied for specific subsidies for mentally ill individuals in need of housing and was reinforced for this follow-through.

F. The client has been able to obtain subsidies to assist with his/her payment for housing, and the implications of this progress were processed.

G. The client has not pursued available subsidies for housing for mentally ill individuals and was redirected to do so.

22. Encourage or Assist with Regular Employment (22)

A. The client was encouraged to obtain regular employment to increase income and defray housing costs.

B. The client was assisted in seeking and obtaining regular employment.

C. The client has found regular employment, and the economic benefits for his/her employment were reviewed.

D. The client has not obtained regular employment; he/she continues to struggle with his/her income level and was redirected in this area.

23. Develop a Budget (23)

A. The client was requested to develop a basic budget, including income, necessary expenses, additional spending, and savings plans.

B. The client has developed a basic budget, and this material was reviewed.

C. The client was given positive feedback for his/her comprehensive, realistic budget.

D. The client has not developed a basic budget and was redirected to do so.

24. Assist in Obtaining a Bank Account (24)

A. The client was assisted in obtaining a low-interest, no-fee bank account with a participating bank.

B. The waiving of basic fees was coordinated with the participating bank to assist the client in stabilizing his/her financial concerns.

C. The client has refused to use a bank account and was redirected in this area.

25. Obtain Emergency Funds (25)

A. Emergency funds were obtained for payment of the client's rent, mortgage, or utilities in order to prevent eviction.

B. The client was directed as to how to seek out emergency funds for payment of rent, mortgage, or utilities to prevent eviction.

C. The client has assertively accessed emergency funds for payment of rent, mortgage, or utilities, which has helped him/her to prevent eviction, and this was reviewed with him/her.

D. The client has failed to follow through on obtaining emergency funds that support housing expenses, and he/she was again encouraged to do so.

26. Plan Discharge Housing Early in Inpatient Hospitalization (26)

A. The discharge-planning coordinator of the client's current inpatient psychiatric setting was contacted to coordinate discharge planning regarding housing.

B. Although the client has recently been psychiatrically hospitalized and is not ready to be discharged, his/her housing upon discharge has been strongly emphasized and is being coordinated.

C. Although the client remains in an inpatient psychiatric setting, arrangements for his/her housing have been made, and the housing is waiting for him/her upon discharge.

D. Efforts to coordinate housing for the client upon discharge from the inpatient psychiatric setting have not resulted in a specific discharge plan, and these plans continue to be developed.

27. Develop Housing Plans for After Incarceration (27)

A. While the client has been incarcerated, regular meetings have occurred to develop housing plans for him/her subsequent to his/her release from incarceration.

B. A specific plan was developed for the client to have stable housing subsequent to his/her release from incarceration.

C. The client has not developed a housing plan for his/her release from incarceration and was redirected to focus on this area and ask for assistance as needed.

28. Coordinate Visits to a Less Restrictive Setting (28)

A. As the client is planning a move to a new, less restrictive setting, he/she was provided with ample visits to the new setting.

B. The client's questions regarding his/her new, less restrictive setting were answered, and he/she was provided with ongoing reassurance.

C. The client was supported as he/she has become more comfortable with the use of the new, less restrictive setting.

D. The client continues to feel uncertain about the new, less restrictive setting, despite ample visitation, and was provided with additional support.

29. Refer for Substance Abuse Treatment (29)

A. The client was referred to a 12-step recovery program (e.g., Alcoholics Anonymous or Narcotics Anonymous).

B. The client was referred to a substance abuse treatment program.

C. The client has been admitted to a substance abuse treatment program and was supported for this follow-through.

D. The client has refused the referral to a substance abuse treatment program, and this refusal was processed.

30. Refer to a Drug-Free Housing Program (30)

A. The client was referred to a drug-free housing program.

B. The client reports that he/she has been more able to remain substance-free through the use of a residence in a drug-free housing program, and he/she was provided with positive feedback for this progress.

C. As the client has continued to use mind-altering substances, his/her residence has not been as stable, and this was processed.

31. Coordinate Mental Health and Substance Abuse Treatment (31)

A. The client's mental health and substance abuse services were coordinated within his/her residential setting.

B. The client was reinforced for participating more fully in both the mental health and substance abuse services provided within his/her residential setting.

C. The client has terminated the substance abuse that has interfered in maintaining his/her residence and was provided with positive feedback for this progress.

D. The client has continued to use substances, despite the use of coordinated mental health and substance abuse services.

32. Encourage the Family and Friends to Support, Teach, and Monitor (32)

A. The client's family members and friends were encouraged to support, teach, and monitor him/her regarding his/her progress with basic living needs, medication administration, and financial management.

B. Family members were provided with positive feedback for their support, teaching, and monitoring of the client.

C. Despite extensive support from the client's support network, he/she continues to experience significant concerns related to his/her basic living needs, medication administration, and financial management and was given further feedback in these areas.

33. Refer to a Support Group (33)

A. The client was referred to a support group for individuals with severe and persistent mental illness.

B. The client has attended the support group for individuals with severe and persistent mental illness, and the benefits of this support group were reviewed.

C. The client reported that he/she has not experienced any positive benefit from the use of a support group but was encouraged to continue to attend.

D. The client has not used the support group for individuals with severe and persistent mental illness and was redirected to do so.

34. Match with a Mentor (34)

A. The client agreed to be matched with a mentor who has already successfully moved from homelessness to a stable living environment.

B. A specific mentor was coordinated for the client to provide him/her with feedback about how to successfully move from homelessness to a stable living environment.

C. The client's contact with his/her mentor was processed, and he/she described that this contact was helpful in providing insight into moving from homelessness to a stable living environment.

D. The client has not regularly met with his/her housing mentor and was redirected to do so.

35. Teach Housekeeping Skills (35)

A. The client was taught about basic housekeeping skills.

B. Sources such as *Mary Ellen's Complete Home Reference Book* by Pinkham and Burg or *The Cleaning Encyclopedia: Your A–Z Illustrated Guide to Cleaning Like the Pros* by Aslett were used to teach the client specific housekeeping skills.

C. The client was provided with positive feedback about his/her increased understanding of basic housekeeping skills.

D. The client's use of basic housekeeping skills has noticeably improved, and he/she was provided with support for this.

E. The client has not improved his/her basic housekeeping skills and was provided with additional feedback in this area.

36. Refer for Training (36)

A. The client was referred to a structured program to obtain hands-on training in basic skills for transitioning to more independent care.

B. The client was taught many of the basic skills needed for transitioning to more independent care.

C. The client has failed to learn the basic skills needed for transitioning to more independent care and was provided with additional remedial training in this area.

37. Obtain Homemaker Assistance (37)

A. The client was offered the use of homemaker assistance because he/she is not capable of doing basic housekeeping activities.

B. The client was assisted in applying for homemaker assistance because he/she is not capable of performing basic housekeeping activities.

C. The client has been provided with homemaker assistance.

D. The client's overall ability to maintain an independent home or apartment has improved through the use of a visiting homemaker.

38. Meet with the Housing Manager (38)

A. A meeting was held with the client's housing manager to provide education about mental illness issues and the client's rights, to mitigate his/her problematic behaviors, and to assist in rent reviews and dwelling inspections.

B. Regular meetings continue to be held with the client's housing manager to train about mental illness issues and the client's rights, to mitigate his/her problematic behaviors, and to assist in rent reviews and dwelling inspections.

C. The client's increased level of communication with his/her housing manager has helped to avert crises that could have threatened his/her residential status, and he/she was directed to continue this pattern of communication.

D. The client's housing manager was provided with 24-hour access to the clinician or agency staff should emergencies arise.

E. The client's housing manager was urged to contact the clinician or agency staff with questions or crisis concerns.

F. The client's potential decompensation has been arrested through the use of immediate contact with his/her housing manager, and this was reflected to the manager and the client.

39. Provide Emergency Health Information Card (39)

A. The client was provided with an emergency health information card, which includes individualized information about whom to call in a crisis situation, including the case manager and physicians.

B. The client was reinforced for using the emergency health information card to help avert crisis situations.

C. The client has failed to use the emergency health information card when experiencing a crisis and was reminded about this resource.

40. Coordinate Funds to Maintain Residence during Decompensation (40)

A. Funds were coordinated to maintain the client's residence during times when he/she would be unable to obtain resources for paying his/her bills (e.g., hospitalization or when he/she briefly loses eligibility for benefits).

B. The client has been able to maintain stability, as he/she has been able to keep his/her regular residence even during periods of brief decompensation, and this was reviewed with him/her.

41. Provide Training Regarding Rights (41)

A. The client was provided with training about his/her rights as related to the Americans with Disabilities Act, including reasonable accommodations that must be made for him/her.

B. The client was reinforced for displaying an understanding of his/her rights and the reasonable accommodations that must be made for him/her.

C. The client displayed a poor understanding of his/her rights and reasonable accommodations and was provided with additional education and guidance in this area.

42. Educate about Tenant's Rights (42)

A. The client was educated about tenant's rights.

B. The client was referred to information about tenant's rights described in *Renter's Rights* by Portman and Stewart.

C. The client displayed increased understanding about tenant's rights and was urged to assert these with his/her landlord.

D. The client was provided with positive feedback regarding his/her assertion of tenant's rights to maintain a more regular and stable living environment.

E. The client has failed to assert his/her rights as a tenant and was provided with additional encouragement to do so.

43. Coordinate Legal Assistance (43)

A. Contact with legal assistance programs was coordinated due to the client's rights continuing to be violated.

B. Legal assistance has been provided to the client to assist in enforcing his/her basic rights and needed accommodations.

C. Legal assistance programs have declined to assist the client, and further advocacy was provided.

INDEPENDENT ACTIVITIES OF DAILY LIVING (IADL)

CLIENT PRESENTATION

1. Lack of Access to IADLs (1)*

A. The client has had limited access to IADLs (e.g., transportation, banking, shopping, or use of community services).

B. The client has often been barred from using IADLs due to his/her mental illness.

C. The client has begun to access IADLs.

D. The client displays an increased pattern of independence through engaging in IADLs.

2. Lack of Experience with IADLs (1)

A. The client described a pattern of inexperience with IADLs (e.g., transportation, banking, shopping, or use of community services).

B. The client has often relied on others for IADLs.

C. The client reports increased experience with IADLs.

D. The client displays more independence as he/she gains experience with IADLs.

3. Poor Functioning on IADLs (1)

A. The client described poor functioning on IADLs, despite his/her regular access to and experience with areas such as transportation, banking, shopping, or use of community services.

B. As the client's severe and persistent mental illness symptoms have stabilized, he/she has improved his/her functioning relative to IADLs.

C. The client regularly takes care of his/her own IADLs in a functional manner.

4. Anxiety Regarding Increasing IADLs (2)

A. The client described feelings of anxiety regarding becoming more independent.

B. The client reported feelings of uncertainty and fear regarding specific areas of IADLs.

C. The client is avoidant of areas in which he/she could increase his/her IADLs.

D. The client has become more confident regarding performing his/her IADLs.

5. Lack of Community Resource Knowledge (3)

A. The client has limited information regarding available community resources.

B. The client often fails to use community resources due to his/her ignorance in this area.

C. As the client has gained increased knowledge of community resources, he/she has increased his/her independence.

6. Poor Emergency Response (4)

A. The client has failed to respond appropriately in emergency situations.

---

* The numbers in parentheses correlate to the number of the Behavioral Definition statement in the companion chapter with the same title in *The Severe and Persistent Mental Illness Treatment Planner,* 2nd ed. (Berghuis and Jongsma) by John Wiley & Sons, 2008.

B. The client displayed a lack of knowledge about emergency services, their function, or how to access them.

C. The client's severe and persistent mental illness symptoms have affected his/her ability to respond appropriately to emergency situations.

D. As the client has stabilized his/her severe and persistent mental illness symptoms, he/she has learned more about appropriate emergency responses.

E. The client has appropriately used emergency resources.

7. Symptoms Affect Independent Use of Community Resources (5)

A. Experiences of severe and persistent mental illness symptoms have affected the client's ability to use community resources independently.

B. As the client has stabilized his/her severe and persistent mental illness symptoms, his/her ability to use community resources has increased.

C. The client reports that he/she is regularly using community resources on an independent basis.

8. Unfamiliarity with Services (6)

A. The client described that he/she has not had experience with resources such as banking, stores, and other services.

B. The client has increased his/her familiarity with resources such as banking, stores, and other services.

C. The client displays independent functioning regarding the use of banking, stores, and other services.

9. Poor Organization (7)

A. The client reported a pattern of poor attention to and organization of personal responsibilities.

B. The client has displayed poor attention to and organization of personal responsibilities, as evidenced by unpaid bills and unkept appointments.

C. As the client has become more organized, he/she has regularly met his/her personal responsibilities (e.g., paying bills and keeping appointments).

10. Limited Access of Community Resources (8)

A. The client has failed to access community resources such as worship centers, libraries, recreational areas, or businesses.

B. The client's failure to access community resources has resulted in his/her decreased involvement within the community.

C. As the client's severe and persistent mental illness symptoms have stabilized, he/she has increased his/her access to community resources.

D. The client regularly uses community resources such as worship centers, libraries, recreational areas, or businesses.

11. Restricted from Community Resources (9)

A. The client's access to community resources has been restricted due to his/her bizarre behaviors.

B. The client has been banned from using specific community resources due to his/her history of bizarre behavior related to his/her severe and persistent mental illness symptoms.

C. As the client's severe and persistent mental illness symptoms have improved, his/her behavior has been more stable.

D. The client has gained access to previously restricted community resources due to his/her regular pattern of stability.

12. Others Take Responsibility for IADLs (10)

A. The client described a history of allowing others to take responsibility for performing IADLs for him/her.

B. The client's family members were noted to have been taking responsibility for performing his/her IADLs.

C. As the client has stabilized his/her severe and persistent mental illness symptoms, he/she has been able to take increased responsibility for performing IADLs.

D. The client's family members have ceased taking inappropriate responsibility for performing his/her IADLs.

INTERVENTIONS IMPLEMENTED

1. Assign an Inventory of IADLs (1)*

A. The client was asked to prepare an inventory of positive and negative functioning regarding his/her IADLs.

B. The client prepared his/her inventory of positive and negative functioning regarding IADLs, and this inventory was reviewed.

C. The client was given positive feedback regarding his/her accurate inventory of positive and negative functioning regarding IADLs.

D. The client has prepared his/her inventory of positive and negative functioning regarding IADLs but needed assistance to develop a more accurate assessment.

E. The client has not prepared an inventory of positive and negative functioning regarding IADLs and was redirected to do so.

2. Examine Problematic IADL Areas (2)

A. The client's problematic IADL areas were examined with him/her.

B. Specific patterns of behavior and thought that contribute to the client's failure at independent functioning were identified.

C. The client described increased understanding of his/her problematic behaviors and cognitions subsequent to reviewing his/her problematic IADL areas.

D. The client has no insight as to failures regarding IADLs or the causes for those failures; additional realistic feedback was provided.

3. Obtain Feedback from a Support Network (3)

A. A proper authorization to release confidential information was obtained in order to review IADLs with the client's support network.

---

* The numbers in parentheses correlate to the number of the Therapeutic Intervention statement in the companion chapter with the same title in *The Severe and Persistent Mental Illness Treatment Planner,* 2nd ed. (Berghuis and Jongsma) by John Wiley & Sons, 2008.

B. Specific feedback was obtained from the client's family members, friends, and caregivers about his/her performance of IADLs.

C. The client's support network's feedback about his/her performance of IADLs was reviewed with the client.

D. The client displayed increased understanding of IADL issues subsequent to reviewing feedback from the support network.

E. The client rejected the IADL feedback provided by his/her support network and was urged to consider this important information.

4. Identify Needed IADLs (4)

A. The client was assisted in identifying those IADLs that are desired but are not present in his/her current repertoire.

B. The client received feedback regarding his/her description of IADLs that he/she wishes to increase.

C. The client was unable to identify specific IADLs that he/she wishes to increase and was assisted in reviewing this area.

5. Refer for Psychological Testing (5)

A. The client was referred for an assessment of cognitive abilities and deficits.

B. The client underwent objective psychological testing to assess his/her cognitive strengths and weaknesses.

C. The client cooperated with the psychological testing, and feedback about the results was given to him/her.

D. The psychological testing confirmed the presence of specific cognitive abilities and deficits.

E. The client has not complied with taking the psychological evaluation and was encouraged to participate completely.

6. Recommend Remediating Programs (6)

A. The client was referred to remedial programs that are focused on removing deficits for performing IADLs, including skill-building groups, token economies, and behavior-shaping programs.

B. The client was assisted in remediating his/her deficits for performing IADLs through the use of skill-building groups, token economies, and behavior-shaping programs.

C. As specific programs have assisted the client in removing deficits for performing IADLs, his/her activities of daily living (ADLs) have gradually increased.

D. The client has not complied with the referral to skill-building groups and was again encouraged to do so.

7. Explore Social Anxiety (7)

A. The client's experience of social anxiety related to increased independence and social contacts was explored.

B. The client was provided with support and empathy as he/she described his/her experience of anxiety.

C. The client denied any anxiety related to increased independence, and this was noted.

8. Teach and Reinforce Social Skills (8)

A. The client was taught some skills that are necessary for appropriate social behavior.

B. The client was provided with feedback regarding his/her use of social skills.

C. As the client has developed more appropriate social skills, his/her social interaction has been more appropriate, and he/she was provided with positive feedback about this progress.

D. The client was confronted about not learning appropriate social skills, and not increasing the frequency and appropriateness of his/her social interactions.

9. Develop IADL Completion Schedule (9)

A. The client was assisted in developing a specific schedule for completing IADLs (e.g., arranging finances on Monday mornings or going to the grocery store on Tuesday).

B. The client has developed his/her own schedule for completing IADLs, and this schedule was reviewed.

C. The client's use of scheduling IADLs has helped him/her complete these on a regular basis, and he/she was provided with positive feedback for this follow-through.

D. The client was taught about situations in which he/she should break from his/her established routine.

E. The client acknowledged specific situations in which he/she should break from his/her established routine (e.g., do the banking on a different day due to a holiday or do the weekly cleaning one day earlier to attend a desired social function) and was provided with support for this flexible approach.

F. The client has not used his/her schedule for completing IADLs and was redirected to do so.

10. Educate about Mental Illness (10)

A. The client was educated about the expected or common symptoms of his/her mental illness, which may negatively impact IADL functioning.

B. As the client's symptoms of mental illness were discussed, he/she displayed an understanding of how these symptoms may affect his/her IADL functioning.

C. The client struggled to identify how symptoms of his/her mental illness may negatively impact IADL functioning and was given additional feedback in this area.

11. Interpret Psychiatric Decompensation (11)

A. The client's poor performance on IADLs was interpreted as an indicator of psychiatric decompensation.

B. The client's pattern of poor IADLs and psychiatric decompensation was shared with him/her, along with caregivers and medical staff.

C. The client acknowledged his/her poor performance on IADLs as prodromals of his/her psychiatric decompensation, and this was supported.

D. The client, caregivers, and medical staff concurred regarding his/her general psychiatric decompensation.

E. The client denied psychiatric decompensation, despite being told that his/her poor performance on IADLs is an indication of psychiatric decompensation.

12. Refer to a Physician (12)

A. The client was referred to a physician for an evaluation for a prescription of psychotropic medications.

B. The client was reinforced for following through on a referral to a physician for an assessment for a prescription of psychotropic medications, but none were prescribed.

C. The client has been prescribed psychotropic medications.

D. The client declined evaluation by a physician for a prescription of psychotropic medications and was redirected to cooperate with this referral.

13. Educate about Psychotropic Medications (13)

A. The client was taught about the indications for and the expected benefits of psychotropic medications.

B. As the client's psychotropic medications were reviewed, he/she displayed an understanding about the indications for and expected benefits of the medications.

C. The client displayed a lack of understanding of the indications for and expected benefits of psychotropic medications and was provided with additional information and feedback regarding his/her medications.

14. Monitor Medications (14)

A. The client was monitored for compliance with his/her psychotropic medication regimen.

B. The client was provided with positive feedback about his/her regular use of psychotropic medications.

C. The client was monitored for the effectiveness and side effects of his/her prescribed medications.

D. Concerns about the client's medication effectiveness and side effects were communicated to the physician.

E. Although the client was monitored for medication side effects, he/she reported no concerns in this area.

15. Review/Model Procurement of Medications (15)

A. Protocol for procuring the client's medications was reviewed with him/her.

B. The procurement of the client's medication was modeled to him/her.

C. The client was shadowed for support as he/she procured his/her own medications.

D. The client does not appropriately and regularly procure his/her own medications and was provided with additional training in this area.

16. Develop Agreement Regarding Monitoring of Medications (16)

A. An agreement was developed with the client regarding the level of responsibility and independence that he/she must display to trigger a decrease in the clinician's monitoring of medications.

B. The closeness with which the clinician monitors the client's medications has been decreased as he/she has displayed increased responsibility and independence.

C. The client's medications continue to be closely monitored as he/she has failed to display the needed level of responsibility and independence.

17. Coordinate an Agreement with the Pharmacist (17)

A. An agreement was coordinated between the client, the pharmacist, and the clinician regarding circumstances that would trigger a transfer of medication monitoring back to the clinician.

B. The client was supported for his/her understanding of circumstances in which the pharmacist would contact the clinician (e.g., failure to pick up the monthly prescription or trying to refill the prescription too soon).

C. The client was provided with positive feedback regarding his/her appropriate use of the pharmacy to obtain medications.

D. As the client has failed to appropriately use the pharmacy to obtain his/her medications, his/her medication usage has been more closely monitored.

18. Brainstorm Transportation Resources (18)

A. The client was assisted in brainstorming possible transportation resources available for his/her use.

B. Specific transportation resources (e.g., public transportation, personal vehicle, agency resources, friends and family, walking, or bicycling) were identified.

C. The client was encouraged to independently use available transportation resources.

D. The client was verbally reinforced for his/her independent use of transportation resources.

E. The client continues to be uncertain about what type of transportation resources to use and was provided with additional feedback in this area.

19. Teach about Public Transportation Options (19)

A. The client was taught about available public transportation options by discussing these options and reviewing written schedules.

B. The client was accompanied on the use of community transportation services, which has helped to teach him/her the safe, socially appropriate use of public transportation.

C. The typical expectations for using public transportation were reviewed, including paying for the transportation, time schedules, and social norms for behavior.

D. The client was praised for his/her understanding of typical expectations for using public transportation.

E. The client has displayed appropriate adherence to social and other expectations while using public transportation and received positive feedback for this.

F. The client has failed to understand the typical expectations for using public transportation and was given further education in this area.

G. The client declined to be accompanied on his/her use of public transportation services, and this choice was accepted.

20. Predict Severe and Persistent Mental Illness Influences and Brainstorm Remedial Techniques (20)

A. The client's pattern of severe and persistent mental illness symptoms was reviewed.

B. Possible influences of the client's severe and persistent mental illness symptoms on his/her ability to use community services were predicted.

C. The client was supported as he/she realistically identified the effects of his/her severe and persistent mental illness symptoms on his/her ability to use community services.

D. The client was assisted in brainstorming techniques to decrease the effects of his/her severe and persistent mental illness symptoms (e.g., relaxation techniques, escape/avoidance plans, and graduated steps to independence).

E. The client was realistic in his/her identification of techniques to decrease the effects of his/her severe and persistent mental illness symptoms on his/her ability to use community services and was provided with encouragement in this area.

F. The client was in a state of denial regarding his/her severe and persistent mental illness symptoms and their effect on his/her ability to use community services and was redirected in this area.

21. Ride Along on Public Transportation (21)

A. The client was accompanied on public transportation to a variety of destinations.

B. The client has identified that he/she is more comfortable with using public transportation without accompaniment and was provided with positive feedback about this.

22. Develop and Budget Income Sources (22)

A. The client was assisted in obtaining, completing, and filing forms for Social Security Disability benefits or other public aid.

B. The client was assisted in identifying ways to increase income through obtaining employment.

C. The client has obtained regular income and is now able to afford the use of resources within the community, and he/she was provided with positive feedback for this progress.

D. The client has not developed any regular sources of income and was redirected to do so.

E. The client was requested to develop a basic budget, including income, necessary expenses, additional spending, and savings plans.

F. The client was given positive feedback for his/her comprehensive, realistic budget.

G. The client has not developed a basic budget and was redirected to do so.

23. Review Banking Pros and Cons (23)

A. The advantage of using the banking system to assist with IADLs was reviewed with the client, including increased security, financial organization, and convenience for paying bills.

B. The client was cautioned about the hazards related to banking (e.g., credit debt, overdrawn checking account charges).

C. The procedures used within the banking system were reviewed.

D. The client was reinforced for his/her verbalization of an increased understanding of the issues related to using a banking system for IADLs.

E. The client displayed a poor understanding of the use of the banking system to assist with IADLs and was provided with further information in this area.

24. Coordinate a Helping Relationship with Bank Staff (24)

A. A helping relationship was coordinated between the client and specific members of the banking staff.

B. Permission to release information to the bank staff was obtained.

C. The staff of the bank was informed about the client's needs and disabilities.

D. The client reported feeling more comfortable through the use of a helpful relationship with specific bank staff, and this experience was processed.

25. Encourage the Use of a Specific Employee at Bank (25)

A. The client was encouraged to select and use a specific staff member at a specific bank branch in order to develop a more personal and understanding relationship.

B. The client has regularly sought out a specific employee at the bank, and this was noted to be helping the client feel more comfortable and to know what to expect in the interaction.

C. The client continues to approach his/her use of the banking system in a rather haphazard manner, and he/she was provided with redirection in this approach.

26. Coordinate a Notification Agreement (26)

A. An agreement was coordinated between the client, a specified bank staff member, and the clinician regarding the circumstances under which the clinician should be notified of an irregularity.

B. Specific situations were identified within an agreement with the banking staff about when to notify the clinician, such as a manic attempt by the client to withdraw his/her entire savings account.

C. The client has agreed to allow the bank staff to contact the clinician under certain circumstances.

D. The client has declined the use of an agreement between himself/herself, a specified bank staff member, and the clinician regarding when the clinician should be notified, and this was accepted.

27. Familiarize with Commercial Resources (27)

A. The client was familiarized with commercial resources that are available in his/her area through a review of newspaper advertisements and a tour of the business districts within the community.

B. The client was provided with positive feedback regarding his/her understanding about the commercial resources available in his/her area.

C. The client continues to have a poor understanding of the commercial resources available in his/her area and was provided with additional information about this topic.

28. Role-Play Shopping Situations (28)

A. Role-playing was used to teach the client how to handle commonly occurring shopping situations.

B. The client was assisted in role-playing specific shopping situations (e.g., asking for assistance, declining a pushy salesperson, or returning a defective item).

C. The client was provided with feedback about his/her functioning in commonly occurring shopping situations.

D. The client has not been able to increase his/her understanding of the needed response in typical shopping situations and was provided with additional information in this area.

29. Accompany to Local Businesses (29)

A. The client was accompanied on visits to local businesses where he/she has felt anxious or unsure.

B. The client has identified that he/she is now more comfortable with using area businesses without accompaniment and was reinforced for this progress.

30. Support Assertiveness and Advocate Regarding Discrimination (30)

A. The client was provided with support and feedback as he/she identified instances in which he/she was discriminated against due to his/her mental illness symptoms.

B. The client was taught assertive steps to respond to discrimination due to his/her mental illness symptoms.

C. The client was supported as he/she implemented assertive responses to instances of discrimination due to his/her mental illness symptoms.

D. Further education and encouragement were provided to the client, as he/she has not used assertive responses to the situations in which he/she has been discriminated against due to his/her mental illness symptoms.

E. The client was provided with support as he/she identified area businesses or service providers who have restricted access to him/her due to concerns over his/her mental illness symptoms.

F. Advocacy was provided on the client's behalf with area businesses or service providers who have restricted his/her access due to his/her mental illness symptoms.

31. Link to Advocacy and Support Groups (31)

A. The client was referred to an advocacy group that will directly assist him/her in developing open access to community businesses and services.

B. The client was reinforced for attending a support group focused on assisting him/her in developing more open access to community businesses and services.

C. The client's greater access to community businesses and services was processed.

D. The client has not taken advantage of support and advocacy groups to develop greater access to community businesses and services and was provided with encouragement to do so.

32. Explore Contacts with Emergency Response Professionals (32)

A. The client's history of prior contacts with emergency response professionals was explored.

B. The client was assisted in identifying situations in which emergency response staff was required to coerce the client (e.g., a prior involuntary hospitalization).

C. The client was assisted in identifying situations in which he/she may have manipulated emergency response staff (e.g., threatened to harm himself/herself for some secondary gain such as obtaining food or a place to sleep).

D. The client was provided with positive feedback as he/she accurately reviewed his/her history of contact with emergency response professionals.

E. The client tended to deny his/her pattern of past involvement with emergency response professionals and was redirected to review these areas.

33. List Preferred Emergency Response Professionals (33)

A. The client was assisted in developing a list of specific emergency response professionals who respond effectively to mentally ill individuals (e.g., a police unit mental health liaison or a specific nurse/orderly at the emergency room).

B. The client was directed to seek out specific professionals when he/she contacts certain agencies or facilities.

C. Regular contact has been maintained with the identified professionals to facilitate greater understanding of the client's needs.

D. The client has not used the identified professionals and continues to misuse the emergency response system; he/she was redirected in this area.

34. Provide 24-Hour Crisis Consultation (34)

A. The area emergency response professionals were provided with 24-hour crisis consultation to assist in responding to the client's use of emergency systems.

B. Provision of the 24-hour crisis consultation has helped to decrease inappropriate use of the emergency response system and inappropriate response to the client by the emergency system.

35. Teach Appropriate Use of Emergency Services (35)

A. The client was taught about the appropriate use of specific emergency service professionals, including their responsibilities and limitations.

B. The client was provided with positive feedback for his/her accurate understanding of responsible use of emergency service professionals, their responsibilities, and limitations.

C. The client was assisted in brainstorming alternative resources that are available to him/her for use instead of nuisance calls to emergency response staff.

D. The client was assisted in developing specific alternatives to use instead of nuisance calls to emergency response staff (e.g., contact a crisis line rather than the police for psychotic symptom development; contact a support group member when feeling lonely instead of going to the emergency room; contact family first if feeling ill).

E. The client has decreased his/her pattern of nuisance calls to emergency response staff and was provided with positive feedback for this progress.

F. The client has not used alternative resources instead of nuisance calls to emergency response staff and was urged to modify this practice.

36. Discuss Making Amends (36)

A. The client was taught regarding the need for making amends to businesses or service providers who have been affected by his/her past inappropriate behavior.

B. The form of restitution to businesses, service providers, or others who have been affected by the client's past inappropriate behavior was brainstormed.

C. Specific areas of the restitution plan were reviewed (e.g., how to approach the business owner, what service could be offered in restitution, where the client would get the money to pay the business owner for debt).

D. The client has made amends to businesses or service providers who have been affected by his/her past inappropriate behavior, and he/she was provided with positive feedback in this area.

E. The client denied the need to make amends with businesses or service providers who have been affected by his/her past inappropriate behavior and was accepted for this position.

F. The client resisted endorsing a specific plan for how to implement restitution to those affected by his/her past inappropriate behavior and was provided with additional feedback in this area.

37. Develop a List of Resources for IADLs (37)

A. The client was asked to identify a list of personal resources that he/she can use for assistance in carrying out IADLs.

B. The client was assisted in identifying specific resources that he/she can use for carrying out IADLs (e.g., family and friends, support group members, neighbors).

C. The client has failed to identify a list of personal resources to assist him/her in carrying out IADLs and was urged to do so.

38. Role-Play Asking for Assistance (38)

A. Role-playing was used to help the client practice how to approach strangers for basic assistance (e.g., asking for directions).

B. Feedback was provided to the client about his/her approach, personal hygiene, and dress, plus how appearance and manner affect a stranger's comfort level.

C. The client displayed an understanding of the issues related to asking others for assistance and was praised for this insight.

D. The client displayed poor understanding of how his/her appearance and manner affect others' comfort level and was provided with additional feedback in this area.

39. Develop a Written Plan for Decompensation (39)

A. The client was assisted in developing a written plan for use when he/she is at risk of decompensation.

B. The client's written plan regarding decompensation includes telephone numbers of resources and how to obtain clinical assistance, and this was noted to be a rather comprehensive plan.

C. The client was praised for the development of his/her written plan for resources and assistance when he/she is at risk for decompensation.

D. The client was reinforced for his/her use of his/her plan when he/she feels to be at risk of decompensation.

E. The client has not used his/her written plan for early responding to decompensation and was reminded of how and when to use this resource.

40. Refer to an Activity Therapist (40)

A. The client was referred to an activity therapist for recommendations regarding physical fitness activities that are available in the community.

B. The client was referred to community physical fitness resources (e.g., health clubs and other recreational programs).

C. The client has been actively participating in community physical fitness programs and was reinforced for this.

D. The client has declined involvement in community physical fitness programs and was redirected to do so.

41. Assist in Identifying and Learning about Recreational Activities (41)

A. The client was assisted in identifying a variety of recreational activities in which he/she might be interested in participating.

B. The client was provided with educational material regarding his/her chosen activities.

C. The client displayed an increased understanding regarding how to access chosen activities as a result of reviewing the information provided to him/her.

D. The client has been reluctant to identify or learn about recreational activities and was redirected to do so.

42. Shadow at Recreational Activities (42)

A. As the client attended his/her chosen recreational activities, he/she was shadowed in order to provide support and direction.

B. To decrease stigma and increase independent functioning, the client was allowed to determine how closely the clinician was involved as he/she was shadowed at his/her selected activity.

C. The client has been able to increase his/her involvement and comfort level at his/her chosen activities because of the support and encouragement provided by the shadowing clinician.

D. The client declined to have the clinician shadow him/her at the chosen activities, and he/she was accepted for this position.

43. Coordinate a Mentor (43)

A. Contact between the client and another mentally ill individual who is further along in his/her recovery was coordinated in order to help the client process how others have achieved increased independence.

B. The client has followed up on his/her contact with another mentally ill individual who is further along in his/her recovery, and this contact was processed.

C. The client has not followed up on contact with another mentally ill individual in recovery and was redirected to do so.

44. Explore Spiritual Interests (44)

A. The client's interest in involvement with spiritual activities was explored.

B. The client was accepted for his/her identified interest in spiritual activities.

C. The potential for the client to experience confusion regarding spiritual messages and imagery due to his/her severe and persistent mental illness symptoms was acknowledged.

D. The client was assisted in differentiating between spiritual concerns and symptoms of mental illness.

E. The client was provided with positive feedback regarding his/her ability to differentiate between legitimate spiritual concerns and his/her spiritually oriented hallucinations and delusions.

F. The client was provided with specific direction and feedback as he/she displayed difficulty understanding and accepting the difference between spiritual concerns and severe and persistent mental illness symptoms.

G. The client indicated no interest in spiritual activities and was accepted for this decision.

45. Coordinate Worship Attendance (45)

A. The client's attendance at his/her preferred place of worship was coordinated.

B. The client was accompanied to his/her preferred place of worship to assist in increasing his/her comfort level.

C. The client's attendance at his/her preferred place of worship was reviewed and processed.

INTIMATE RELATIONSHIP CONFLICTS

CLIENT PRESENTATION

1. Indifferent to Emotional Needs (1)*

A. The client displayed a pattern of indifference toward the emotional needs of his/her partner.

B. The client's partner has complained about the client's pattern of indifference toward the partner's emotional needs.

C. When the client's partner expresses emotional needs, the client becomes critical, frustrated, and overly reactive.

D. The client reported an increased focus on his/her partner's needs.

E. The client consistently takes notice of and considers the emotional needs of his/her partner.

2. Distrust Due to Paranoia (2)

A. The client described a pattern of consistent distrust of his/her partner.

B. The client offered no sufficient basis for his/her pattern of distrust of his/her partner.

C. The client's level of distrust toward his/her partner has diminished.

D. The client verbalized trust in his/her partner despite the previously held extreme distrust.

3. Relationship Stress (3)

A. The effects of the client's erratic behavior (e.g., legal problems, impulsive spending, inability to work) have led to increased levels of stress within the relationship.

B. The client's intimate relationship is at risk for dissolution due to the increased levels of stress relating to the effects of his/her erratic behavior.

C. Stress levels have decreased significantly for the client and his/her partner as the effects of the client's erratic behavior have decreased.

D. As the client's erratic behavior has decreased, his/her relationship with his/her partner has become significantly more stable.

4. Pattern of Discontinuation of Relationships (4)

A. The client described a pattern of repeated discontinuation of relationships due to personal deficiencies in problem solving, social skills, or assertion.

B. The client's current relationship is at risk of dissolution due to his/her personal deficiencies in problem solving, social skills, or assertion.

C. As the client has gained conflict resolution and social skills to help relationship problems, his/her relationship has become more stable.

5. Impulsive Sexual Involvement (5)

A. The client described a pattern of impulsive sexual involvement outside of the committed relationship.

---

* The numbers in parentheses correlate to the number of the Behavioral Definition statement in the companion chapter with the same title in *The Severe and Persistent Mental Illness Treatment Planner*, 2nd ed. (Berghuis and Jongsma) by John Wiley & Sons, 2008.

B. The client described a pattern of impulsive sexual involvement outside of the committed relationship and subsequent regret.

C. The client acknowledged that he/she has developed an unhealthy pattern of impulsive sexual involvement outside of the committed relationship.

D. The client has terminated his/her pattern of impulsive sexual involvement outside of the committed relationship.

6. Increased Spousal Discontent (6)

A. The client reported that his/her partner has identified increased discontent with the changes that have occurred in the relationship due to his/her severe and persistent mental illness symptoms.

B. The client's partner reported discontent with the changes in the relationship due to the client's severe and persistent mental illness symptoms.

C. As the client has stabilized his/her pattern of severe and persistent mental illness symptoms, he/she describes a more contented relationship with his/her partner.

7. Violence or Abuse between Partners (7)

A. The client reported incidents of verbal abuse that occur within the relationship.

B. The client described incidents of physical abuse that occur within the relationship.

C. The client has taken steps to remove himself/herself from the abusive relationship.

D. The client reported that the pattern of abusive behavior has been terminated.

INTERVENTIONS IMPLEMENTED

1. Explore Relationship History (1)*

A. The client's history of intimate relationships was explored.

B. The client was assisted in identifying the positive and negative outcomes of his/her history of intimate relationships.

C. The client was provided with positive feedback as he/she displayed insight into his/her pattern of intimate relationships.

D. The client failed to identify positive and negative outcomes related to his/her pattern of intimate relationships and was provided with additional feedback in this area.

2. Develop a Time line (2)

A. A graphic time line display was used to help the client chart his/her pattern of intimate relationship conflicts.

B. The client was assisted in identifying his/her precursors, triggers, intimate relationship conflicts, and outcomes on a time line to review how he/she experiences and is affected by the relationship conflicts.

C. The client displayed a greater understanding of his/her pattern of intimate relationship conflicts and was given support and positive feedback for this insight.

---

* The numbers in parentheses correlate to the number of the Therapeutic Intervention statement in the companion chapter with the same title in *The Severe and Persistent Mental Illness Treatment Planner,* 2nd ed. (Berghuis and Jongsma) by John Wiley & Sons, 2008.

D. The client failed to understand his/her pattern of intimate relationship conflicts and was redirected in this area.

3. Obtain Family Feedback (3)

A. The client's partner was consulted about the history of their relationship conflicts.

B. The client's extended family was solicited for feedback about his/her history of relationship successes and problems.

C. The client's family members supplied feedback regarding their relationship conflicts; this was presented to the client.

D. Each partner has demonstrated a tendency to project blame onto the other for his/her conflicts, and this was reflected to him/her.

E. Although the client's partner was asked to provide perceptions regarding the relationship, no information was forthcoming.

F. The client was praised for his/her increased understanding of his/her pattern of relationship successes and problems.

G. The client was provided with additional feedback as he/she indicated poor understanding of his/her pattern of relationship successes and problems.

4. Identify Current Relationship Successes and Challenges (4)

A. The client was requested to identify the successes and challenges in his/her current relationship.

B. The client's pattern of successes and challenges in his/her current relationship was reviewed and processed.

C. The client failed to identify current successes and challenges in his/her relationship and was redirected to review this area more closely.

5. Assess Marital Satisfaction (5)

A. The administration of marital satisfaction surveys was coordinated for the client and his/her partner.

B. *The Marital Satisfaction Inventory* (Snyder) or *The Marital Status Inventory* (Weiss and Correto) was administered to the client and his/her partner.

C. The results of the marital satisfaction survey were shared with the client and his/her partner.

D. The marital satisfaction survey results indicated a significant degree of dissatisfaction on the part of the partners.

6. Educate about Mental Illness, Emphasizing Accurate Causes (6)

A. The client and his/her partner were taught about the expected or common symptoms of his/her mental illness that may negatively impact his/her intimate relationships.

B. The client and his/her partner were referred to specific books for further information about mental illness (e.g., *Schizophrenia: The Facts* by Tsuang and Faraone or *Bipolar Disorder: A Guide for Patients and Families* by Mondimore).

C. As the client's mental illness symptoms were discussed, he/she and his/her partner displayed an understanding of how these symptoms may affect their relationship.

D. Emphasis was placed on the fact that neither the family nor the partner are the cause of the client's mental illness.

E. The client, his/her partner, and his/her family were supported as they displayed an accurate understanding about the causes for his/her mental illness.

F. The client failed to identify how symptoms of his/her mental illness may negatively impact his/her intimate relationships and was given additional feedback in this area.

G. The client, his/her partner, and his/her family members continue to inappropriately place blame for the client's mental illness and were provided with additional feedback and information in this area.

7. Request Examples of Symptoms' Effects on Relationship (7)

A. The client and his/her partner were requested to identify at least two ways in which their relationship has been affected by the severe and persistent mental illness symptoms.

B. The client and his/her partner identified ways in which their relationship has been affected by the severe and persistent mental illness symptoms, and these effects were reviewed.

C. The client and his/her partner failed to identify ways in which their relationship has been affected by the severe and persistent mental illness symptoms and were encouraged to review this area more thoroughly.

8. Refer to a Physician (8)

A. The client was referred to a physician for an evaluation for a prescription of psychotropic medications.

B. The client was reinforced for following through on a referral to a physician for an assessment for a prescription of psychotropic medications, but none were prescribed.

C. The client has been prescribed psychotropic medications.

D. The client declined evaluation by a physician for a prescription of psychotropic medications and was redirected to cooperate with this referral.

9. Educate about Psychotropic Medications (9)

A. The client and his/her partner were taught about the indications for, the expected benefits of, and the possible side effects from psychotropic medications.

B. As the client's psychotropic medications were reviewed, he/she displayed an understanding about the indications for, expected benefits of, and possible side effects from the medications.

C. The client displayed a lack of understanding of the indications for, expected benefits of, and possible side effects from the psychotropic medications and was provided with additional information and feedback regarding his/her medications.

D. The client's partner was noted to display a clear understanding of the medication concerns.

E. The client's partner was noted to display a poor understanding of the medication concerns.

10. Monitor Medications (10)

A. The client was monitored for compliance with, effectiveness of, and side effects from his/her psychotropic medication regimen.

B. The client was provided with positive feedback about his/her regular use of psychotropic medications.

C. Concerns about the client's medication effectiveness and side effects were communicated to the physician.

D. Although the client was monitored for medication side effects, he/she reported no concerns in this area.

E. The client's partner provided feedback regarding the client's medication compliance and medication efficacy, which was used to help monitor his/her use of medications.

F. The client's partner refused to monitor the client's medication compliance and efficacy; this resistance was processed.

11. Coordinate Medication Agreement (11)

A. An agreement was coordinated between the client and his/her partner about the responsibility for administration and monitoring of the client's medications, including the circumstances under which control of medications will be returned to the client.

B. The client and his/her partner were reinforced for developing a helpful, supportive agreement to make certain that his/her medication is administered and monitored appropriately.

C. As a result of the client's agreement regarding the responsibility for administration and monitoring of his/her medications, he/she has been more regular in his/her use of medications and has stabilized psychiatrically; reinforcement was given for this progress.

D. Specific criteria (e.g., extended period of time in remission) were developed to identify when the client should be able to regain control of administration of his/her medications.

E. The client was reinforced for agreeing to specific plans for regaining control of his/her medications.

F. The client has declined to develop an agreement with his/her partner regarding the administration and monitoring of his/her medications, and additional redirection was given in this area.

12. Assign Reading Material for the Partner (12)

A. The client's partner was assigned to read books on coping with a loved one who has a severe and persistent mental illness.

B. The client's partner was referred to specific texts regarding coping with mental illness (e.g., *When Someone You Love Has a Mental Illness* by Woolis; *Surviving Schizophrenia: A Manual for Families, Consumers, and Providers* by Torrey; or *Bipolar Puzzle Solution: A Mental Health Client's Perspective* by Cort and Nelson).

C. The client's partner has read books on coping with a loved one who has severe and persistent mental illness symptoms, and this information was reviewed and processed.

D. The client's partner has not read books on coping with a loved one who has a mental illness and was redirected to review this information.

13. Teach the Partner Techniques for Managing the Client (13)

A. The client's partner was taught specific techniques to help manage the client when he/she is agitated, psychotic, or manic (e.g., maintaining a calm demeanor, providing basic directives, giving redirection).

B. The client's partner was supported for displaying an understanding of the specific techniques that were taught to help manage the client during agitation, psychosis, or mania.

C. The client's partner was provided with reinforcement for regular use of management techniques when the client is agitated, psychotic, or manic.

D. The client's partner has not used specific techniques to help manage the client when he/she is agitated, psychotic, or manic and was redirected to do so.

14. **Process Emotional Reaction (14)**

A. Emotional reactions from the client's partner due to the client's onset or recurrence of severe and persistent mental illness symptoms were processed.

B. The client's partner was assisted in expressing emotional reactions due to the onset or recurrence of the client's severe and persistent mental illness symptoms.

C. The client's partner refused to express feelings related to the client's illness and was urged to do so when comfortable with such disclosure.

15. **Reassure Accessibility (15)**

A. The client's partner was reassured about how accessible the clinician will be for consultation, questions, or support.

B. The client's partner has accessed the clinician for consultation, questions, or support.

C. The client's partner has not contacted the clinician for support or consultation and was again encouraged to do so.

D. The client's partner was provided with telephone numbers to access 24-hour crisis lines for professional assistance when the clinician is not available.

E. The client's partner was supported for using 24-hour crisis lines for professional assistance when the clinician is not available.

F. The client's partner has refused to use the 24-hour crisis lines and was again encouraged to do so.

16. **Emphasize Outside Interests (16)**

A. The client's partner and family members were urged to maintain interests outside of the mental illness concerns that the client may present.

B. The client's partner and family members have maintained interests outside of the mental illness concerns that the client may present and were provided with positive support for this activity.

C. The client's partner and family members have failed to maintain interests outside of the mental illness concerns that the client may present and were redirected to do so.

17. **Refer Partner to a Support Group (17)**

A. The client's partner was referred to a stress management or support group specifically designed for the family and friends of individuals with severe and persistent mental illness.

B. The client's partner has used the stress management and support groups and was reinforced for this.

C. The client's partner has not used the stress management or support groups and was redirected to do so.

18. **Clarify Emotions (18)**

A. The client was encouraged to share his/her emotions regarding the severe and persistent mental illness symptoms and how these affect the relationship.

B. The client has continued to share his/her feelings and has been assisted in identifying causes for them.

C. Distorted cognitive messages that contribute to the client's emotional response were identified.

D. The client demonstrated a sad affect and tearfulness as his/her emotions were reviewed.

E. As the client has been assisted in developing better coping mechanisms, he/she reports a decrease in his/her negative feelings related to his/her pattern of severe and persistent mental illness symptoms and their effect on the relationships.

F. The client's emotions continue to confuse him/her, and additional support and clarification were given.

19. Facilitate Conjoint Sessions (19)

A. Both partners were asked to commit themselves to a series of conjoint sessions to address issues of communication and problem solving.

B. Both partners were supported for agreeing to the conjoint sessions to work toward strengthening their relationship.

C. Both partners were assisted in clarifying their communication and expression of feelings within conjoint sessions.

D. Both partners have reported that they have increased the quality and frequency of communication with each other due to the conjoint sessions.

E. Both partners have not committed to regularly attending conjoint sessions and were redirected to commit themselves in this area.

20. Teach Healthy Communication Skills (20)

A. The client and his/her partner were taught healthy communication skills (e.g., expressing specific positive and negative emotions, making requests, communicating information clearly, giving "I" messages, and implementing active listening).

B. The client and his/her partner were reinforced for displaying increased understanding of the communication skills that were being taught.

C. The use of healthy communication skills by each partner was reviewed.

D. The client and his/her partner have failed to regularly use appropriate healthy communication skills, and they were redirected to use these types of skills.

21. Identify Mistrust Due to Mental Illness (21)

A. The client and his/her partner were focused on identifying trust issues that are attributable to mental illness symptoms.

B. The client and his/her partner were assisted in identifying how specific mental illness symptoms (e.g., paranoia or mania) have caused mistrust within the relationship.

C. The nonvolitional aspects of the client's mental illness symptoms were emphasized during the discussion of trust issues and mental illness symptoms.

D. The client and his/her partner have not been able to consistently identify trust issues as being attributable to mental illness symptoms and were provided with additional feedback in this area.

22. Explore Closeness Vulnerability (22)

A. Each partner's fears regarding getting too close and feeling vulnerable to hurt, rejection, and abandonment were explored.

B. The partners have clarified their own fears of getting too close to each other out of fear of being hurt and were accepted for this insight.

C. The partners were assisted in identifying experiences in their past that have contributed to their fear of closeness.

D. The partners denied fear of emotional vulnerability and were encouraged to reconsider their denial.

23. Generalize Increased Trust (23)

A. The client and his/her partner were requested to identify specific areas in which they have experienced increased trust.

B. The client and his/her partner were focused on ways in which they can generalize their experience of trust into other areas of their relationship.

C. The client and his/her partner were provided with positive feedback regarding their increased pattern of trust.

D. The client and his/her partner have struggled to generalize trust into other areas and were urged to continue to focus in this area.

24. Identify Relationship Changes Due to Mental Illness (24)

A. The client and his/her partner were requested to identify changes that have occurred in their relationship due to the client's pattern of mental illness symptoms.

B. The client and his/her partner were assisted in identifying the changes that have occurred in the relationship due to the client's mental illness symptoms.

C. The client and his/her partner were provided with positive feedback regarding their insight into the changes that have occurred in their relationship due to the client's mental illness symptoms.

D. The client and his/her partner could not identify changes that have occurred in the relationship due to the client's mental illness symptoms and were requested to review this area more closely.

25. Challenge the Couple to Share Power and Control (25)

A. The client and his/her partner were focused on the need to share power and control, despite the client's mental illness symptoms.

B. The client and his/her partner were challenged to identify specific ways in which power and control within the relationship can be shared, despite the client's mental illness symptoms.

C. The client and his/her partner were given suggestions about specific ways in which power and control can be shared, despite the client's mental illness symptoms (e.g., develop advanced directives regarding treatment expectations, returning responsibility to the mentally ill partner during periods of stabilization).

D. The client and his/her partner could not identify ways to share power and control within the relationship and were given additional feedback in this area.

26. Legitimize Mourning (26)

A. The client and his/her partner were provided with support regarding the legitimate need to mourn the loss of functioning within the relationship due to the client's severe and persistent mental illness symptoms.

B. The client and his/her partner used the support provided to express their grief regarding the loss of functioning in the relationship.

C. The client and his/her partner denied any grief regarding the loss of functioning in the relationship due to the client's severe and persistent mental illness symptoms, and they were given additional feedback regarding grieving.

27. Explore Substance Abuse (27)

A. The role of substance abuse was explored regarding its contribution to conflict within the relationship, as well as contributing to the client's severe and persistent mental illness symptoms.

B. Substance abuse by one of the partners was acknowledged as a strong contributing factor to escalating conflict between them.

C. Although substance abuse appears to be a critical component of relationship conflict, neither partner was willing to acknowledge the fact of substance abuse being a factor.

D. The client was confronted with his/her need for substance abuse treatment in addition to continued treatment for his/her severe and persistent mental illness.

28. Integrate Substance Abuse and Mental Health Treatment (28)

A. The client's mental health and substance abuse treatment were coordinated so they can be provided in an integrated manner.

B. Clinicians focusing primarily on the client's severe and persistent mental health treatment were urged to integrate his/her substance abuse treatment as well.

C. Treatment staff, focusing on the client's substance abuse treatment, were alerted to the need to also treat his/her severe and persistent mental illness.

29. Discuss Closeness versus Distance (29)

A. A discussion was facilitated between the client and his/her partner regarding the factors that contribute to a desire for closeness versus those that promote distance/safety.

B. The client and his/her partner were provided with assistance in identifying factors that contribute to a closeness or for distance/safety.

C. The need for a waiting period for the client's partner to regain trust was acknowledged as a normal expectation.

D. The client and his/her partner were provided with feedback regarding the partner's caution about resuming normal levels of trust, interaction, sexual activity, and so forth, subsequent to the client's symptoms abating.

E. The client was praised for his/her acceptance of his/her partner's need for caution prior to resuming normal closeness.

F. The client and his/her partner have argued over the level of closeness expected after the client's symptoms have abated and were provided with additional feedback in this area.

30. Emphasize the Sexual Relationship as a Mirror (30)

A. Emphasis was placed on the concept of the sexual relationship being a mirror of the rest of the relationship.

B. The need for positive emotional interaction prior to sexual involvement was emphasized.

C. The client was provided with positive reinforcement for his/her focus on positive emotional interaction with his/her intimate partner.

D. The client's partner reported that the client does not focus on positive emotional interaction, and the client was provided with additional education in this area.

31. Physician Evaluation Referral (31)

A. The couple was referred to a physician who specializes in sexual dysfunction to obtain an evaluation of any organic causes for their sexual problems.

B. The physician evaluation did not identify any organic basis for the couple's sexual dysfunction, and the implication of this finding was processed.

C. The medical problems identified by the physician as causes for the sexual dysfunction are being treated.

D. The client was urged to follow up on recommendations from his/her physician regarding treatment for sexual dysfunction (e.g., medications, specialty assessments, or lab work).

E. The client was provided with assistance for following up on the recommendations from the physician regarding sexual dysfunction treatment.

F. The client's treating psychiatrist has been informed about the client's sexual dysfunction concerns, physical exam, and follow-up needs.

G. The client has failed to comply with directives regarding physician assessment, treatment, and follow-up for sexual dysfunction and was redirected to do so.

32. Focus on Sexual Arousal Issues (32)

A. The client was focused on how his/her physical appearance and personal hygiene needs may affect his/her partner's sexual arousal.

B. The client was reinforced for displaying an understanding of the need for better personal hygiene and physical appearance as a way to increase sexual arousal for his/her partner.

C. The client was provided with positive reinforcement for his/her attempts to improve his/her physical appearance and personal hygiene needs.

D. The client has failed to improve his/her personal appearance and personal hygiene needs and was provided with additional direction in this area.

33. Assign Reading on Human Sexual Functioning (33)

A. The client and his/her intimate partner were assigned to read books on human sexual functioning.

B. The client and his/her imitate partner were referred to specific books (e.g., *The New Joy of Sex* by Comfort or *The Reader's Digest Guide to Love and Sex* by Roberts and Padgett-Yawn).

C. The client was referred to watch sexual education videos.

D. The client was referred to specific video programs (e.g., *Better Sex Videos* from the Sinclair Institute).

E. The client and his/her intimate partner have not sought out educational material regarding human sexual functioning and were redirected to do so.

34. Identify and Process a Pattern of Impulsive Sexual Activity (34)

A. The client was assisted in identifying his/her history of impulsive sexual acting out and how it has affected his/her intimate relationship.

B. The client was provided with positive feedback as he/she was realistic and truthful about his/her sexual acting out and the effect it has had on the relationship.

C. The client was in denial regarding his/her pattern of impulsive sexual acting out and was urged to provide a more complete review of this behavior pattern.

D. The client's partner was assisted in identifying feelings related to the client's history of infidelity.

E. The faithful partner was supported in expressing the hurt, disappointment, and anxiety that has resulted from the unfaithful partner's affairs.

F. The client was reinforced for displaying understanding regarding his/her partner's pain related to his/her history of infidelity.

G. The client tended to be quite rejecting of the partner's feelings generated by his/her history of infidelity and was redirected in this area.

35. Manage Impulsivity (35)

A. The client's impulsive behavior was repeatedly reviewed so as to help him/her identify this pattern and the negative consequences that result from it.

B. The negative consequences of the client's self-defeating and impulsive behavior was reviewed.

C. The client was given specific directives about how to manage his/her manic or impulsive behaviors.

D. The client has difficulty identifying his/her impulsive behaviors and was given additional feedback in this area

36. Develop Boundaries (36)

A. The client and his/her intimate partner were assisted in developing a clear set of boundaries for sexual, emotional, and social contact with others.

B. The client and his/her intimate partner were provided with feedback regarding the boundaries they have established for sexual, emotional, and social contact with others.

C. The client and his/her intimate partner have not developed a clear set of boundaries for sexual, emotional, and social contact with others and were redirected to do so.

37. Teach Anger Control Techniques (37)

A. The client was taught some specific anger control techniques.

B. The client and his/her partner were assisted in developing a clear verbal or behavioral signal to be used by either partner to terminate interaction immediately if either of them fears impending abuse.

C. Role-playing and modeling were used to teach how the conflict termination signal could be used in future disagreements between the client and his/her partner.

D. The client was provided with positive feedback as he/she displayed understanding regarding the anger techniques he/she has been taught.

E. The client and his/her partner were provided with positive reinforcement for their use of conflict termination signals.

F. The client has not used the anger control techniques and was redirected to do so.

38. Develop a Safety Plan (38)

A. The client's partner was assisted in developing a safety plan to help manage the client and maintain his/her own safety during periods when the client is emotionally and behaviorally unstable.

B. The client's partner was assisted in developing an understanding of when to contact public safety officials.

C. The client was informed about the safety plan to be implemented when he/she is not in control of his/her behavior.

D. The safety plan has been used, and its effectiveness was reviewed.

E. The safety plan has not been helpful toward containing the client's anger outbursts, and additional plans were developed in this area.

39. Identify Symptom Effects on Children (39)

A. The client and his/her partner were assisted in identifying how mental illness symptoms affect the children in the relationship.

B. The client and his/her partner identified specific effects of mental illness on the children in the relationship (e.g., confusion, embarrassment, or caretaking), and these were processed with the client.

C. The client and his/her partner failed to identify how mental illness symptoms affect the children in the relationship and were provided with general examples in this area.

40. Teach Effective Child Rearing Practices (40)

A. The client and his/her partner were taught effective child rearing practices.

B. The client and his/her partner were referred to specific resources to learn effective child rearing practices.

C. The client was reinforced for a decrease in family problems due to more consistent child rearing practices.

D. The client has not used consistent child rearing practices, continues to have problematic family relationships, and was provided with additional encouragement for change.

41. Develop a Parenting Agreement (41)

A. An agreement was facilitated between the client and his/her partner regarding acceptable parenting practices (e.g., discipline and rewards, or when the partner should become involved).

B. The client and his/her partner were reinforced for using the parenting agreement to become more consistent in their parenting choices.

C. The client and his/her partner have not adhered to their parenting agreement and were provided with feedback in this area.

42. Assist in Obtaining Income (42)

A. The client was assisted in obtaining employment.

B. The client was assisted in obtaining alternative sources of income (e.g., disability payments).

C. The client has obtained regular income and reported that this has helped to decrease some of the relationship conflicts he/she had experienced.

43. Refer to Credit Counseling (43)

A. The client and his/her intimate partner were referred to a credit counseling/budget assistance program.

B. The client and his/her partner were reinforced for following through with the use of budgeting assistance.

C. The client and his/her partner have not used the referral for budgeting counseling and were redirected to do so.

44. Encourage Expressing Emotions about Relationship Loss (44)

A. The client was encouraged to express his/her feelings regarding the loss of his/her relationship.

B. The client was provided with support, feedback, and empathy as he/she expressed his/her emotions regarding the loss of his/her relationship.

C. The client has not expressed his/her emotions regarding the loss of his/her relationship and was provided with additional support and encouragement in this area.

D. The client was assigned to read material regarding how to deal with grief that is associated with the loss of a relationship.

E. The client was assigned to read *How to Survive the Loss of a Love* by Colgrove, Bloomfield, and McWilliams.

F. The client has followed through on reading the assigned grief material associated with the breakup of a relationship, and this material was processed.

G. The client has not read the grief material regarding the loss of a relationship and was encouraged to do so.

45. Refer to a Divorce Support Group (45)

A. The client was referred to a support group for divorced or divorcing people to assist in resolving the loss and adjusting to a new life.

B. The client verbalized the feelings associated with grieving the loss of a relationship, and those feelings were processed.

C. The client was supported for participating in a divorce group where he/she has clarified and expressed his/her feelings associated with the loss of the relationship.

D. The client has not followed through on attending a support group for divorced people and was encouraged to do so.

LEGAL CONCERNS

CLIENT PRESENTATION

1. Illegal Behavior (1)*

A. The client has a long history of illegal behavior, including theft, assault, disorderly conduct, or threats to others.

B. The client described a pattern of engaging in illegal behavior without empathy for the effects of his/her behavior on others.

C. The client showed little remorse for his/her illegal activities.

D. As treatment has progressed, the client has decreased his/her pattern of illegal behavior.

2. Criminal Justice Involvement (2)

A. The client described a history of multiple arrests due to his/her illegal behavior.

B. The client has had numerous convictions for his/her illegal activity.

C. The client has spent extensive time incarcerated in jail or prison due to his/her illegal behaviors.

D. The client has recently been released from incarceration.

3. Current Legal Involvement (3)

A. The client has been arrested and has legal charges pending.

B. The client's legal charges have been processed, and a sentence has been handed down.

C. The client is currently incarcerated.

D. The client is currently receiving oversight through a probation/parole program.

E. The client has completed all legal involvement, and is not under jurisdiction of any court program.

4. Poor Functioning in the Corrections Setting (4)

A. The client displayed a pattern of poor adjustment to the corrections setting due to his/her persistent paranoia, mania, or other severe mental illness symptoms.

B. The client reports numerous problems with corrections staff and other inmates due to his/her severe mental illness symptoms.

C. As the client has stabilized, his/her ability to function within the corrections setting has increased.

5. Vulnerable While Incarcerated (5)

A. Due to his/her mental illness, the client has been vulnerable to attack or manipulation by others while incarcerated.

B. The client described a variety of specific situations in which he/she has been attacked or manipulated by others while incarcerated.

---

* The numbers in parentheses correlate to the number of the Behavioral Definition statement in the companion chapter with the same title in *The Severe and Persistent Mental Illness Treatment Planner,* 2nd ed. (Berghuis and Jongsma) by John Wiley & Sons, 2008.

C. Advocacy with the corrections staff and stabilization in mental illness symptoms has decreased the client's pattern of vulnerability while incarcerated.

6. Addiction Problems (6)

A. The client has engaged in illegal behaviors related to substance use or abuse (e.g., drunk driving, drug possession).

B. The client engages in illegal behaviors to support his/her addiction problems.

C. As treatment has progressed, the client's addiction problems have decreased with a commensurate decrease in his/her illegal behaviors.

7. Guardianship (7)

A. The client is being evaluated for having a guardian placed over him/her.

B. The client has had a guardian dictated by the courts.

C. As the client has stabilized, he/she is pursuing his/her own guardianship.

D. The client has become his/her own guardian.

8. Others Pursuing Guardianship (8)

A. Significant others involved in the client's life have petitioned the court to name a legal guardian over him/her.

B. A temporary guardian has been named over the client.

C. Legal proceedings to name a permanent guardian over the client have been initiated.

D. A permanent guardian has been approved by the court.

E. Although others have sought guardianship over the client, he/she has proved himself/herself capable of being his/her own guardian within the court setting.

9. Court-Ordered Hospitalization (9)

A. As the client was an imminent threat to harm himself/herself or others due to his/her mental illness symptoms, an involuntary hospitalization was ordered by the court.

B. The client has been maintained in a psychiatric hospital on an involuntary basis due to a court order.

C. The client has been released from the court mandate for hospitalization.

10. Legal Representation Needs (10)

A. The client has a need for legal representation due to arrests.

B. The client has a need for legal representation due to guardianship procedures.

C. The client has a need for legal representation due to involuntary hospitalization.

D. The client has been appointed an attorney through the court system to represent him/her.

11. Loss of Personal Rights (11)

A. The client has experienced the loss of basic personal rights due to a lack of advocacy.

B. The client has been limited or restricted due to poor understanding of his/her mental illness symptoms.

C. Advocacy has helped to restore the client's basic personal rights.

INTERVENTIONS IMPLEMENTED

1. Identify Legal Concerns (1)*

A. The client was requested to identify his/her history of illegal behaviors.

B. The client was requested to identify the legal system response to his/her illegal behaviors.

C. The client was provided with positive feedback as he/she gave a complete description of his/her pattern of illegal behaviors.

D. The client appeared to minimize or deny his/her pattern of illegal behaviors, and this tendency was pointed out to him/her.

2. Review Guardianship (2)

A. A copy of the client's guardianship stipulations was reviewed with him/her.

B. As guardianship stipulations were discussed, specific reasons for the stipulations were identified.

C. The client was provided with positive feedback as he/she displayed a good understanding of his/her guardianship and the reasons for the guardianship.

3. Obtain and Compare Criminal History (3)

A. Specific information regarding the client's current legal charges was obtained, including police reports, court documents, or attorney reports.

B. The client's official criminal history was compared with his/her disclosed history.

C. Inconsistencies between the client's disclosed criminal history and his/her official list of arrests and convictions were identified and questioned.

D. More specific information regarding the client's current legal charges has helped to more clearly define his/her current concerns.

E. The client's description of his/her past criminal history and his/her official list of arrests and convictions were quite similar, and the client was praised for his/her honesty.

F. Specific information was provided to the client regarding his/her current legal charges that has helped him/her gain a more complete understanding of his/her situation.

G. Little specific information regarding the client's legal charges was available, despite efforts to get more complete information.

4. Assess for Antisocial Behavior (4)

A. The client's pattern of behavior was assessed for any antisocial traits.

B. The client's antisocial behavior pattern was interpreted as being linked to past emotional conflicts and abusive experiences.

C. The client has accepted the interpretation of his/her antisocial behavior and is beginning to disclose feelings related to past abuse.

D. The client's behavior did not display any pattern of antisocial trends, and this was reflected to him/her.

E. The client rejected any interpretation of his/her behavior as antisocial and was encouraged to reconsider this assessment.

---

* The numbers in parentheses correlate to the number of the Therapeutic Intervention statement in the companion chapter with the same title in *The Severe and Persistent Mental Illness Treatment Planner,* 2nd ed. (Berghuis and Jongsma) by John Wiley & Sons, 2008.

5. Assist in Legal Representation Decisions (5)

A. The client was assisted in making decisions about the need for legal representation.

B. The client was encouraged to meet with an attorney to discuss plans for resolving his/her legal issues.

C. The client was referred to specific attorneys who are knowledgeable about mental illness concerns.

D. The client has obtained counsel and has met with the attorney to make plans for resolving his/her legal conflicts, and this was reviewed.

E. The client does not have financial resources to hire an attorney; therefore, the court was asked to appoint a public defender.

F. The client has declined any legal representation and was strongly urged to reconsider this decision.

6. Review Court Proceedings (6)

A. The basic proceedings and people involved in court hearings were reviewed with the client.

B. The client was quizzed about the role of each person involved in the court proceedings in order to test his/her understanding.

C. The client displayed a more complete understanding of the events that will likely occur in his/her court hearing subsequent to reviewing these proceedings.

D. The client has failed to show a complete understanding of his/her likely court involvement and was provided with remedial information in this area.

7. Graphically Display Criminal Proceedings (7)

A. The steps in a criminal proceeding were graphically displayed, identifying the reasons for each step within the process.

B. The client's legal concerns were broken down into specific steps (e.g., investigation, arrest, arraignment, pretrial conferences, trial, and sentencing).

C. As a result of being provided information in an alternative format, the client has developed an increased understanding of his/her criminal proceedings.

D. The client failed to completely understand the process of his/her legal proceedings and was provided with additional, remedial information in this area.

8. Advocate and Refer for Psychological Testing (8)

A. The court was requested to require a psychological evaluation of the client.

B. The client was referred for an assessment of cognitive abilities and deficits, as well as personality functioning.

C. The client underwent objective psychological testing to assess his/her cognitive strengths and weaknesses, as well as personality functioning.

D. The client cooperated with the psychological testing, and feedback about the results was given to him/her.

E. The psychological testing confirmed the presence of specific cognitive abilities and deficits, and personality dynamics.

F. The client was not compliant with taking the psychological evaluation and was encouraged to participate completely.

9. Coach Preparation for Court Hearings (9)

A. The client was coached regarding his/her need to prepare himself/herself for court hearings (e.g., doing personal grooming, clothing selection, and gathering appropriate documentation).

B. The client was provided with positive feedback regarding his/her giving a positive impression within the court setting.

C. The client was provided with additional direction as he/she displayed poor preparation for his/her court hearings.

10. Review Court Protocol (10)

A. Normal conventions within the court setting were reviewed with the client (e.g., referring to the judge as "Your Honor," standing when the judge enters, and waiting for the appropriate time to speak).

B. The client was provided with instruction on how to be a good witness (e.g., tell the truth, only answer the question asked, be prepared for an opposing attorney to try to increase his/her anxiety).

C. Role-playing techniques were used to help the client practice how to be a good witness.

D. The client displayed a positive understanding of the behavioral expectations within the court setting and was encouraged for his/her mastery of this area.

E. The client displayed a poor understanding of the behavioral expectations within the court setting and was provided with additional, remedial information in this area.

11. Role-Play Court Hearings (11)

A. Role-playing techniques were used to teach the client about the upcoming court hearing, with an emphasis on the expected progression of the hearing, typical conventions in the courtroom, and being an effective witness.

B. During the role-playing, the client displayed a clear grasp of how to make a positive impression within the court setting and was given positive feedback in this area.

C. During the role-playing, the client failed to present a positive impression and was provided with additional feedback.

12. Refer to a Physician (12)

A. The client was referred to a physician for an evaluation for a prescription of psychotropic medications.

B. The client was reinforced for following through on a referral to a physician for an assessment for a prescription of psychotropic medications, but none were prescribed.

C. The client has been prescribed psychotropic medications.

D. The client declined evaluation by a physician for a prescription of psychotropic medications and was redirected to cooperate with this referral.

13. Educate about Psychotropic Medications (13)

A. The client was taught about the indications for and the expected benefits of psychotropic medications.

B. As the client's psychotropic medications were reviewed, he/she displayed an understanding about the indications for and expected benefits of the medications.

C. The client displayed a lack of understanding of the indications for and expected benefits of psychotropic medications and was provided with additional information and feedback regarding his/her medications.

14. Monitor Medications (14)

A. The client was monitored for compliance with his/her psychotropic medication regimen.

B. The client was provided with positive feedback about his/her regular use of psychotropic medications.

C. The client was monitored for the effectiveness and side effects of his/her prescribed medications.

D. Concerns about the client's medication effectiveness and side effects were communicated to the physician.

E. Although the client was monitored for medication side effects, he/she reported no concerns in this area.

15. Review Side Effects of the Medications (15)

A. The possible side effects related to the client's medications were reviewed with him/her.

B. The client identified significant side effects, and these were reported to the medical staff.

C. Possible side effects of the client's medications were reviewed, but he/she denied experiencing any side effects.

16. Advise Jail Staff (16)

A. Appropriate authorization to release confidential information to the corrections staff was obtained.

B. The corrections staff was advised about the client's mental illness symptoms.

C. The corrections staff was provided with information and training regarding how to respond to the client.

D. A jail mental health liaison was contacted regarding the client's mental illness symptoms.

E. The client declined to have any information provided to the jail staff, and this request was honored.

17. Advocate for Alternative Sentencing/Housing (17)

A. Advocacy was provided toward the court and jail system for alternative sentencing/housing options for the mentally ill offender who is unable to cope in the typical jail setting.

B. Alternative options (e.g., an electronic tether or a mental health unit within the corrections facility) were identified as appropriate options for the client.

C. Due to advocacy provided on the client's behalf, corrections and court personnel have identified more appropriate sentencing alternatives for him/her.

D. Despite advocacy with the court and jail system, more appropriate sentencing/housing has not been provided.

18. Review Incarceration Impact on Mental Illness (18)

A. The client was assisted in developing an understanding of how his/her mental illness symptoms may interact with his/her incarceration.

B. The client identified specific ways in which his/her mental illness symptoms may interact with incarceration (e.g., increased paranoia, more acute anxiety, or difficulty managing mania), and this was reviewed.

C. The client's more complete understanding of the interaction of his/her mental illness symptoms with his/her incarceration has assisted in helping him/her complete his/her jail sentence, and he/she was provided with positive feedback in this area.

D. The client displayed poor understanding of the impact of his/her mental illness symptoms interacting with his/her incarceration and was provided with additional feedback in this area.

19. Monitor Medications in Corrections Setting (19)

A. The client was monitored for the appropriate provision and use of his/her medication within the corrections setting.

B. The corrections staff was advised about the potential side effects that should be monitored regarding the client's psychiatric medications.

C. The corrections staff was advised about the potential negative consequences that may result from neglecting the client's medications.

D. As a result of regular advocacy regarding the client's medications, he/she has been more regular in his/her use of the medications.

E. The client has not regularly taken his/her medications, and solutions to this problem were developed.

20. Review Personal Safety While Incarcerated (20)

A. Personal safety considerations were reviewed with the client regarding the time that he/she is incarcerated.

B. The client was assisted in understanding how other inmates may treat him/her, how to get help if threatened or assaulted, and how to respond to others within the corrections setting.

C. As a result of the client's increased understanding of personal safety considerations, he/she has been able to maintain his/her personal safety within the corrections setting.

D. The client has failed to focus on his/her personal safety considerations and was provided with additional feedback in this area.

21. Develop Responses to Hostility in Jail (21)

A. The client was assisted in developing assertive, nonviolent responses to potentially hostile individuals in the corrections setting.

B. The client was provided with positive feedback as he/she displayed increased understanding of how to respond to hostile individuals in the corrections setting.

C. The client displayed poor understanding of how to cope with hostile individuals in the corrections setting and was provided with additional, remedial feedback in this area.

22. Facilitate Appointments with Court Officers (22)

A. The client's attendance at appointments with court officers was monitored.

B. The client was provided with encouragement to make certain that he/she regularly keeps his/her appointments with court officers.

C. The client's regular attendance at appointments with court officers was facilitated.

D. As a result of regular involvement regarding the client's appointments with the court officers, he/she has been able to successfully complete the sentencing requirements imposed upon him/her.

23. Attend Probation Meetings (23)

A. The client's probation meetings were attended on an intermittent basis to facilitate communication.

B. The probation staff working with the client was educated about his/her strengths and limitations.

C. As a result of involvement with the client's probation meetings, he/she has been able to successfully complete probation and other sentencing requirements that have been set forth by the court.

24. Support Involvement in Court-Mandated Activities (24)

A. The client's involvement in court-mandated activities was supported in order to help him/her adhere to probation requirements.

B. The client's involvement in court-mandated activities was facilitated in order to help him/her adhere to probation requirements.

C. As a result of assistance provided to the client, he/she has been able to maintain his/her involvement in court-mandated activities (e.g., mental health treatment, job procurement, stable residence, or community service).

D. The client has failed to complete his/her court-mandated activities, despite support and facilitation in these areas.

25. Educate Support System about the Legal System and Ramifications (25)

A. The client's family, friends, and caregivers were educated about the legal system and the specific legal issues related to the client's current situation.

B. As the client was not actively psychotic during his/her inappropriate behavior, his/her family, friends, and caregivers were encouraged to allow him/her to be appropriately incarcerated.

C. Because the client's mental health symptoms have not been controlled, his/her family, friends, and caregivers were encouraged to allow mandatory hospitalization to occur.

D. The client reported an increased level of assistance from his/her family and support system regarding his/her involvement in the legal system, and the positive effects of this were noted.

E. The client's family, friends, and caregivers were supported for their choice to allow him/her to experience the appropriate legal ramifications of his/her inappropriate behavior.

F. The client's family, friends, and caregivers have not allowed him/her to experience the appropriate legal ramifications of his/her behavior and were challenged to do so.

G. The client's support system has failed to assist him/her through the legal system, and they were provided with redirection in this area.

26. Encourage the Support System Contact during Incarceration (26)

A. The client's support system was challenged to remain in contact with him/her, despite his/her incarceration.

B. Members of the client's support system were encouraged for their regular contact with him/her, despite his/her incarceration.

C. The client's support system has not kept in regular contact with him/her and were encouraged to maintain more regular contact.

27. Identify the Effect of Illegal Behaviors (27)

A. The client was requested to identify ways in which his/her illegal behaviors have affected others.

B. The client was assisted in empathizing with others by identifying his/her own emotional responses to prior instances of being victimized.

C. The client was provided with positive feedback regarding his/her ability to relate his/her experiences of victimization with how his/her illegal behaviors have affected others.

D. The client denied any connection between his/her own victimization and the effects of his/her illegal behaviors on others and was redirected in this area.

28. Encourage Restitution (28)

A. The client was encouraged to provide restitution to those whom he/she has victimized.

B. The client was assisted in identifying options for restitution to those to whom he/she has victimized (e.g., financial reimbursement or community service).

C. The client was provided with positive feedback regarding his/her provision of restitution to those whom he/she has victimized.

D. The client has declined any use of restitution to those whom he/she has victimized and was urged to reconsider this decision.

29. Relate Mental Illness Symptoms to Illegal Behaviors (29)

A. The client's pattern of mental illness symptoms was explored as to how it has contributed to his/her legal conflicts.

B. The client acknowledged that his/her mental illness symptoms have played an important part in his/her legal problems, and specific concerns in this area were developed.

C. The client denied any connection between his/her mental illness symptoms and illegal behaviors and was provided with additional feedback in this area.

30. Refer for Therapy (30)

A. The client was referred for individual therapy to assist in developing alternatives to acting out when facing stressful circumstances.

B. The client was referred to a group therapy program to assist in developing alternatives to acting out when facing stressful circumstances.

C. The client and his/her significant other were referred to marital therapy to assist in developing adaptive relationship patterns to help decrease acting out.

D. As a result of the client's psychotherapy, he/she has decreased his/her pattern of acting out in stressful circumstances.

E. The client continues to act out in stressful circumstances, despite the use of psychotherapy.

31. Coordinate Substance Abuse Assessment (31)

A. The client was assessed for substance abuse problems that may contribute to his/her legal concerns.

B. The client was identified as having a concomitant substance abuse problem.

C. Upon review, the client does not display evidence of a substance abuse problem.

D. The client's mental health and substance abuse treatment services were coordinated in an integrated fashion.

E. The client's substance abuse treatment providers have been furnished with increased information about the client's mental health diagnosis and treatment.

F. The client's mental health treatment providers have been provided with increased information about the client's substance abuse diagnosis and treatment.

32. Coordinate Guardianship Assessment (32)

A. A psychological evaluation was coordinated to facilitate a guardianship hearing, including an assessment of functional decision-making abilities (e.g., regarding treatment, finances).

B. The client has participated in the psychological evaluation to facilitate a guardianship hearing, and the results of this evaluation were shared with him/her.

C. The client's psychological evaluation was shared with the court to assist in the decision-making process for guardianship.

D. The client has declined involvement in a psychological evaluation and was redirected to complete this evaluation.

33. Assist in the Guardianship Process (33)

A. Family members or other interested parties were assisted in obtaining guardianship of the client in order to increase supervision and monitoring of his/her behavior and treatment.

B. The client has agreed to have a guardian placed over him/her in order to monitor his/her behavior and treatment.

C. Guardianship procedures have been instituted to assist family members or others in obtaining guardianship of the client, despite his/her belief that he/she does not need a guardian.

34. Educate the Potential Guardian about Person-Centered Planning (34)

A. The client's potential guardian was educated about issues related to person-centered planning.

B. The client's potential guardian was educated about the ability of mentally ill people to manage many aspects of their lives, despite serious and persistent symptoms.

C. The client's potential guardian was provided with positive feedback regarding understanding of person-centered planning issues and the client's ability to manage many aspects of his/her life.

D. The client's potential guardian was urged to seek more information regarding the person-centered needs of the client.

35. Advocate against Unnecessary Guardianship Practices (35)

A. Advocacy was provided for the client regarding unnecessary or overly restrictive guardianship orders or practices.

B. Specific information and education was provided to the guardian and court personnel regarding the unnecessary or overly restrictive guardianship orders or practices that have been implemented.

C. As a result of advocacy for the client against unnecessary or overly restrictive guardianship orders, the least restrictive, legally necessary guardianship was implemented.

36. Assist in Developing Advanced Directives (36)

A. The client was assisted in developing an advanced directive should he/she decompensate and become unable to legally make such decisions.

B. The client was assisted in developing specific wishes for treatment, emergency contact, medication needs, and other issues in case of his/her severe decompensation.

C. The client was provided with positive feedback regarding his/her development of the advanced directive.

D. The client has not developed an advanced directive and was redirected in this area.

37. Discuss End-of-Life Wishes (37)

A. The client was engaged in a discussion regarding his/her wishes for end-of-life issues, including funeral arrangements, estate dispersal, and financial needs.

B. The client has participated in developing specific arrangements for his/her end-of-life issues.

C. The client has avoided any review of his/her end-of-life issues and was urged to apply himself/herself to this area.

38. Focus on Responsibilities Regarding Treatment (38)

A. The client was focused on his/her responsibilities regarding treatment.

B. The client was assisted in understanding his/her responsibilities (e.g., attendance at appointments, providing the clinician with accurate information, and confidentiality) regarding other clients in treatment.

C. The client displayed an increased understanding of his/her responsibilities regarding treatment and was provided with positive feedback in this area.

D. The client has failed to display a clear understanding regarding his/her responsibilities for treatment and was provided with remedial information for this progress.

39. Advocate for the Client's Rights (39)

A. Advocacy was provided for the client with other clinicians, family members, and legal personnel to adhere to his/her rights.

B. The client was assisted in advocating with other clinicians, family members, and legal personnel to adhere to his/her rights.

C. The client reported an increased experience of empowerment due to the client rights advocacy provided on his/her behalf.

MANIA OR HYPOMANIA

CLIENT PRESENTATION

1. Increased, Pressured Speech (1)*

A. The client gave evidence of increased, pressured speech within the session.

B. The client reported that his/her speech rate increases as he/she feels stressed.

C. The client's pressured speech has shown evidence of a decrease in intensity.

D. The client showed no evidence of pressured speech in today's session.

2. Racing Thoughts (2)

A. The client demonstrated a pattern of racing thoughts, moving from one subject to another without maintaining focus.

B. The client reported that he/she experiences racing thoughts, including difficulty concentrating on one thought as other thoughts interfere.

C. The client reported that at times of quiet reflection, he/she is disturbed by thoughts racing through his/her mind.

D. The client reported that his/her thoughts are not racing as they had been, and he/she is able to stay focused.

3. Inflated Sense of Self (3)

A. The client gave evidence of an inflated sense of self-esteem and an exaggerated, euphoric belief in capabilities that denies any limitations or realistic obstacles.

B. The client appears oblivious to his/her inflated sense of self-esteem or euphoric beliefs but sees others as standing in his/her way.

C. In spite of attempts to try to get the client to be more realistic, his/her inflated self-esteem and exaggerated, euphoric beliefs have persisted.

D. The client's sense of self-esteem and beliefs in his/her capabilities have become more reality based.

E. There has been no recent evidence of inflated self-esteem or exaggerated, euphoric beliefs.

4. Persecutory Delusions (3)

A. The client described a pattern of persecutory delusions, including suspiciousness of others without reasonable cause.

B. The client demonstrated a pattern of misinterpretation of benign events as having threatening personal significance.

C. The client's history is replete with incidents in which he/she believed he/she was persecuted by others.

D. The client is beginning to accept a more reality-based interpretation of events and relationships, which is much less threatening.

---

* The numbers in parentheses correlate to the number of the Behavioral Definition statement in the companion chapter with the same title in *The Severe and Persistent Mental Illness Treatment Planner,* 2nd ed. (Berghuis and Jongsma) by John Wiley & Sons, 2008.

E. The client no longer demonstrates a pattern of bizarre, persecutory delusions and has verbalized not feeling personally threatened.

5. Lack of Sleep (4)

A. The client described a pattern of attaining far less sleep than would ordinarily be needed.

B. The client has gone through periods of time when he/she did not sleep for 24 consecutive hours or more because his/her energy level was so high.

C. As the client's mania has begun to diminish, he/she has begun to return to a more normal sleeping pattern.

D. The client is getting six to eight hours of sleep per night.

6. Psychomotor Agitation (5)

A. The client was restless and agitated within the session and reports an inability to sit quietly and relax.

B. The client's high energy level is reflected in increased motor activity, restlessness, and agitation.

C. The client's motor activity has decreased, and the level of agitation has diminished.

D. The client demonstrated normal motor activity and reports being able to stay calm and relaxed.

7. Loss of Inhibitions/Self-Damaging Activities (6)

A. The client reported a behavior pattern that reflected a lack of normal inhibition and an increase in potentially self-damaging activities.

B. The client's impulsivity has been reflected in sexual acting out, poor financial decisions, and committing social offenses.

C. The client has gained more control over his/her impulses and has returned to a normal level of inhibition and social propriety.

8. Expansive/Variable Mood (7)

A. The client gave evidence of a very expansive mood that could easily turn to impatience and irritability if his/her behavior is blocked or confronted.

B. The client related instances of feeling angry when others tried to control his/her expansive, grandiose ideas and mood.

C. As the client's expansive mood has been controlled, his/her impatience and irritable anger have diminished.

9. Lack of Follow-Through (8)

A. The client described a behavior pattern that portrayed a lack of follow-though on many projects, even though his/her energy level is high, since he/she lacks discipline and goal directiveness.

B. The client's lack of follow-through has resulted in frustration on the part of others.

C. The client has begun to exercise more discipline and goal directiveness in his/her behavior, resulting in the completion of projects.

10. Disregard for Social Mores (9)

A. The client's behavior pattern confirmed his/her disregard for social mores within academic, social, or employment settings.

B. The client verbalized that he/she sees social rules or mores as applying to others but not to himself/herself.

C. The client is beginning to accept the need for rules within any society and to apply them to himself/herself.

D. The client has not had a recent incident of disregard for social mores and is more compliant.

11. Bizarre Dress and Grooming (10)

A. The client displays bizarre patterns of dressing.

B. The client displays an unusual grooming pattern.

C. The client's clothing is much more revealing that he/she normally wears.

D. As the client is stabilized his/her mania/hypomania, his/her grooming and dressing pattern has returned to normal.

INTERVENTIONS IMPLEMENTED

1. Explore for Manic Signs (1)*

A. The client's thoughts, feelings, and behavior were explored for classic signs of mania (e.g., pressured speech, impulsive behavior, euphoric mood, flight of ideas, high energy level, reduced need for sleep, and inflated self-esteem).

B. The clinical assessment confirmed the presence of the classic signs of mania.

C. The clinical assessment did not find adequate evidence to diagnose mania.

2. Assess Mania Intensity (2)

A. The client was assessed for his/her current stage of elation: none, hypomanic, manic, or psychotic.

B. The client's assessment indicated no current symptoms of mania.

C. The client was assessed to be hypomanic.

D. The client was assessed to be manic.

E. The client's mania was so severe that periods of psychosis have been present.

3. Assess Ability to Remain Safe (3)

A. An assessment was performed of the client's ability to remain safe within the community.

B. The client was assessed in regard to his/her level of manic behavior, impulsivity, and propensity toward potentially unsafe situations.

C. The natural and programmatic supports that can assist the client to remain safe within the community were assessed.

D. Due to programmatic supports, the client has been assessed as being able to remain safe within the community, despite his/her symptoms of mania/hypomania.

E. The client was judged to be unable to remain safe within the community due to his/her symptoms of mania and was referred for a more restrictive setting.

* The numbers in parentheses correlate to the number of the Therapeutic Intervention statement in the companion chapter with the same title in *The Severe and Persistent Mental Illness Treatment Planner,* 2nd ed. (Berghuis and Jongsma) by John Wiley & Sons, 2008.

4. Arrange for a More Restrictive Setting (4)

A. Arrangements were made for the client to be hospitalized in a psychiatric setting based on the fact that his/her mania is so intense that he/she could be harmful to himself/herself or others or unable to care for his/her own basic needs.

B. The client was not willing to submit voluntarily to hospitalization; therefore, commitment procedures were initiated.

C. The client was supported for acknowledging the need for hospitalization and voluntarily admitting himself/herself to the psychiatric facility.

5. Develop a Short-Term Crisis Plan (5)

A. A short-term, round-the-clock crisis plan was developed.

B. It was determined that components of the client's short-term, round-the-clock crisis plan must include multiple caregivers, psychiatric involvement, and crisis assistance in order to maintain him/her within the community.

C. With the implementation of the crisis plan, the client has been able to remain within the community as he/she stabilizes from his/her period of mania/hypomania.

D. The client continues to decompensate and is not safe to maintain within the community, despite the use of the crisis plan, and arrangements for a more restrictive setting were initiated.

6. Remove Dangerous Items (6)

A. Significant others were encouraged to remove dangerous items (e.g., sharp objects, weapons, and access to motor vehicles).

B. Permission was obtained from the client to remove potentially dangerous items.

C. Contact was made with significant others within the client's life to monitor his/her behavior and remove potential means of suicide or impulsive harm.

7. Provide a Calm Setting (7)

A. A plan was developed with the client that focused on reducing the level of stress that he/she receives in his/her environment.

B. The client was assisted in developing a calmer setting for himself/herself, including low lighting and decreased stimulation.

C. Steps have been taken to change the environment in such a way as to reduce the client's feelings of agitation associated with it.

D. Arrangements have been made for the client to be visited, monitored, supervised, and encouraged more frequently by supportive people.

8. Refer for Psychiatric Evaluation (8)

A. The client was referred for a psychiatric evaluation to consider psychotropic medication to control the manic state.

B. The client has followed through with the psychiatric evaluation and pharmacotherapy has begun.

C. The client has been resistive to cooperating with a psychiatric evaluation and was encouraged to follow through on this recommendation.

9. Monitor Medication Reaction (9)

A. The client's reaction to the medication in terms of side effects and effectiveness were monitored.

B. The client reported that the medication has been effective at reducing energy levels, flight of ideas, and the decreased need for sleep; he/she was urged to continue this medication regimen.

C. The client has been reluctant to take the prescribed medication for his/her manic state, but was urged to follow through on the prescription.

D. As the client has taken his/her medication, which has been successful in reducing the intensity of the mania, he/she has begun to feel that it is no longer necessary and has indicated a desire to stop taking it; he/she was urged to continue the medication as prescribed.

10. Monitor Ability to Participate in Psychotherapy (10)

A. The client's pattern of symptom improvement was monitored, with a focus on how stable he/she is in regard to participation in psychotherapy.

B. The client was judged to be significantly improved and capable of participating in psychotherapy.

C. The client was judged to still be too manic to allow helpful participation in psychotherapy.

11. Conduct Family-Focused Treatment (11)

A. The client and significant others were included in the treatment model.

B. Family-focused treatment was used with the client and significant others as indicated in *Bipolar Disorder: A Family-Focused Approach* (Miklowitz and Goldstein).

C. As family members were not available to participate in therapy, the family-focused treatment model was adapted to individual therapy.

12. Assess Family Communication Patterns (12)

A. Objective instruments were used to assess the family communication patterns.

B. The level of expressed emotions within the family was specifically assessed.

C. The *Perceived Criticism Scale* (Hooley and Teasdale) was used to assess family communication problems.

D. The family was provided with feedback about their pattern of communication.

E. The family has not been involved in the assessment of communication patterns, and the focus of treatment was diverted to this resistance.

13. Educate about Mood Episodes (13)

A. A variety of modalities were used to teach the family about signs and symptoms of the client's mood episodes.

B. The phasic relapsing nature of the client's mood episodes was emphasized.

C. The client's mood episode concerns were normalized.

D. The client's mood episodes were destigmatized.

14. Teach Stress Diathesis Model (14)

A. The client was taught a stress diathesis model of Bipolar Disorder

B. The biological predisposition to mood episodes was emphasized.

C. The client was taught about how stress can make him/her more vulnerable to mood episodes.

D. The manageability of mood episodes was emphasized.

E. The client was reinforced for his/her clear understanding of the stress diathesis model of Bipolar Disorder.

F. The client struggled to display a clear understanding of the stress diathesis model of Bipolar Disorder and was provided with additional remedial information in this area.

15. Provide Rationale for Treatment (15)

A. The client was provided with the rationale for treatment involving ongoing medication and psychosocial treatment.

B. The focus of treatment was emphasized, including recognizing, managing, and reducing biological and psychological vulnerabilities that could precipitate relapse.

C. A discussion was held about the rationale for treatment.

D. The client was reinforced for his/her understanding of the appropriate rationale for treatment.

E. The client was redirected when he/she displayed a poor understanding of the rationale for treatment.

16. Identify Relapse Triggers (16)

A. Sources of the client's stress and triggers of potential relapse were identified.

B. Negative events, cognitive interpretations, aversive communication, poor sleep hygiene, and medication noncompliance were investigated as potential stressors or triggers of potential relapse.

C. Cognitive-behavioral techniques were used to address the sources of stress and triggers for potential relapse.

17. Enhance Engagement in Medication Use (17)

A. Motivational approaches were used to help enhance the client's level of engagement in his/her medication use and compliance to the medication regimen.

B. Modeling, role-playing, and behavioral rehearsal were used to help the client use problem-solving skills to work through several current conflicts.

C. The client was taught about the risk for relapse when medication is discontinued.

D. Commitment was obtained to continuous prescription adherence.

E. As a result of motivational approaches for medication compliance, the subject's use of medication has significantly improved.

F. The client continues to be medication noncompliant despite use of motivational approaches; the client was refocused on this task.

18. Assess Prescription Noncompliance Factors (18)

A. Factors that have precipitated the client's prescription noncompliance were assessed.

B. The client was checked for specific thoughts, feelings, and stressors that might contribute to his/her prescription noncompliance.

C. The client was assigned "Why I Dislike Taking My Medication" from the *Adult Psychotherapy Homework Planner,* 2nd ed. (Jongsma).

D. A plan was developed for recognizing and addressing the factors that have precipitated the client's prescription noncompliance.

19. Educate about Lab Work (19)

A. The client was educated about the need to stay compliant with necessary lab work involved in regulating his/her medication levels.

B. The client was encouraged to stay compliant with necessary lab work.

C. The client was reinforced for his/her compliance to completing necessary lab work to help regulate his/her medication levels.

D. The client has not been regular in his/her compliance to lab work for regulating his/her medication levels and was redirected to do so.

20. Teach about Sleep Hygiene Importance (20)

A. The client was taught about the importance of good sleep hygiene.

B. The client was assigned the "Sleep Pattern Record" from the *Adult Psychotherapy Homework Planner,* 2nd ed. (Jongsma).

C. The client's sleep pattern was routinely assessed.

D. Interventions for the client's sleep pattern were provided, as he/she has been noted to have a dysfunctional sleep pattern.

21. Educate about Symptoms of Relapse (21)

A. The client was educated about the signs and symptoms of pending relapse.

B. The client's family was educated about the signs and symptoms of pending relapse.

22. Develop Relapse Drill (22)

A. The client and family were assisted in drawing up a "relapse drill," detailing roles and responsibilities.

B. Family members were asked to take responsibility for specific roles (e.g., who will call a meeting of the family to problem solve potential relapse; who will call physician, schedule a serum level, or contact emergency services, if needed).

C. Obstacles to providing family support to the client's potential relapse were reviewed and problem solved.

D. The family was asked to make a commitment to adherence to the plan.

E. The family was reinforced for their commitment to the adherence to the plan.

F. The family has not developed a clear commitment to the relapse prevention plan and was redirected in this area.

23. Assess and Educate about Aversive Communication (23)

A. The family was assessed for the role of aversive communication in family distress and in the risk for the client's manic relapse.

B. The family was educated about the role of aversive communication (e.g., highly expressed emotion) in developing greater family stress and in increasing the client's risk for manic relapse.

C. The family displayed a clear understanding of the effects of aversive communication and this was reinforced.

D. The family was provided with remedial feedback, as they did not display a clear understanding of the risk for relapse due to aversive communication.

24. **Teach Communication Skills (24)**

A. Behavioral techniques were used to teach communication skills.

B. Communication skills such as offering positive feedback, active listening, making positive requests for behavioral change, and giving negative feedback in an honest, respectful manner were taught to the client and family.

C. Behavioral techniques were used to teach the family healthy communication skills.

D. Education, modeling, role-playing, corrective feedback, and positive reinforcement were used to teach communication skills.

25. **Assign Communication Skills Homework (25)**

A. The client and family were assigned homework exercises to use and record newly learned communication skills.

B. Family members have used newly learned communication skills, and the results were processed within the session.

C. Family members have not used the newly learned communication skills and were redirected to do so.

26. **Differentiate Losses, Abilities, and Expectations (26)**

A. The client was assisted in differentiating between actual losses, abilities, and expectations, and imagined or exaggerated losses, abilities, and expectations.

B. The client verbalized grief, fear, and anger regarding imagined losses in life and was provided with support and redirection in this area.

C. The client was able to differentiate between his/her real and imagined losses, abilities, and expectations and was provided with positive feedback in this area.

D. The client continues to focus on imagined, exaggerated losses, abilities, and expectations and was focused on being more reality oriented in this area.

27. **Confront Grandiosity (27)**

A. The client's grandiosity and demandingness were kindly but firmly confronted.

B. The client has become less expansive in his/her mood and more socially appropriate due to the consistent confrontation of his/her grandiosity and demandingness.

C. The client has reacted with anger and irritability when his/her grandiosity was confronted.

28. **Focus on Impulsive Behavior Consequences (28)**

A. The client's impulsive behavior was repeatedly reviewed in order to help him/her identify the negative consequences that result from this pattern.

B. The impulsive nature of the client's manic/hypomanic episode was reviewed regarding its negative consequences.

C. The client was focused onto the need to identify his/her impulsive, manic/hypomanic symptoms as early as possible.

D. The client was helped to identify the impulsive nature and negative consequences of his/her manic/hypomanic episodes and not to be so focused on just the here and now, and he/she was provided with additional feedback in this area.

29. Increase Sensitivity to Effects of Behavior (29)

A. Role-playing, role reversal, and behavioral rehearsal were used to increase the client's sensitivity to the negative effects of his/her impulsive behavior.

B. The client was reinforced for his/her increased sensitivity to the negative effects of his/her impulsive behavior on others.

C. The client has had significant difficulty identifying negative consequences for his/her impulsive behavior, despite the use of role-playing, role reversal, and behavioral rehearsal.

30. Confront Mania and Enforce Rules (30)

A. Unhealthy, impulsive, or manic behaviors that occur during contacts with the clinician were identified and confronted.

B. Clear rules and roles in the relationship were identified and enforced with immediate, short-term consequences for breaking such boundaries.

C. The client's unhealthy, impulsive, or manic behaviors have diminished in response to limit setting within the session.

31. Address Problem Solving (31)

A. The client was asked to identify conflicts that can be addressed through problem-solving techniques.

B. The family members were asked to give input about conflicts that could be addressed with problem-solving techniques.

C. The client and family arrived at a list of conflicts that could be addressed with problem-solving techniques.

32. Teach Problem-Solving Skills (32)

A. Behavioral techniques such as education, modeling, role-playing, corrective feedback, and positive reinforcement were used to teach the client and family problem-solving skills.

B. Specific problem-solving skills were taught to the family, including defining the problem constructively and specifically, brainstorming options, evaluating options, choosing options, implementing a plan, evaluating the results, and reevaluating the plan.

C. Family members were asked to use the problem-solving skills on specific situations.

D. The family was reinforced for positive use of problem-solving skills.

E. The family was redirected for failures to properly use problem-solving skills.

33. Assign Problem-Solving Homework (33)

A. The client and family were assigned to use newly learned problem-solving skills and record their use.

B. The client and family were assigned "Plan Before Acting" in the *Adult Psychotherapy Homework Planner,* 2nd ed. (Jongsma).

C. The results of the family members' use of problem-solving skills were reviewed within the session.

34. Reinforce Control Over Thought Process (34)

A. The client was reinforced for controlling his/her slower speech.

B. The client was reinforced for his/her more deliberate thought process.

35. Reinforce Agitation Control (35)

A. The client was reinforced for controlling his/her motor agitation and helped to set goals for and limits on his/her behavior.

B. The client was taught relaxation techniques to help him/her reduce the level of agitation and restlessness.

C. The "Plan Before Acting" assignment from the *Adult Psychotherapy Homework Planner,* 2nd ed. (Jongsma) was used to help model and teach increased behavioral control.

D. It was noticed that the client has become less agitated and more relaxed.

36. Monitor Energy Level (36)

A. The client's energy level was monitored, and he/she was reinforced for increased control over behavior, pressured speech, and expression of ideas.

B. The client has responded favorably to placing more structure and control over his/her behavior and reported less agitation and flight of ideas.

C. The client continues to have periods of increased agitation, pressured speech, and flight of ideas and was provided with remedial feedback in this area.

37. Schedule Maintenance Session (37)

A. The client was scheduled for a maintenance session between 1 and 3 months after therapy ends.

B. The client was advised to contact the therapist if he/she needs to be seen prior to the maintenance session.

C. The client's maintenance session was held, and he/she was reinforced for his/her successful implementation of therapy techniques.

D. The client's maintenance session was held, and he/she was coordinated for further treatment, as his/her progress has not been sustained.

38. Test/Treat for Sexually Transmitted Diseases (STDs)/Pregnancy (38)

A. Testing was arranged for STDs.

B. The client was tested to determine if she is pregnant.

C. Follow-up treatment for the client's STDs was coordinated.

D. The client has tested positive for pregnancy and was assisted in processing this development.

E. The client has tested negatively for STDs, and this information was passed on to him/her.

F. The client was informed that she is not pregnant.

39. Assist through Criminal Justice System (39)

A. The client was assisted in working through the requirements of the criminal justice system.

B. Advocacy and support were provided as the client is negotiating the criminal justice system.

C. The client has been able to meet the requirements of the criminal justice system through the use of support and advocacy from the clinician.

40. List Relationships Affected by Mental Illness (40)

A. The client was assisted in developing a list of relationships that have been affected by his/her severe and persistent mental illness symptoms.

B. The client's list of relationships affected by his/her severe and persistent mental illness symptoms was processed.

C. The client has minimized or denied that relationships have been affected by his/her symptoms and was redirected to reconsider this issue.

41. Provide Feedback about Behavior (41)

A. The client was provided with feedback about how his/her behavior or verbal messages have an impact on others.

B. The client was taught more effective and sensitive social skills.

C. The client was able to accept the feedback provided and has improved in his/her relationship skills.

D. The client denied any problems with his/her behavior or verbal messages, despite feedback, and has not improved his/her relationships with others.

42. Assign Reading on Bipolar Disorder (42)

A. The client was assigned to read a book on Bipolar Disorder.

B. The client was assigned to read *The Bipolar Disorder Survival Guide* (Miklowitz).

C. The client has read the assigned information on Bipolar Disorder, and key concepts were reviewed.

D. The client has not read the assigned information on Bipolar Disorder and was redirected to do so.

MEDICATION MANAGEMENT

CLIENT PRESENTATION

1. Failure to Take Medications (1)*

A. The client has failed to consistently take his/her psychotropic medications as prescribed.

B. A review of the client's medications indicates that he/she has not used the expected amounts.

C. The client has become more regular in his/her use of his/her psychotropic medications.

D. The client has been regularly taking his/her psychotropic medications as prescribed.

2. Negative Side Effects (2)

A. The interactions from the client's medications are causing negative side effects.

B. The client reported that he/she has great difficulty tolerating the side effects from his/her medication interaction.

C. As the client's medications have been adjusted, he/she reported a decrease in the negative side effects.

D. The side effects of the client's medications have been sufficiently decreased such as to increase his/her consistent use of medications.

3. Verbalized Fears of Side Effects (3)

A. The client has verbalized his/her fears related to physical and/or emotional side effects of prescribed medications.

B. The client dislikes the side effects of his/her prescribed medications.

C. As the side effects of the client's medications have been decreased, he/she has become more comfortable and regular in using the medications.

D. The client verbalized his/her acceptance of the side effects of the medications, which are outweighed by the beneficial aspects.

4. Failure to Respond to Medications (4)

A. The client has not responded as expected to his/her prescribed medication regimen.

B. The client's failure to respond as expected to his/her medications has been traced to his/her erratic use of them.

C. The client's failure to respond as expected to prescribed medications has been traced to the confounding effects of polypharmacy.

D. The client is now responding as expected to his/her prescribed medication regimen.

5. Lack of Medication Knowledge (5)

A. The client displayed a lack of knowledge about his/her medications and their usefulness or potential side effects.

---

* The numbers in parentheses correlate to the number of the Behavioral Definition statement in the companion chapter with the same title in *The Severe and Persistent Mental Illness Treatment Planner,* 2nd ed. (Berghuis and Jongsma) by John Wiley & Sons, 2008.

B. The client's lack of knowledge regarding his/her medications has led to poor decisions about using them.

C. As the client has gained more knowledge about his/her medications, their usefulness, and potential side effects, he/she has been more regular with his/her use of them.

6. Unwilling to Take Prescribed Medications (6)

A. The client has indicated reluctance to take his/her prescribed medications.

B. The client has made specific statements about his/her unwillingness to take prescribed medications.

C. The client has refused any medications.

D. As treatment has progressed, the client has become more willing to take his/her prescribed medications.

E. The client is regularly taking his/her medications.

7. Alcohol/Drug Use (7)

A. The client has been consuming alcohol along with his/her psychotropic medications, which has negatively affected the usefulness of his/her medications.

B. The client has been using illicit street drugs along with his/her psychotropic medications, which has altered the benefits of his/her medications.

C. As the client's substance abuse has decreased, the benefits of his/her psychotropic medications have increased.

D. The client is free from drugs and alcohol, which has helped his/her medications to be more beneficial.

INTERVENTIONS IMPLEMENTED

1. Request a List of Medications (1)*

A. The client was asked to identify all of his/her currently prescribed medications, including names, times administered, and dosage.

B. The client was provided with feedback regarding the accuracy of his/her list of medications.

2. Request a Description of Medication Compliance to Compare with Data (2)

A. The client was requested to provide an honest, realistic description of his/her medication compliance.

B. The client's description of his/her medication usage was compared with information from his/her medical chart, information from his/her personal physician/psychiatrist, and other objective data.

C. An objective data review indicates a substantial pattern of compliance.

D. An objective data review indicates poor medication compliance.

E. The client was praised for his/her realistic description of his/her medication compliance.

F. The client reported complete medication compliance, and this description was accepted.

---

* The numbers in parentheses correlate to the number of the Therapeutic Intervention statement in the companion chapter with the same title in *The Severe and Persistent Mental Illness Treatment Planner,* 2nd ed. (Berghuis and Jongsma) by John Wiley & Sons, 2008.

G. The client seemed to minimize his/her noncompliance with prescribed medications and was confronted about this.

3. Obtain Blood Levels (3)

A. A blood draw was conducted, and the client's blood levels for specific medications have been assessed.

B. The analysis of the client's blood chemistry indicates substantial compliance with his/her medication regimen.

C. An analysis of the client's blood chemistry indicates substantial noncompliance with his/her medication regimen.

D. The client's suspected pattern of medication use (based on blood chemistry studies) was reflected to him/her.

4. Conduct Motivational Interviewing (4)

A. Motivational interviewing techniques were used to help assess the client's preparation for change.

B. The client was assisted in identifying his/her stage of change regarding his/her substance abuse concerns.

C. It was reflected to the client that he/she is currently building motivation for change.

D. The client was assisted in strengthening his/her commitment to change.

E. The client was noted to be participating actively in treatment.

5. Review and Supplement Medication Knowledge (5)

A. The client was requested to identify the reason for each of his/her medications.

B. The client was provided with positive feedback as he/she displayed a clear understanding of the reasons for each of his/her medications.

C. The client was provided with written information about his/her medications, the acceptable dosage levels, and the side effects.

D. The client reported that he/she has read the written information provided to him/her and has gained a better understanding of his/her medications.

E. The client has not read the written information provided to him/her and was redirected to do so.

6. Process Fears Regarding Medication (6)

A. The client was requested to describe the fears that he/she may experience regarding the use of his/her medications.

B. Myths and misinformation regarding the client's understanding and fears of his/her medications were corrected.

C. The client's fears were reviewed, discussed, and processed to conclusion.

D. The client was provided with positive feedback regarding his/her increased comfort with his/her use of medications.

E. The client tended to minimize or deny his/her fears regarding his/her medications, and he/she was encouraged to be more open about these concerns.

7. Behavioral Experiments (7)

A. The client was directed to conduct "behavioral experiments" in which bias predictions about medications are tested against the client's past, present, and/or future experience using the medication.

B. The client was assisted in identifying the criteria against which to test his/her experience with medication.

C. The client has conducted the behavioral experiments to test his/her predictions about the medication, and these conclusions were reviewed.

D. The client has not engaged in the behavioral experiments and this resistance was problem-solved.

8. Reinforce Positive Cognitive Messages (8)

A. The client was reinforced for positive, reality-based cognitive messages that enhance medication prescription compliance.

B. The client used positive, reality-based cognitive messages, he/she was taught to use those messages to enhance his/her medication prescription compliance.

C. The client has not engaged in positive, reality-based cognitive message to enhance his/her medication prescription compliance, and was provided with specific examples in this area.

9. Refer to Family Psycho-Educational Program (9)

A. The family was referred to a psycho-educational program to help learn about the client's severe and persistent mental illness and the need for medication.

B. The client was referred to a multi-group family psycho-educational program to help learn about the client's severe and persistent mental illness and the need for medication.

C. The family was engaged in the psycho-educational program and has identified ways in which they have learned about the client's severe and persistent mental illness and the need for medication.

D. The client's family has not engaged in the psycho-educational program and was redirected to do so.

10. Use Family-Focused Treatment Therapy Model (10)

A. The client was referred to therapy program based on the principles of family-focused treatment, as noted in *Bipolar Disorder: A Family-Focused Treatment Approach (Miklowitz and Goldstein)*.

B. Family-focused treatment was conducted to assist in improving communication patterns between the client and his/her family.

C. The family and the client have engaged in the family-focused treatment, and the positive results of this treatment were reviewed.

D. The family and the client have not engaged in the family-focused treatment and were encouraged to do so.

11. Refer to a Physician (11)

A. The client was referred to a physician for an evaluation for a prescription of psychotropic medications.

B. The client was reinforced for following through on a referral to a physician for an assessment for a prescription of psychotropic medications, but none were prescribed.

C. The client has been prescribed psychotropic medications.

D. The client declined evaluation by a physician for a prescription of psychotropic medication and was redirected to cooperate with this referral.

12. Review Side Effects of the Medications (12)

A. The possible side effects related to the client's medications were reviewed with him/her.

B. The client identified significant side effects, and these were reported to the medical staff.

C. Possible side effects of the client's medications were reviewed, but he/she denied experiencing any side effects.

13. Inform Other Health Care Providers about the Medications (13)

A. A written authorization to release confidential information was obtained to allow communication with the client's primary physician and other health care providers.

B. The client's primary physician and other health care providers were informed of the medications he/she is currently using, their expected side effects, risks, and benefits.

14. Encourage or Assist with Regular Employment (14)

A. The client was encouraged to obtain regular employment to increase income and defray medication costs.

B. The client was assisted in seeking and obtaining regular employment.

C. The client has found regular employment, and the economic benefits for his/her employment were reviewed.

D. The client has not obtained regular employment and continues to struggle with his/her ability to pay for medications and was redirected in this area.

E. The client was assisted in obtaining, completing, and filing forms for Social Security Disability benefits or other public aid.

F. The client has completed all necessary documentation for filing for Social Security Disability benefits or other public aid, and this material was reviewed.

G. The client's application for Social Security Disability benefits and other public aid has been incomplete, and he/she received assistance in completing these applications.

15. Coordinate Generic or Reduced-Cost Medication Programs (15)

A. Free or low-cost medication programs through drug manufacturers or other resources were requested for the client.

B. The client was assisted in accessing free or low-cost medication programs.

C. The client was directed to specific programs for obtaining free or low-cost medications from drug manufacturers or other resources.

D. The client has not followed through on accessing reduced-cost medication programs and was redirected to do so.

E. When appropriate, the use of generic drugs was advocated for as a way to decrease the client's cost for medications.

F. The client's physician was consulted regarding the use of generic drugs rather than brand-name drugs.

G. Generic drugs were contraindicated in this client's situation, and this was reflected to him/her and the pharmacist.

16. Assess Suicidal Ideation (16)

A. The client was asked to describe the frequency and intensity of his/her suicidal ideation, the details of any existing suicide plan, the history of any previous suicide attempts, or any family history of depression or suicide.

B. The client was encouraged to be forthright regarding the current strength of his/her suicidal feelings and the ability to control such suicidal urges.

C. The client was assessed as being at low risk of suicide.

D. The client was assessed at being at high risk of suicide, and further intervention was necessary.

17. Remove Medications (17)

A. As the client was assessed to be at risk for suicide, his/her medications were removed from his/her immediate access.

B. Significant others were encouraged to remove medications or other potentially lethal means of suicide from the client's easy access.

C. Arrangement was made to coordinate regular delivery of the client's medications as they have been removed from his/her immediate access.

D. Due to the client's suicide risk, he/she was monitored in the actual taking of his/her medications.

E. As the client has decreased his/her suicide risk, he/she has been provided with increased control over his/her medications.

18. Refer to a Supervised Environment (18)

A. Because the client was judged to be uncontrollably harmful to himself/herself, arrangements were made for psychiatric hospitalization.

B. Due to concerns about the client's inability to manage himself/herself within a less restrictive setting, he/she was referred to a crisis residential facility.

C. The client was supported for cooperating voluntarily with admission to a more supervised environment.

D. The client refused to voluntarily admit himself/herself to a more supervised environment; therefore, civil commitment procedures were initiated.

19. Refer for Personality Testing (19)

A. The client was referred for psychological testing to assist in obtaining a more complete clinical picture.

B. The client was compliant with the testing, which indicated a specific diagnosis.

C. The psychological test results confirm previous diagnostic expectations.

D. The psychological testing results indicate that the client's mental illness concerns have significantly abated, and this was reviewed.

E. The client was not compliant with the psychological testing and was redirected to this referral.

20. Educate about Lifestyle Effects on the Medications (20)

A. The client was educated about lifestyle habits (e.g., tobacco use, diet) that can be modified to decrease the side effects of the medications.

B. The client displayed an understanding of the effects of his/her lifestyle habits on the efficacy of his/her medications and was provided with positive feedback.

C. The client has made substantial changes in his/her lifestyle habits, which have increased the efficacy of his/her medications, and this was reinforced.

D. The client has failed to make any lifestyle changes to assist with medication efficacy and was redirected to do so.

21. Coordinate Dosing in Ranges to Facilitate Client Control (21)

A. The client's prescribing physician was approached regarding writing dosages to be within a certain range, when possible, in order to increase the client's authority over his/her own medication regimen.

B. In an effort to increase the client's authority over and investment in the medication process, the physician has written orders so that the client can make minimal modifications in his/her medications, in consultation with the clinician.

C. The client's authority over his/her own regimen of medications was emphasized.

D. The client described increased investment in and authority over his/her medication process as he/she has been allowed to vary his/her medications within the confines of the physician's order, and this was reinforced.

E. The client was assisted in learning how to vary his/her medications within the prescribed dosage range, depending on his/her own daily needs.

F. The client does not display increased investment in the medication process, despite being provided with an increased allowance to modify his/her medications, and this was reflected to him/her.

22. Assess Ability to Administer Medications (22)

A. The client's ability to properly self-administer medications was assessed.

B. The client displayed the ability to self-administer medications and was provided with this authority over his/her own medications.

C. The client was judged to be unable to self-administer his/her medications; therefore, appropriate supervision was arranged.

23. Recruit Support Network to Administer Medications (23)

A. An appropriate authorization to release confidential information was obtained from the client in order to recruit members of his/her support network to administer medications to him/her.

B. Specific members of the client's support network have agreed to administer medications to him/her, and the benefits of this were reviewed.

C. No specific individuals from within the client's support network will agree to administer medications to him/her, so alternative supports were recruited.

24. Arrange Daily Medication Drop-Offs (24)

A. Daily medication drop-offs were arranged, with instructions for the client on which dosages to take at each time of day.

B. The client has been more regular with his/her medications as a result of the daily medication drop-offs, and the benefits were reflected to him/her.

C. The client continues to take medication on a sporadic basis, despite daily medication drop-offs; redirection was provided on this practice.

25. Encourage a Consistent Place and Time for Taking Medications (25)

A. The client was encouraged to take his/her medications at a specific, consistent place and time every day.

B. The client was encouraged for his/her use of a specific, consistent place and time for taking his/her medications.

C. The client continues to take his/her medications on a sporadic basis and was provided with additional encouragement to be more consistent.

26. Arrange Prescription Distribution in a Compartmentalized Medication Box (26)

A. Arrangements were made for the client's prescriptions to be distributed in a multidose, compartmentalized daily medication box.

B. The client was monitored for his/her accurate usage of the compartmentalized daily medication box.

C. The client was reinforced for the appropriate use of the compartmentalized daily medication box.

D. The client has failed to properly take his/her medications, despite the use of a compartmentalized daily medication box, and this was reflected to him/her.

27. Monitor Expected Use of Medications (27)

A. The number of pills left in the client's prescription of psychotropic medications was counted and compared with the expected amount that should remain.

B. Discrepancies within the expected and actual amounts of the medications remaining were reviewed with the client and medical staff.

C. The client's remaining medications correspond with the amount expected to remain, and this was reviewed with him/her.

28. Coordinate All Prescriptions from One Pharmacy (28)

A. Arrangements were made to transfer all of the client's prescriptions, including nonpsychiatric medications, to one pharmacy.

B. The client's variety of prescribing clinicians were requested to use the same pharmacy for all of his/her prescriptions.

C. The client described that he/she finds it easier to obtain all of his/her medications from the same pharmacy, and the benefits of this simplified process were reviewed.

29. Coordinate Family/Couple's Therapy (29)

A. Conjoint sessions with the client's significant other and other family members were coordinated to promote an understanding of his/her illness and the impact of the illness on his/her and the family's needs.

B. The client's family members were supported for participating in the conjoint sessions and increasing their understanding of his/her illness and the impact on his/her and the family's needs.

C. The client reported an increased understanding from his/her significant other or family members subsequent to conjoint sessions and was urged to allow family members to assist him/her in his/her medication management.

D. The client, his/her significant other, and other family members have not regularly participated in conjoint sessions and were redirected to do so.

30. Train the Support Network in Medication Management (30)

A. The client's family members, peers, and others in his/her support network were trained in the proper use and administration of medications.

B. The client's support network was directed to encourage and reinforce him/her when he/she complies with his/her medication regimen.

C. The client's support system has been more involved in helping him/her manage his/her medications, and the effects of this were processed with him/her.

D. The client's support network has not been regularly involved with his/her medication management, despite training and encouragement, and they were encouraged again to provide support in this area.

31. Coordinate Family Transportation for Client (31)

A. Family members were asked to provide the client with transportation to the clinic or pharmacy.

B. Family members have regularly provided the client with transportation to the clinic or pharmacy and were encouraged to continue this.

C. Family members have not regularly coordinated transportation for the client and were urged to become more consistent in this area.

32. Process Social Concerns Regarding Medications (32)

A. The client was requested to identify social concerns that he/she may experience regarding medication uses (e.g., stigmatization and loss of independence).

B. The client identified his/her social concerns related to medication usage, and these were processed to resolution.

C. The client failed to identify his/her social or emotional concerns that affect his/her medication usage and was provided with common concerns that others have experienced, including stigmatization or loss of independence.

33. Advocate for Less Complicated Dosing Times (33)

A. Advocacy was provided to the client's physician for less complicated dosing times for his/her medications.

B. The client's physician has agreed to use less complicated dosing times for his/her medications.

C. The client's physician has not agreed to less complicated dosing times for the client's medications, despite advocacy.

34. Explore Substance Use (34)

A. The client was assessed for substance abuse that may affect his/her medication efficacy.

B. The client was identified as having a concomitant substance abuse problem.

C. Upon review, the client does not display evidence of a substance abuse problem.

35. Educate about Substance Abuse (35)

A. The client was educated about the negative effects of substance abuse on his/her symptoms.

B. The client was educated about the depotentiating effects of mood-altering substances on his/her medications.

C. The client was provided with positive feedback regarding his/her understanding of the effects of mood-altering substance use on his/her medications.

D. The client continues to use substances despite the effects on his/her symptoms and medication efficacy and was provided with additional confrontation in this area.

36. Refer for Substance Abuse Treatment (36)

A. The client was referred to a 12-step recovery program (e.g., Alcoholics Anonymous or Narcotics Anonymous).

B. The client was referred to a substance abuse treatment program.

C. The client has been admitted to a substance abuse treatment program and was supported for this follow-through.

D. The client has refused the referral to a substance abuse treatment program, and this refusal was processed.

37. Process Improvement Due to Medications (37)

A. The client was requested to identify how his/her reduction in mental illness symptoms has improved his/her social or family system.

B. The client identified ways in which his/her mental illness symptoms have decreased and how this has improved his/her social and family relationships, and he/she was provided with positive feedback in this area.

C. The client failed to identify ways in which his/her medications have improved his/her symptoms and relationships and was provided with examples of these changes.

OBSESSIVE-COMPULSIVE DISORDER (OCD)

CLIENT PRESENTATION

1. Recurrent/Persistent Thoughts (1)*

A. The client described recurrent and persistent thoughts or impulses that are viewed as senseless, intrusive, and time consuming and that interfere with his/her daily routine.

B. The intensity of the recurrent and persistent thoughts and impulses is so severe that the client is unable to efficiently perform daily duties or interact in social relationships.

C. The strength of the client's obsessive thoughts has diminished, and he/she has become more efficient in his/her daily routine.

D. The client reported that the obsessive thoughts are under significant control and he/she is able to focus attention and effort on the task at hand.

2. Failed Control Attempts (2)

A. The client reported failure at attempts to control or ignore his/her obsessive thoughts or impulses.

B. The client described many different failed attempts at learning to control or ignore his/her obsessions.

C. The client is beginning to experience some success at controlling and ignoring his/her obsessive thoughts and impulses.

3. Recognize Internal Source of Obsessions (3)

A. The client has a poor understanding that his/her obsessive thoughts are a product of his/her own mind.

B. The client reported that he/she recognizes the obsessive thoughts are a product of his/her own mind and are not coming from some outside source or power.

C. The client acknowledged that the obsessive thoughts are related to anxiety and are not a sign of any psychotic process.

4. Compulsive Behaviors (4)

A. The client described repetitive and intentional behaviors that are performed in a ritualistic fashion.

B. The client's compulsive behavior pattern follows rigid rules and has many repetitions to it.

C. The repetitive and intentional behaviors of the client are performed in response to obsessive thoughts.

D. The client's repetitive and compulsive behavior is engaged in to prevent some dreaded situation from occurring, which the client is often not able to define clearly.

E. The client's repetitive and compulsive behavior rituals are not connected in any realistic way with what the client is trying to prevent or neutralize.

---

* The numbers in parentheses correlate to the number of the Behavioral Definition statement in the companion chapter with the same title in *The Severe and Persistent Mental Illness Treatment Planner,* 2nd ed. (Berghuis and Jongsma) by John Wiley & Sons, 2008.

F. The client's anxiety over some dreaded event has diminished significantly, and his/her compulsive rituals have also decreased in frequency.

G. The client has not engaged in any ritualistic behaviors designed to prevent some dreaded situation.

5. Compulsions Seen as Unreasonable (5)

A. The client acknowledged that his/her repetitive and compulsive behaviors are excessive and unreasonable.

B. The client's recognition of his/her compulsive behaviors as excessive and unreasonable has provided good motivation for cooperation with treatment and follow-through on attempt to change.

INTERVENTIONS IMPLEMENTED

1. Develop Trust (1)*

A. Today's clinical contact focused on building the level of trust with the client through consistent eye contact, active listening, unconditional positive regard, and warm acceptance.

B. Empathy and support were provided for the client's expression of thoughts and feelings during today's clinical contact.

C. The client was provided with support and feedback as he/she described his/her maladaptive pattern of anxiety.

D. As the client has remained mistrustful and reluctant to share his/her underlying thoughts and feelings, he/she was provided with additional reassurance.

E. The client verbally recognized that he/she has difficulty establishing trust because he/she has often felt let down by others in the past, and he/she was accepted for this insight.

2. Assess OCD History (2)

A. Active listening was used as the client described the nature, history, and severity of his/her obsessive thoughts and compulsive behaviors.

B. Through a clinical interview, the client described a severe degree of interference in his/her daily routine and ability to perform a task efficiently because of the significant problem with obsessive thoughts and compulsive behaviors.

C. *The Anxiety Disorder's Interview Schedule for DSM-IV* (DiNardo, Brown, and Barlow) was used to assess the client's frequency, intensity, duration, and history of obsessions and compulsions.

D. The client was noted to have made many attempts to ignore or control the compulsive behaviors and obsessive thoughts, but without any consistent success.

E. It was noted that the client gave evidence of compulsive behaviors within the interview.

---

* The numbers in parentheses correlate to the number of the Therapeutic Intervention statement in the companion chapter with the same title in *The Severe and Persistent Mental Illness Treatment Planner,* 2nd ed. (Berghuis and Jongsma) by John Wiley & Sons, 2008.

3. Conduct Psychological Testing (3)

A. Psychological testing was administered to evaluate the nature and severity of the client's obsessive-compulsive problem.

B. *The Yale-Brown Obsessive-Compulsive Scale* (Goodman and colleagues) was used to assess the depth and breadth of the client's OCD symptoms.

C. The psychological testing results indicate that the client experiences significant interference in his/her daily life from obsessive-compulsive rituals.

D. The psychological testing indicated a rather mild degree of Obsessive-Compulsive Disorder within the client.

E. The results of the psychological testing were interpreted to the client.

4. Refer for Physical Evaluation (4)

A. The client was referred to a physician to undergo a thorough examination to rule out any medical etiologies for anger outbursts and to receive recommendations for further treatment options.

B. The client has followed through on the physician evaluation referral and specific medical etiologies for anger outbursts were reviewed.

C. The client was supported as he/she is seeking medical treatment that may decrease his/her anger outbursts.

D. The client has followed through on the physician evaluation referral but no specific medical etiologies for anger outbursts have been identified.

E. The client declined evaluation by a physician for a prescription of psychotropic medication, and was redirected to cooperate with this referral.

5. Follow Up on Physical Evaluation Recommendations (5)

A. The client was supported in following up on the recommendations from the medical evaluation.

B. The client's follow-up on the recommendations from the medical evaluation has been monitored.

C. The client has been following up on the recommendations from the medical evaluation, and the benefits and trials of this were reviewed.

D. The client has not regularly followed up on his/her medical evaluation recommendations, and was redirected to do so.

6. Review Psychoactive Chemicals (6)

A. The client's use of psychoactive chemicals, such as nicotine, caffeine, alcohol, or street drugs was reviewed.

B. The client's pattern of psychoactive chemical use was connected to his/her symptoms.

C. The client was supported as he/she identified that his/her psychoactive chemical use is affecting his/her anxiety symptoms.

D. As the client has decreased his/her psychoactive chemical use, anxiety symptoms have been noted to decrease as well.

E. The client denies any connection between his/her psychoactive chemical use and his/her anxiety symptoms and has continued to utilize psychoactive chemicals, despite encouragement to discontinue this.

7. Recommend Substance Abuse Evaluation and/or Termination (7)

A. It was recommended to the client that he/she terminate the consumption of substances that could contribute to anxiety.

B. The client was referred for a substance abuse evaluation to more completely assess his/her substance abuse concerns and how they may trigger anxiety.

C. The client was referred for substance abuse treatment to assist him/her in discontinuing his/her consumption of substances.

D. As the client has decreased his/her use of trigger substances, he/she has experienced a decrease in anxiety, and this was reviewed.

E. The client has declined any evaluation or treatment related to his/her substance use, and was encouraged to seek this out at a later time.

8. Differentiate Anxiety Symptoms (8)

A. The client was assisted in differentiating anxiety symptoms that are a direct affect of his/her severe and persistent mental illness, as opposed to a separate diagnosis of an anxiety disorder.

B. The client was provided with feedback regarding his/her differentiation of symptoms that are related to his/her severe and persistent mental illness, as opposed to a separate diagnosis.

C. The client has identified a specific anxiety disorder, which is freestanding from his/her severe and persistent mental illness, and this was reviewed within the session.

D. The client has been unsuccessful in identifying ways in which his/her anxiety symptoms are related to his/her mental illness versus a separate anxiety disorder and was provided with some examples of each area.

9. Acknowledge Anxiety Related to Delusional Experiences (9)

A. It was acknowledged that both real and delusional experiences could cause anxiety.

B. The client was provided with support regarding his/her anxieties and worries, which are related to both the real experiences and delusional experiences.

C. The client described a decreased pattern of anxiety due to the support provided to him/her.

10. Identify Diagnostic Classification (10)

A. The client was assisted in identifying a specific diagnostic classification for his/her anxiety symptoms.

B. Utilizing a description of anxiety symptoms such as that found in Bourne's *The Anxiety and Phobia Workbook,* the client was taken through a detailed review of his/her anxiety symptoms, diagnosis, and treatment needs.

C. The client has failed to clearly understand and classify his/her anxiety symptoms and was given additional feedback in this area.

11. Refer to Physician (11)

A. A referral to a physician was made for the purpose of evaluating the client for a prescription of psychotropic medications.

B. The client was reinforced for following through on a referral to a physician for an assessment for a prescription of psychotropic medications, but none were prescribed.

C. The client has been prescribed psychotropic medications.

D. The client declined evaluation by a physician for a prescription of psychotropic medication, and was redirected to cooperate with this referral.

12. Educate about Psychotropic Medication (12)

A. The client was taught about the indications for and the expected benefits of psychotropic medications.

B. As the client's psychotropic medications were reviewed, he/she displayed an understanding about the indications for and expected benefits of the medication.

C. The client displayed a lack of understanding of the indications for and expected benefits of psychotropic medications and was provided with additional information and feedback regarding his/her medications.

13. Monitor Medications (13)

A. The client was monitored for compliance with his/her psychotropic medication regimen.

B. The client was provided with positive feedback about his/her regular use of psychotropic medication.

C. The client was monitored for the effectiveness and side effects of his/her prescribed medications.

D. Concerns about the client's medication effectiveness and side effects were communicated to the physician.

E. Although the client was monitored for medication side effects, he/she reported no concerns in this area.

14. Enroll in Group Therapy (14)

A. The client was enrolled in intensive (e.g., daily) group therapy for exposure and ritual prevention.

B. The client was enrolled in a nonintensive (e.g., weekly) group for exposure and ritual prevention therapy.

C. The client was enrolled in a small (closed enrollment) group for exposure and ritual prevention for OCD, as described in *Obsessive-Compulsive Disorder* (Foa and Franklin).

D. The client has been enrolled in group therapy; the benefits of this program were reviewed.

E. The client has not participated in group therapy, and the barriers to this treatment were reviewed.

15. Assign Reading Materials (15)

A. The client was assigned to read psychoeducational chapters of books or treatment manuals on the rationale for exposure and ritual prevention therapy.

B. The client was assigned to read psychoeducational chapters of books or treatment manuals for the rationale for cognitive restructuring for OCD.

C. The client was assigned to read information from *Mastery of Obsessive-Compulsive Disorder* (Kozak and Foa).

D. The client was assigned to read information from *Stop Obsessing* (Foa and Wilson).

E. The client has read the assigned material on the rationale for OCD treatment; key points were reviewed.

F. The client has not read the assigned information on the rationale for OCD treatment and was redirected to do so.

16. Discuss Usefulness of Treatment (16)

A. A discussion was held about how treatment serves as an arena to desensitize learned fear, reality test obsessional fears and underlying beliefs, and build confidence in managing fears without compulsions.

B. The client was provided with a rationale for treatment as described in *Mastery of Obsessive-Compulsive Disorder* (Kozak and Foa).

C. Positive feedback was provided to the client as he/she displayed a clear understanding about the usefulness of treatment.

D. The client did not display a clear understanding of the usefulness of treatment and was provided with additional feedback in this area.

17. Explore Schema and Self-Talk (17)

A. The client was assisted in exploring how his/her schema and self-talk mediate his/her obsessional fears and compulsive behaviors.

B. The client's schema and self-talk were reviewed as described in *Mastery of Obsessive-Compulsive Disorder* (Kozak and Foa).

C. The client's schema and self-talk were reviewed as described in *Obsessive-Compulsive Disorder* (Salkovskis and Kirk).

D. The client was reinforced for his/her insight into his/her self-talk and schema that support his/her obsessional fears and compulsive behaviors.

E. The client struggled to develop insight into his/her own self-talk and schema and was provided with tentative examples of these concepts.

18. Teach Thought-Stopping Techniques (18)

A. The client was taught to interrupt obsessive thoughts by shouting "STOP" to himself/herself silently while picturing a red traffic signal and then thinking about a calming scene.

B. The client was assisted in developing his/her own thought-stopping techniques and images.

C. Positive feedback was provided to the client for his/her helpful use of thought-stopping techniques.

D. The client does not regularly use thought-stopping techniques and was redirected to do so.

19. Assign Thought-Stopping Techniques between Sessions (19)

A. The client was assigned the use of thought-stopping techniques on a daily basis between sessions.

B. The client was assigned "Making Use of the Thought-Stopping Technique" from the *Adult Psychotherapy Homework Planner,* 2nd ed. (Jongsma).

C. The client's implementation of thought-stopping techniques was reviewed and successes were reinforced.

D. The client's use of thought-stopping techniques was reviewed; successes were reinforced and failures were redirected.

20. Assess Cues (20)

A. The client was assessed in regard to the nature of any external cues (e.g., persons, objects, situations) that precipitate the client's obsessions and compulsions.

B. The client was assessed in regard to the nature of any internal cues (e.g., thoughts, images, impulses) that precipitate the client's obsessions and compulsions.

C. The client was provided with feedback about his/her identification of cues.

21. Construct a Hierarchy of Fear Cues (21)

A. The client was directed to construct a hierarchy of feared internal and external cues.

B. The client was assisted in developing a hierarchy of internal and external fear cues.

22. Select Likely Successful Imaginal Exposure (22)

A. The client was assisted in identifying initial imaginal exposures with a bias toward those that have a likelihood of being successful experiences for the client.

B. Cognitive restructuring techniques were used within and after the imaginal exposure of the OCD cues.

C. Imaginal exposure and cognitive restructuring techniques were used as described in *Mastery of Obsessive-Compulsive Disorder* (Kozak and Foa).

D. Imaginal exposure and cognitive restructuring techniques were used as described in *Treatment of Obsessive-Compulsive Disorder* (McGran and Sanderson).

E. The client was provided with feedback about his/her use of imaginal exposures.

23. Assign Cue Exposure Practice (23)

A. The client was assigned a homework exercise in which he/she repeats the exposure to the internal and/or external OCD cues.

B. The client was instructed to use restructured cognitions between sessions and to record his/her responses.

C. The client was assigned to use "Reducing the Strength of Compulsive Behaviors" from the *Adult Psychotherapy Homework Planner,* 2nd ed. (Jongsma).

D. The client's use of the cue exposure homework was reviewed and his/her success was reinforced.

E. Corrective feedback was provided to the client for his/her struggles in using restructured cognitions during exposure to OCD cues.

F. The client was assisted in using restructured cognitions as described in *Mastery of Obsessive-Compulsive Disorder* (Kozak and Foa).

24. Differentiate between Lapse and Relapse (24)

A. A discussion was held with the client regarding the distinction between a lapse and a relapse.

B. A lapse was associated with an initial and reversible return of symptoms, fear, or urges to avoid.

C. A relapse was associated with the decision to return to fearful and avoidant patterns.

D. The client was provided with support and encouragement as he/she displayed an understanding of the difference between a lapse and a relapse.

25. Discuss Management of Lapse Risk Situations (25)

A. The client was assisted in identifying future situations or circumstances in which lapses could occur.

B. The session focused on rehearsing the management of future situations or circumstances in which lapses could occur.

C. The client was reinforced for his/her appropriate use of lapse management skills.

D. The client was redirected in regard to his/her poor use of lapse management skills.

26. Encourage Routine Use of Strategies (26)

A. The client was instructed to routinely use the strategies that he/she has learned in therapy (e.g., cognitive restructuring, exposure).

B. The client was urged to find ways to build his/her new strategies into his/her life as much as possible.

C. The client was reinforced as he/she reported ways in which he/she has incorporated coping strategies into his/her life and routine.

D. The client was redirected about ways to incorporate his/her new strategies into his/her routine and life.

27. Schedule Maintenance Sessions (27)

A. Maintenance sessions were proposed to help maintain therapeutic gains and adjust to life without anger outbursts.

B. The client was reinforced for agreeing to the scheduled maintenance sessions.

C. The client refused to schedule maintenance sessions, and this was processed.

28. Enlist Support System (28)

A. The client's support system was enlisted in the implementation of specific stress reduction techniques.

B. The client's support system was enthusiastic and supportive of the client's stress reduction techniques, and the client was encouraged to utilize this support on a regular basis.

C. The client's support system has declined significant involvement in helping the client to implement specific stress reduction techniques, so alternative means of development support for stress reduction were developed.

D. The client has declined support from his/her family, friends, and caretakers and was urged to utilize this support.

29. Explore Unresolved Conflicts (29)

A. As the client's unresolved life conflicts were explored, he/she verbalized and clarified feelings connected to those conflicts.

B. The client was supported as he/she identified key life conflicts that raise his/her anxiety level and intensify the OCD symptoms.

C. As the client was helped to clarify and share his/her feelings regarding current unresolved life conflicts, his/her level of anxiety diminished and the OCD symptoms were reduced.

D. The client has been guarded about his/her feelings regarding current life conflicts and was encouraged to be more open in this area.

30. Encourage Feelings Sharing (30)

A. The client was encouraged, supported, and assisted in identifying and expressing feelings related to key unresolved life issues.

B. As the client shared his/her feelings regarding life issues, he/she reported a decreased level of emotional intensity around these issues; he/she was reinforced for this progress.

C. It was difficult for the client to get in touch with, clarify, and express emotions, as his/her pattern is to detach himself/herself from feelings; this pattern was reflected to the client.

31. Assign Ericksonian Task (31)

A. The client was assigned an Ericksonian task of performing a behavior that is centered around the obsession or compulsion instead of trying to avoid it.

B. As the client has faced the issue directly and performed a task, bringing feelings to the surface, the results of this were processed.

C. As the client has processed his/her feelings regarding the anxiety-provoking issue, the intensity of those feelings has been noted to be diminishing.

D. The client has not used the Ericksonian task and was redirected to do so.

32. Develop Ritual Interruption (32)

A. The client was helped to develop a ritual of a very unpleasant task that he/she agrees to perform each time he/she experiences obsessive thoughts.

B. The client has begun to implement the distasteful ritual at the times of experiencing obsessive thoughts; his/her experience was reviewed.

C. The client reports that engaging in the distasteful ritual has interrupted the obsessive thoughts and the current pattern of compulsion; his/her progress was reinforced.

D. The client has not used the ritual interruption technique and was reminded to use this helpful technique.

PANIC/AGORAPHOBIA

CLIENT PRESENTATION

1. Severe Panic Symptoms (1)*

A. The client has experienced sudden and unexpected severe panic symptoms that have occurred repeatedly and have resulted in persistent concern about additional attacks.

B. The client has significantly modified his/her normal behavior patterns in an effort to avoid panic attacks.

C. The frequency and severity of the panic attacks have diminished significantly.

D. The client reported that he/she has not experienced any recent panic attack symptoms.

2. Fear of Environmental Situations Triggering Anxiety (2)

A. The client described fear of environmental situations that he/she believes may trigger intense anxiety symptoms.

B. The client's fear of environmental situations has resulted in his/her avoidance behavior directed toward those environmental situations.

C. The client has a significant fear of leaving home and being in open or crowded public situations.

D. The client's phobic fear has diminished, and he/she has left the home environment without being crippled by anxiety.

E. The client is able to leave home normally and function within public environments.

3. Recognition That Fear Is Unreasonable (3)

A. The client's phobic fear has persisted in spite of the fact that he/she acknowledges that the fear is unreasonable.

B. The client has made many attempts to ignore or overcome his/her unreasonable fear, but has been unsuccessful.

4. Increasing Isolation (4)

A. The client described situations in which he/she has declined involvement with others due to a fear of traveling or leaving a safe environment, such as his/her home.

B. The client reported that he/she has become increasingly isolated due to his/her fear of traveling or leaving a safe environment.

C. The client has severely constricted his/her involvement with others.

D. Although the client experiences some symptoms of panic, he/she still feels capable of leaving home.

E. The client has been able to leave his/her safe environment on a regular basis.

---

* The numbers in parentheses correlate to the number of the Behavioral Definition statement in the companion chapter with the same title in *The Severe and Persistent Mental Illness Treatment Planner,* 2nd ed. (Berghuis and Jongsma) by John Wiley & Sons, 2008.

5. Avoids Public Places and Large Groups (5)

A. The client avoids public places, such as malls or large stores.

B. The client avoids large groups of people.

C. The client has constricted his/her involvement with others in order to avoid social situations.

D. The client has begun to reach out socially and feels more comfortable in public places or with large groups of people.

E. The client reported enjoying involvement with large groups of people and feels comfortable going to public places.

6. Panic without Agoraphobia (6)

A. The client does not display evidence of Agoraphobia.

B. Although the client experiences symptoms of panic, he/she still feels capable of leaving home.

INTERVENTIONS IMPLEMENTED

1. Develop Trust (1)*

A. Today's clinical contact focused on building the level of trust with the client through consistent eye contact, active listening, unconditional positive regard, and warm acceptance.

B. Empathy and support were provided for the client's expression of thoughts and feelings during today's clinical contact.

C. The client was provided with support and feedback as he/she described his/her maladaptive pattern of anxiety.

D. As the client has remained mistrustful and reluctant to share his/her underlying thoughts and feelings, he/she was provided with additional reassurance.

E. The client verbally recognized that he/she has difficulty establishing trust because he/she has often felt let down by others in the past and was accepted for this insight.

2. Assess Nature of Panic Symptoms (2)

A. The client was asked about the frequency, intensity, duration, and history of his/her panic symptoms, fear, and avoidance.

B. *The Anxiety Disorder's Interview Schedule for DSM-IV* (DiNardo, Brown, and Barlow) was used to assess the client's panic symptoms.

C. The assessment of the client's panic symptoms indicated that his/her symptoms are extreme and severely interfere with his/her life.

D. The assessment of the client's panic symptoms indicates that these symptoms are moderate and occasionally interfere with his/her daily functioning.

E. The results of the assessment of the client's panic symptoms indicate that these symptoms are mild and rarely interfere with his/her daily functioning.

F. The results of the assessment of the client's panic symptoms were reviewed with the client.

---

* The numbers in parentheses correlate to the number of the Therapeutic Intervention statement in the companion chapter with the same title in *The Severe and Persistent Mental Illness Treatment Planner,* 2nd ed. (Berghuis and Jongsma) by John Wiley & Sons, 2008.

3. Explore Panic Stimulus Situations (3)

A. The client was assisted in identifying specific stimulus situations that precipitate panic symptoms.

B. The client could not describe any specific stimulus situations that produce panic; he/she was helped to identify that they occur unexpectedly and without any pattern.

C. The client was helped to identify that his/her panic symptoms occur when he/she leaves the confines of his/her home environment and enters public situations where there are many people.

4. Administer Assessments for Agoraphobia Symptoms (4)

A. The client was administered psychological instruments designed to objectively assess his/her level of Agoraphobia symptoms.

B. The client administered *The Mobility Inventory for Agoraphobia* (Chambless, Coputo, and Gracely).

C. The client was provided with feedback regarding the results of the assessment of his/her level of Agoraphobia symptoms.

D. The client declined to participate in the objective assessment of his/her level of Agoraphobia symptoms, and this resistance was processed.

5. Administer Assessments for Anxiety Symptoms (5)

A. The client was administered psychological instruments designed to objectively assess his/her level of anxiety symptoms.

B. The client was administered *The Anxiety Sensitivity Index* (Reiss, Peterson, and Grusky).

C. The client was provided with feedback regarding the results of the assessment of his/her level of anxiety symptoms.

D. The client declined to participate in the objective assessment of his/her level of anxiety symptoms, and this resistance was processed.

6. Refer for Physical Evaluation (6)

A. The client was referred to a physician to undergo a thorough examination to rule out any medical etiologies for his/her anxiety symptoms and to receive recommendations for further treatment options.

B. The client has followed through on the physician evaluation referral and specific medical etiologies for anxiety symptoms were reviewed.

C. The client was supported as he/she is seeking out medical treatment that may decrease his/her anxiety symptoms.

D. The client has followed through on the physician evaluation referral but no specific medical etiologies for anxiety symptoms have been identified.

E. The client declined evaluation by a physician for a prescription of psychotropic medication and was redirected to cooperate with this referral.

7. Follow Up on Physical Evaluation Recommendations (7)

A. The client was supported in following up on the recommendations from the medical evaluation.

B. The client's follow-up on the recommendations from the medical evaluation has been monitored.

C. The client has been following up on the recommendations from the medical evaluation.

D. The client has not regularly followed up on his/her medical evaluation recommendations and was redirected to do so.

8. Review Psychoactive Chemicals (8)

A. The client's use of psychoactive chemicals, such as nicotine, caffeine, alcohol, or street drugs was reviewed.

B. The client's pattern of psychoactive chemical use was connected to his/her symptoms.

C. The client was supported as he/she identified that his/her psychoactive chemical use is affecting his/her anxiety symptoms.

D. As the client has decreased his/her psychoactive chemical use, anxiety symptoms have been noted to decrease as well.

E. The client denies any connection between his/her psychoactive chemical use and his/her anxiety symptoms and has continued to utilize psychoactive chemicals, despite encouragement to discontinue this.

9. Recommend Substance Abuse Evaluation and/or Termination (9)

A. It was recommended to the client that he/she terminate the consumption of substances that could contribute to anxiety.

B. The client was referred for a substance abuse evaluation to more completely assess his/her substance abuse concerns and how they may trigger anxiety.

C. The client was referred for substance abuse treatment to assist him/her in discontinuing his/her consumption of substances.

D. As the client has decreased his/her use of trigger substances, he/she has experienced a decrease in anxiety, and this was reviewed.

E. The client has declined any evaluation or treatment related to his/her substance use and was encouraged to seek this out at a later time.

10. Differentiate Anxiety Symptoms (10)

A. The client was assisted in differentiating anxiety symptoms that are a direct affect of his/her severe and persistent mental illness, as opposed to a separate diagnosis of an anxiety disorder.

B. The client was provided with feedback regarding his/her differentiation of symptoms that are related to his/her severe and persistent mental illness, as opposed to a separate diagnosis.

C. The client has identified a specific anxiety disorder, which is freestanding from his/her severe and persistent mental illness, and this was reviewed within the session.

D. The client has been unsuccessful in identifying ways in which his/her anxiety symptoms are related to his/her mental illness or a separate anxiety disorder.

11. Acknowledge Anxiety Related to Delusional Experiences (11)

A. It was acknowledged that both real and delusional experiences could cause anxiety.

B. The client was provided with support regarding his/her anxieties and worries, which are related to both the real experiences and delusional experiences.

C. The client described a decreased pattern of anxiety due to the support provided to him/her.

12. Identify Diagnostic Classification (12)

A. The client was assisted in identifying a specific diagnostic classification for his/her anxiety symptoms.

B. Utilizing a description of anxiety symptoms such as that found in Bourne's *The Anxiety and Phobia Workbook,* the client was taken through a detailed review of his/her anxiety symptoms, diagnosis, and treatment needs.

C. The client has failed to clearly understand and classify his/her anxiety symptoms and was given additional feedback in this area.

13. Refer to Physician (13)

A. A referral to a physician was made for the purpose of evaluating the client for a prescription of psychotropic medications.

B. The client was reinforced for following through on a referral to a physician for an assessment for a prescription of psychotropic medications, but none were prescribed.

C. The client has been prescribed psychotropic medications.

D. The client declined evaluation by a physician for a prescription of psychotropic medication and was redirected to cooperate with this referral.

14. Educate about Psychotropic Medication (14)

A. The client was taught about the indications for and the expected benefits of psychotropic medications.

B. As the client's psychotropic medications were reviewed, he/she displayed an understanding about the indications for and expected benefits of the medication.

C. The client displayed a lack of understanding of the indications for and expected benefits of psychotropic medications and was provided with additional information and feedback regarding his/her medications.

15. Monitor Medications (15)

A. The client was monitored for compliance with his/her psychotropic medication regimen.

B. The client was provided with positive feedback about his/her regular use of psychotropic medication.

C. The client was monitored for the effectiveness and side effects of his/her prescribed medications.

D. Concerns about the client's medication effectiveness and side effects were communicated to the physician.

E. Although the client was monitored for medication side effects, he/she reported no concerns in this area.

16. Discuss Nature of Panic Symptoms (16)

A. A discussion was held about how panic attacks are "false alarms" of danger, but are not medically dangerous.

B. A discussion was held about how panic attacks are not a sign of weakness or craziness.

C. The client's panic attacks were discussed, including how they are a common symptom but can lead to unnecessary avoidance, thereby reinforcing the panic attack.

17. Assign Information on Panic Disorders and Agoraphobia (17)

A. The client was assigned to read psychoeducational chapters of books or treatment manuals about Panic Disorders and Agoraphobia.

B. The client was assigned specific chapters from *Mastery of Your Anxiety and Panic* (Barlow and Craske).

C. The client was assigned to read chapters from *Don't Panic: Taking Control of Anxiety Attacks* (Wilson).

D. The client was assigned to read *Living with Fear* (Marks).

E. The client has read the assigned information on Panic Disorders and Agoraphobia, and key points were discussed.

F. The client has not read the assigned information on Panic Disorders and Agoraphobia and was redirected to do so.

18. Discuss Benefits of Exposure (18)

A. The client was taught about how exposure can serve as an arena to desensitize learned fear, build confidence, and create success experiences.

B. A discussion was held about the use of exposure to decrease fear, build confidence, and feel safer.

C. The client was reinforced as he/she indicated a clear understanding of how exposure can help to conquer panic and Agoraphobia symptoms.

D. The client did not display understanding about how exposure can help overcome his/her Agoraphobia and panic symptoms and was provided with remedial feedback in this area.

19. Assign Reading on Exposure (19)

A. The client was assigned to read about exposure in books or treatment manuals on social anxiety.

B. The client was assigned to read excerpts from *Mastery of Your Anxiety and Panic* (Barlow and Craske).

C. The client was assigned portions of *Living with Fear* (Marks).

D. The client's information about exposure was reviewed and processed.

E. The client has not read the information on exposure and was redirected to do so.

20. Train about Coping Strategies (20)

A. The client was taught progressive relaxation methods and debriefing exercises.

B. The client was trained in the use of coping strategies to manage symptoms of panic attacks.

C. The client was taught coping strategies such as staying focused on behavioral goals, muscular relaxation, evenly paced diaphragmatic breathing, and positive self-talk in order to manage his/her symptoms.

D. The client has become proficient in coping techniques for his/her panic attacks; he/she was reinforced for the regular use of these techniques.

E. The client has not regularly used coping techniques for panic attacks and was provided with additional training in this area.

21. Urge External Focus (21)

A. The client was urged to keep his/her focus on external stimuli and behavioral responsibilities rather than be preoccupied with internal states and physiological changes.

B. The client was reinforced as he/she had made a commitment to not allow panic symptoms to take control of his/her life and to not avoid and escape normal responsibilities and activities.

C. The client has been successful at turning his/her focus away from internal anxiety states and toward behavioral responsibilities; he/she was reinforced for this progress.

D. The client has not maintained an external focus in order to keep panic symptoms from taking control of his/her life and was reminded about this helpful technique.

22. Assign Information on Breathing and Relaxation (22)

A. The client was assigned to read information about progressive muscle relaxation.

B. The client was assigned information on paced diaphragmatic breathing.

C. The client was directed to read portions of *Mastery of Your Anxiety and Panic* (Barlow and Craske).

D. The client has read the assigned information on progressive muscle relaxation and paced diaphragmatic breathing, and his/her key learnings were reviewed.

E. The client has not read the assigned information on progressive muscle relaxation and paced diaphragmatic breathing and was redirected to do so.

23. Counteract Panic Myths (23)

A. The client was consistently reassured of the fact that there is no connection between panic symptoms and heart attack, loss of control over behavior, or serious mental illness.

B. The client was reinforced as he/she verbalized an understanding that panic symptoms do not promote serious physical or mental illness.

24. Utilize Modeling/Behavioral Rehearsal (24)

A. Modeling and behavioral rehearsal were used to train the client in positive self-talk that reassured him/her of the ability to work through and endure anxiety symptoms without serious consequences.

B. The client has implemented positive self-talk to reassure himself/herself of the ability to endure anxiety without serious consequences; he/she was reinforced for this progress.

C. The client has not used positive self-talk to help endure anxiety and was provided with additional direction in this area.

25. Identify Distorted Thoughts (25)

A. The client was assisted in identifying the distorted schemas and related automatic thoughts that mediate anxiety responses.

B. The client was taught the role of distorted thinking in precipitating emotional responses.

C. The client was reinforced as he/she verbalized an understanding of the cognitive beliefs and messages that mediate his/her anxiety responses.

D. The client was assisted in replacing distorted messages with positive, realistic cognitions.

E. The client failed to identify his/her distorted thoughts and cognitions and was provided with tentative examples in this area.

26. Assign Reading Materials (26)

A. The client was assigned to read psychoeducational chapters of books or treatment manuals on cognitive restructuring.

B. The client was assigned to read psychoeducational chapters of books or treatment manuals for the rationale for cognitive restructuring for panic/Agoraphobia.

C. The client was assigned information from *Mastery of Your Anxiety and Panic* (Barlow and Craske).

D. The client has read the assigned material on cognitive restructuring; key points were reviewed.

E. The client has not read the assigned information on the rationale for panic/Agoraphobia treatment and was redirected to do so.

27. Assign Exercises on Self-Talk (27)

A. The client was assigned homework exercises in which he/she identifies fearful self-talk and creates reality-based alternatives.

B. The client was directed to do assignments from *10 Simple Solutions to Panic* (Antony and McCabe).

C. The client was directed to complete assignments from *Mastery of Your Anxiety and Panic* (Barlow and Craske).

D. The client was reinforced for his/her successes at replacing fearful self-talk with reality-based alternatives.

E. The client was provided with corrective feedback for his/her failures to replace fearful self-talk with reality-based alternatives.

F. The client has not completed his/her assigned homework regarding fearful self-talk and was redirected to do so.

28. Teach Sensation Exposure Techniques (28)

A. The client was taught about sensation exposure techniques.

B. The client was taught about generating feared physical sensations through exercise (e.g., breathing rapidly until slightly light-headed) and the use of coping strategies to keep himself/herself calm.

C. The client was assigned information about sensation exposure techniques in *10 Simple Solutions to Panic* (Antony and McCabe).

D. The client was assigned information about sensation exposure techniques in *Mastery of Your Anxiety and Panic—Therapist's Guide* (Craske, Barlow, and Meadows).

E. The client displayed a clear understanding of the sensation exposure technique and was reinforced for his/her understanding.

F. The client struggled to understand the sensation exposure technique and was provided with remedial feedback.

29. Assign Material on Sensation Exposure (29)

A. The client was assigned to read about sensation (interceptive) exposure in books or treatment manuals on Panic Disorder and Agoraphobia.

B. The client was assigned to read *Mastery of Your Anxiety and Panic* (Barlow and Craske).

C. The client was asked to read *10 Simple Solutions to Panic* (Antony and McCabe).

D. The client has read the assigned information on the sensation exposure techniques and was reinforced for his/her understanding of these concepts.

E. The client does not display an understanding of the sensation exposure technique and was provided with remedial feedback in this area.

30. Assign Homework on Sensation Exposure (30)

A. The client was assigned homework exercises to perform sensation exposure and record his/her experiences.

B. The client was assigned sensation exposure homework from *Mastery of Your Anxiety and Panic* (Barlow and Craske).

C. The client was assigned sensation exposure homework from *10 Simple Solutions to Panic* (Antony and McCabe).

D. The "Panic Attack Rating Form" from the *Adolescent Psychotherapy Homework Planner,* 2nd ed. (Jongsma, Peterson, and McInnis) was used to help the client's experiences of anxiety during sensation exposure.

E. The client's use of sensation exposure techniques was reviewed and reinforced.

F. The client has struggled in his/her implementation of sensation exposure techniques and was provided with corrective feedback.

G. The client has not attempted to use the sensation exposure techniques and was redirected to do so.

31. Construct Anxiety Stimuli Hierarchy (31)

A. The client was assisted in constructing a hierarchy of anxiety-producing situations associated with two or three spheres of worry.

B. It was difficult for the client to develop a hierarchy of stimulus situations, as the causes of his/her anxiety remains quite vague; he/she was assisted in completing the hierarchy.

C. The client was successful at creating a focused hierarchy of specific stimulus situations that provoke anxiety in a gradually increasing manner; this hierarchy was reviewed.

32. Select Initial Exposures (32)

A. Initial exposures were selected from the hierarchy of anxiety-producing situations, with a bias toward likelihood of being successful.

B. A plan was developed with the client for managing the symptoms that may occur during the initial exposure.

C. The client was assisted in rehearsing the plan for managing the exposure-related symptoms within his/her imagination.

D. Positive feedback was provided for the client's helpful use of Symptom management techniques.

E. The client was redirected for ways to improve his/her symptom management techniques.

33. Assign Information on Situational Exposure (33)

A. The client was assigned to read information about situational (exteroceptive) exposure in books or treatment manuals on Panic Disorder and Agoraphobia.

B. The client was assigned to read *Mastery of Your Anxiety and Panic* (Barlow and Craske).

C. The client was assigned to read *Living with Fear* (Marks).

D. The client has read the assigned information on situational exposure and his/her key learnings were reviewed.

E. The client has not read the assigned information on situational exposure and was redirected to do so.

34. Assign Homework on Situational Exposures (34)

A. The client was assigned homework exercises to perform situational exposures and record his/her experiences.

B. The client was assigned "Gradually Facing a Phobic Fear" from the *Adolescent Psychotherapy Homework Planner,* 2nd ed. (Jongsma, Peterson, and McInnis).

C. The client was assigned situational exposures homework from *Mastery of Your Anxiety and Panic* (Barlow and Craske).

D. The client was assigned situational exposures homework from *10 Simple Solutions to Panic* (Antony and McCabe).

E. The client's use of situational exposure techniques was reviewed and reinforced.

F. The client has struggled in his/her implementation of situational exposure techniques and was provided with corrective feedback.

G. The client has not attempted to use the situational exposure techniques and was redirected to do so.

35. Differentiate between Lapse and Relapse (35)

A. A discussion was held with the client regarding the distinction between a lapse and a relapse.

B. A lapse was associated with an initial and reversible return of symptoms, fear, or urges to avoid.

C. A relapse was associated with the decision to return to fearful and avoidant patterns.

D. The client was provided with support and encouragement as he/she displayed an understanding of the difference between a lapse and a relapse.

E. The client struggled to understand the difference between a lapse and a relapse and was provided with remedial feedback in this area.

36. Discuss Management of Lapse Risk Situations (36)

A. The client was assisted in identifying future situations or circumstances in which lapses could occur.

B. The session focused on rehearsing the management of future situations or circumstances in which lapses could occur.

C. The client was reinforced for his/her appropriate us of lapse management skills.

D. The client was redirected in regard to his/her poor use of lapse management skills.

37. Encourage Routine Use of Strategies (37)

A. The client was instructed to routinely use the strategies that he/she has learned in therapy (e.g., cognitive restructuring, exposure).

B. The client was urged to find ways to build his/her new strategies into his/her life as much as possible.

C. The client was reinforced as he/she reported ways in which he/she has incorporated coping strategies into his/her life and routine.

D. The client was redirected about ways to incorporate his/her new strategies into his/her routine and life.

38. Develop a Coping Card (38)

A. The client was provided with a coping card on which specific coping strategies were listed.

B. The client was assisted in developing his/her coping card in order to list his/her helpful coping strategies.

C. The client was encouraged to use his/her coping card when struggling with anxiety-producing situations.

39. Explore Secondary Gain (39)

A. Secondary gain was identified for the client's panic symptoms because of his/her tendency to escape or avoid certain situations.

B. The client denied any role for secondary gain that results from his/her modification of life to accommodate panic; he/she was provided with tentative examples.

C. The client was reinforced for accepting the role of secondary gain in promoting and maintaining the panic symptoms and encouraged to overcome this gain through living a more normal life.

40. Differentiate Current Fear from Past Pain (40)

A. The client was taught to verbalize the separate realities of the current fear and the emotionally painful experience from the past that has been evoked by the phobic stimulus.

B. The client was reinforced when he/she expressed insight into the unresolved fear from the past that is linked to his/her current phobic fear.

C. The irrational nature of the client's current phobic fear was emphasized and clarified.

D. The client's unresolved emotional issue from the past was clarified.

41. Encourage Sharing of Feelings (41)

A. The client was encouraged to share the emotionally painful experience from the past that has been evoked by the phobic stimulus.

B. The client was taught to separate the realities of the irrationally feared object or situation and the painful experience from his/her past.

42. Support Activity Rather than Escape (42)

A. The client was urged to engage in activities rather than escape into a pattern of avoidance.

B. The client was reinforced as he/she reviewed his/her pattern of engagement rather than escape.

C. The client continues to focus on escape and was urged to increase his/her engagement in small steps.

43. Enlist Support System (43)

A. The client's support system was enlisted in the implementation of specific stress reduction techniques.

B. The client's support system was enthusiastic and supportive of the client's stress reduction techniques, and the client was encouraged to utilize this support on a regular basis.

C. The client's support system has declined significant involvement in helping the client to implement specific stress reduction techniques, so alternative means of development support for stress reduction were developed.

D. The client has declined support from his/her family, friends, and caretakers, and was urged to utilize this support.

44. Schedule a Booster Session (44)

A. The client was scheduled for a booster session between 1 and 3 months after therapy ends.

B. The client was advised to contact the therapist if he/she needs to be seen prior to the booster session.

C. The client's booster session was held, and he/she was reinforced for his/her successful implementation of therapy techniques.

D. The client's booster session was held, and he/she was encouraged to attend further treatment, as his/her progress has not been sustained.

PARANOIA

CLIENT PRESENTATION

1. Fixed Persecutory Delusions (1)*

A. The client described a pattern of fixed persecutory delusions regarding others, their intentions, and possible harm.

B. The client described beliefs that others are persecuting him/her or intend to do him/her harm, but was unable to identify these as delusions.

C. As treatment has progressed, the client reports a decrease in persecutory thoughts.

D. The client reported that he/she now understands that his/her former persecutory beliefs were due to his/her mental illness.

2. Extreme Distrust (2)

A. The client described a pattern of consistent distrust of others generally.

B. The client described an extreme distrust of a significant other in his/her life without sufficient basis.

C. The client's level of distrust toward others has diminished.

D. The client verbalized trust in the significant other that he/she had previously held in extreme distrust.

E. The client displayed normal levels of trust toward others.

3. Expectation of Harm by Others (3)

A. The client described an expectation of being exploited or harmed by others.

B. The client displayed an animated fear of being exploited or harmed by others.

C. The client's fear of being harmed by others has diminished.

D. The client no longer holds to an irrational belief that he/she is being plotted against by others.

4. Misinterpretation of Benign Events (4)

A. The client demonstrated a pattern of misinterpretation of benign events as having threatening personal significance.

B. The client is beginning to accept a more reality-based interpretation of benign events as nonthreatening.

C. The client no longer demonstrates a pattern of misinterpretation of benign events and has verbalized not feeling personally threatened.

5. Auditory/Visual Hallucinations (5)

A. The client has experienced auditory hallucinations suggesting harm, threats to safety, or disloyalty.

---

* The numbers in parentheses correlate to the number of the Behavioral Definition statement in the companion chapter with the same title in *The Severe and Persistent Mental Illness Treatment Planner,* 2nd ed. (Berghuis and Jongsma) by John Wiley & Sons, 2008.

B. The client has experienced visual hallucinations suggesting harm, threats to safety, or disloyalty.

C. The client's hallucinations have decreased in intensity and frequency.

D. The client reported no longer experiencing hallucinations of any type.

6. Avoids Others (6)

A. The client acknowledged that he/she is inclined to keep an emotional and social distance from others for fear of being hurt or being taken advantage of by them.

B. The client is beginning to show some trust of others as demonstrated by increased social interaction.

C. The client described relationships with others that involve a degree of vulnerability and intimacy with which he/she has become comfortable.

7. Easily Offended/Quick to Anger (7)

A. The client's history is replete with incidents in which he/she has become easily offended and was quick to anger.

B. The client described a pattern of defensiveness in which he/she easily feels threatened by others and becomes angry with them.

C. The client described a pattern of projection of threatening motivations onto others to which he/she reacts with irritability, defensiveness, and anger.

D. The client has become less defensive and has not shown any recent incidents of unreasonable anger.

8. Suspicious of Treatment (8)

A. The client described irrational persecutory beliefs regarding his/her treatment.

B. The client displayed a pattern of unwillingness to take advantage of treatment due to his/her irrational persecutory beliefs.

C. As a more trusting therapeutic relationship has been developed, the client reports decreased suspiciousness of his/her treatment.

D. The client displayed a willingness to take advantage of treatment regardless of persecutory beliefs.

E. The client has displayed no persecutory beliefs associated with his/her treatment.

9. Violence Potential (9)

A. The client described urges to become violent as a defensive reaction to his/her delusion or hallucination that some person or agency is a threat to self or others.

B. The client reported that he/she has initiated physical encounters that have injured others as a defensive reaction to his/her delusions or hallucinations.

C. The client has decreased his/her pattern of violence as a defensive reaction to delusions or hallucinations.

D. As the client's delusions and hallucinations have decreased, his/her potential for being violent has decreased as well.

E. The client shows no current evidence of irrational urges to become violent.

INTERVENTIONS IMPLEMENTED

1. Review History of Paranoia Symptoms (1)*

A. The client was requested to identify his/her history of persecutory hallucinations, delusions, or other paranoia symptoms.

B. The client was provided with positive feedback as he/she gave a description of his/her history of persecutory hallucinations, delusions, or other paranoia symptoms.

C. The client tended to minimize his/her history of paranoia symptoms and was provided with gentle confrontation in this area.

2. Assess Paranoia (2)

A. The nature and extent of the client's current paranoia were assessed with special attention to severely delusional components.

B. The client identified those people and/or agencies that are distrusted and was allowed to give his/her irrational explanation for this distrust.

C. The client was accepted as he/she demonstrated a pattern of severe delusional aspects to his/her paranoia, although his/her delusions were not endorsed.

D. The client was gently confronted regarding being extremely guarded and defensive, refusing to openly describe the nature and severity of his/her distrust.

E. The client was supported for demonstrating a decrease in his/her level of paranoia.

3. Conduct Antecedent and Coping Interview (3)

A. The Antecedent and Coping Interview (ACI) was used to identify the factors relevant to each symptom related to paranoid ideation.

B. Emotional and behavioral reactions were identified for the client's paranoid ideation.

C. Coping strategies were identified for the client's paranoid ideation.

4. Arrange for Psychological Testing (4)

A. The client was referred for psychological testing to evaluate the extent and severity of his/her paranoia.

B. The client was compliant with the testing, which indicated a significant pattern of paranoia.

C. The psychological test results indicate only mild levels of paranoia, and this was reviewed.

D. The psychological testing results indicate that the client's paranoia has significantly abated, and this was reviewed.

E. The client was not compliant with the psychological testing and was redirected to this referral.

5. Obtain Information from Other Sources (5)

A. A proper authorization to release information was obtained in order to seek out information about the client.

B. Family members have been asked to provide information about the client's pattern of paranoia.

C. Other sources (e.g., police officers) have been sought out for additional information.

---

* The numbers in parentheses correlate to the number of the Therapeutic Intervention statement in the companion chapter with the same title in *The Severe and Persistent Mental Illness Treatment Planner,* 2nd ed. (Berghuis and Jongsma) by John Wiley & Sons, 2008.

D. Based on the information obtained, the conclusion is drawn that the client displays significant paranoia.

E. Based on the information obtained, the conclusion is drawn that the client does not display significant paranoia.

6. Assess Reality Orientation (6)

A. The client's immediate ability to maintain reality orientation was assessed.

B. The client was assessed regarding his/her threat to safety of himself/herself and others.

C. The client was judged to be reality-oriented and not a significant threat to the safety of himself/herself and others.

D. Due to the client's poor reality orientation, he/she was judged to be a threat to the safety of himself/herself and others, and steps were coordinated to place the client in a more structured environment.

7. Provide Direct Instructions (7)

A. The client was provided with direct, basic instructions and with firm reassurance of his/her safety and maintenance of confidentiality.

B. The client has become less agitated as he/she has felt reassured and was encouraged to maintain this stability.

C. The client continues to be quite agitated, despite being provided with direct, basic instructions and firm reassurances.

8. Refer for an Evaluation for Hospitalization (8)

A. The client was immediately referred for an evaluation by a psychiatrist or other clinician regarding his/her psychotic symptoms and the need for psychiatric hospitalization.

B. The client was not judged to be in need of psychiatric hospitalization.

C. The client was judged to be in need of psychiatric hospitalization, and this was immediately coordinated.

9. Coordinate Hospitalization (9)

A. The client was referred for a voluntary admission to a psychiatric hospital, as he/she is so out of touch with reality as to pose a threat to himself/herself or others.

B. As the client has refused the necessary admission to a psychiatric hospital, steps were taken for the client to be hospitalized involuntarily.

C. The client has been admitted to a psychiatric hospital and was encouraged to use this treatment to stabilize himself/herself.

10. Arrange for a Stable, Supervised Setting (10)

A. A stable, supervised setting was arranged for the client to remain in at least until the acute psychotic episode is stabilized.

B. The client has been admitted to a crisis adult foster care placement in order to provide a stable, supervised setting.

C. The client is using a friend or family member's home to provide a stable, supervised setting until his/her psychotic episode is stabilized and was assisted with coordinating the details of this arrangement.

11. Provide Empathetic Acceptance (11)

A. Empathetic listening was provided to the client, displaying respect for him/her by accepting him/her, despite his/her angry or delusional presentation.

B. Acceptance was communicated to the client, despite his/her angry or delusional presentation, but the client's paranoid delusions were not confirmed.

C. As the client has been provided with unconditional acceptance, his/her anger, agitation, and paranoia have subsided.

12. Demonstrate Calm Demeanor (12)

A. A calm demeanor was demonstrated to the client when he/she disclosed bizarre or antagonistic beliefs.

B. As a result of the calm demeanor demonstrated to the client, he/she appears to have decreased his/her fear of rejection.

C. The client continues to display fears related to rejection, despite the calm acceptance with which he/she has been provided, and additional feedback was provided to him/her in this area.

13. Reflect Emotions (13)

A. Indicators of the client's intense emotions (e.g., posture, facial expression, or general presentation) were reflected to him/her.

B. Empathy was displayed for the client who was experiencing significant distress related to his/her paranoid delusions.

C. The client acknowledged his/her emotions related to paranoid delusions, and these were processed.

D. The client tended to deny or minimize emotions related to his/her pattern of delusions, and these were tentatively presented to him/her.

14. Ask Open-Ended Questions (14)

A. The client was asked open-ended questions about some of his/her delusions or paranoid beliefs.

B. The client's paranoid beliefs were accepted as his/her thoughts, although not confirmed.

C. Arguing with the client about his/her paranoid beliefs was consistently avoided.

D. The client has been more open about his/her delusions or paranoid beliefs and was provided with positive feedback about this openness.

15. Physician Referral (15)

A. The client was referred to a physician to undergo a thorough examination to rule out any medical etiologies for his/her paranoia and to receive recommendations for further treatment options.

B. The client has followed through on the physician evaluation referral, and specific medical etiologies for his/her experience of paranoia were reviewed.

C. The client was supported as he/she is seeking out treatment for the medical concerns that are leading to his/her experience of paranoid thoughts.

D. The client has followed through on the physician evaluation referral, but no specific medical etiologies for his/her paranoia have been identified.

E. The client declined evaluation by a physician regarding his/her paranoia and was redirected to cooperate with this referral.

16. Refer for Vision/Hearing Exams (16)

A. The client was referred to an audiologist for a clinical assessment of his/her hearing abilities.

B. The client was referred to an ophthalmologist for a specific evaluation of his/her vision needs.

C. Expert clinical review of the client's hearing and vision indicated deficits in these areas, as well as suggestions for remediation.

D. No concerns were identified through the expert clinical evaluations of hearing and vision.

17. Support/Monitor Physical Evaluation Recommendations (17)

A. The client was supported in following up on the recommendations from the medical evaluation.

B. The client's follow-up on the recommendations from the medical evaluation has been monitored.

C. The client was reinforced for following up on the recommendations from the medical evaluation.

D. The client has not regularly followed up on his/her medical evaluation recommendations and was redirected to do so.

18. Refer for Psychological Evaluation (18)

A. The client was referred for a complete psychological evaluation in order to rule out cognitive disorders (e.g., dementia) as a cause for the paranoia.

B. The client has completed his/her psychological evaluation, and the results of this evaluation were processed.

C. The client has not submitted to a psychological evaluation and was redirected to do so.

19. Evaluate Substance Abuse (19)

A. The client was evaluated for his/her use of substances, the severity of his/her substance abuse, and treatment needs/options.

B. The client was referred to a clinician knowledgeable in both substance abuse and severe and persistent mental illness treatment in order to assess his/her substance abuse concerns and treatment needs.

C. The client was compliant with the substance abuse evaluation, and the results of the evaluation were discussed with him/her.

D. The client did not participate in the substance abuse evaluation and was encouraged to do so.

20. Refer for Substance Abuse Treatment (20)

A. The client was referred to a 12-step recovery program (e.g., Alcoholics Anonymous or Narcotics Anonymous).

B. The client was referred to a substance abuse treatment program.

C. The client has been admitted to a substance abuse treatment program and was supported for this follow-through.

D. The client has refused the referral to a substance abuse treatment program, and this refusal was processed.

21. Identify Delusions as Symptoms (21)

A. The client was gently informed that his/her delusional, persecutory beliefs are based in a mental illness and not in reality.

B. The client was educated about the symptoms of and the treatment for his/her mental illness.

C. The client was provided with positive feedback, as he/she was able to accept the assertion that his/her delusional, persecutory beliefs are symptoms of his/her mental illness.

D. The client denied that his/her delusional, persecutory beliefs are symptoms of his/her mental illness and was provided with additional feedback in this area.

22. Refer to a Physician (22)

A. The client was referred to a physician for an evaluation for a prescription of psychotropic medications.

B. The client was reinforced for following through on a referral to a physician for an assessment for a prescription of psychotropic medications, but none were prescribed.

C. The client has been prescribed psychotropic medications.

D. The client was assisted in filling his/her prescription for psychotropic medications.

E. The client declined evaluation by a physician for a prescription of psychotropic medication and was redirected to cooperate with this referral.

23. Educate about Psychotropic Medications (23)

A. The client was taught about the indications for and the expected benefits of psychotropic medications.

B. As the client's psychotropic medications were reviewed, he/she displayed an understanding about the indications for and expected benefits of the medications.

C. An emphasis was placed on the safety the client should be able to experience about his/her medications and that it is not intended to be harmful to him/her.

D. The client displayed a lack of understanding of the indications for and expected benefits of psychotropic medications and was provided with additional information and feedback regarding his/her medications.

24. Monitor Medications (24)

A. The client was monitored for compliance with his/her psychotropic medication regimen.

B. The client was provided with positive feedback about his/her regular use of psychotropic medications.

C. The client was monitored for the effectiveness and side effects of his/her prescribed medications.

D. Concerns about the client's medication effectiveness and side effects were communicated to the physician.

E. Although the client was monitored for medication side effects, he/she reported no concerns in this area.

25. Ensure Medication Adherence (25)

A. Direct, supervised administration of the client's medications was arranged.

B. Liquid forms of medications were requested to ensure the client's regular adherence to his/her regimen.

C. The client has become more regular with his/her medications, and the positive psychiatric benefits of his/her adherence were reviewed.

D. The client continues to have significant symptoms, despite regular medication adherence, and additional psychiatric evaluation was arranged.

26. Review Side Effects of Medications (26)

A. The possible side effects related to the client's medications were reviewed with the client.

B. The client identified significant side effects, and these were reported to the medical staff.

C. Possible side effects of the client's medications were reviewed, but he/she denied experiencing any side effects.

D. The client was monitored for signs of tardive dyskinesia.

27. Advocate for Medications to Reduce Side Effects (27)

A. Advocacy was provided with the client's physician/psychiatrist for an adjustment in his/her medications to reduce or eliminate tardive dyskinesia.

B. The client's physician has been able to modify his/her medications in order to maintain efficacy and decrease the likelihood of long-term side effects (e.g., tardive dyskinesia).

C. The client's medications cannot be modified to reduce the likelihood of long-term side effects (e.g., tardive dyskinesia) without reducing efficacy, and this was presented to him/her.

D. The client has identified his/her willingness to have reduced efficacy of his/her medications in order to reduce the likelihood of long-term side effects (e.g., tardive dyskinesia), and this was processed.

E. The client has elected to accept the risk for long-term side effects (e.g., tardive dyskinesia) in order to have greater efficacy in his/her medications, and the risks and benefits of this decision were reviewed.

28. Assess Tardive Symptoms (28)

A. Arrangements were made for assessment of the client's tardive symptoms, using the client, the staff, or personal observation.

B. Objective measurement of the client's tardive symptoms was performed by qualified personnel using a specific instrument (e.g., the Abnormal Involuntary Movement Scale [AIMS]).

C. The client displayed no evidence of tardive symptoms, and this was reflected to him/her.

D. The client displayed both subjective and objective evidence of tardive symptoms, and this was reported to the physician who prescribed his/her psychotropic medications.

29. Explore Paranoid Thinking (29)

A. The client was referred for cognitive-behavioral therapy to explore his/her paranoid thoughts.

B. The client was provided with cognitive-behavioral therapy to educate him/her about his/her paranoid thoughts.

C. Skills training was provided to the client regarding his/her paranoid thoughts.

D. Behavioral experiments were conducted in order to help the client understand more about his/her paranoid thoughts.

E. As a result of the therapy, the client has come to understand more about his/her paranoid thoughts.

F. Despite significant therapy to help understand his/her paranoid thinking, the client does not display any insight in this area.

30. Teach about Cognitive Restructuring and Behavioral Experiments (30)

A. The client was taught about how cognitive restructuring can be used to reality test delusional thoughts, decrease fears, develop personal skills, and build confidence.

B. Behavioral experiments were used to help test the reality of the client's delusional thoughts.

C. As a result of Cognitive Restructuring and Behavioral Experiments the client is less fearful, more confident, and more reality oriented.

D. Despite the use of Cognitive Restructuring and Behavioral Experiments the client continues to display significant delusional thoughts, fearfulness, skill deficits, and a lack of confidence; he/she was provided with remedial assistance in this area.

31. Explore Schema (31)

A. The client was assisted in exploring his/her schema and self-talk that mediate his/her paranoid thoughts.

B. The client was assisted in challenging the biases that support his/her paranoid thoughts.

C. The client was assisted in generating alternative appraisals that could be tested for truthfulness.

D. The client has gained greater reality orientation through exploring and testing his/her schema and self talk.

E. Despite exploring the client's schema and self-talk, he/she continues to have significant paranoid thoughts; this pattern was summarized to him/her.

32. Assign Reality-Testing Homework (32)

A. The client was given a homework exercise in which he/she identifies a few biased beliefs and creates reality-based alternatives.

B. The client was directed to utilize the "Check Suspicions Against Reality" task in the *Adult Psychotherapy Homework Planner,* 2nd ed. (Jongsma).

C. The client's success in becoming more reality oriented though the homework exercises was reinforced.

D. The client was provided with corrective feedback toward improving his/her skills and being reality oriented.

33. Identify Reality Testing Activities (33)

A. The client was encouraged to participate in activities that can help him/her to test his/her paranoid predictions against reality-based alternatives.

B. The client was assisted in listing activities that may help him/her to test his/her predictions against reality-based alternatives.

C. The client has engaged in activities that can help to test his/her paranoid predictions against reality-based alternatives, and the results of his/her experiments were reviewed.

D. The client has not engaged in activities that can help to test his/her paranoid predictions and was redirected to do so.

34. Select Successful Behavioral Experiments (34)

A. The client was assisted in selecting initial behavioral experiments that will have a high likelihood of being successful.

B. Cognitive restructuring techniques were used within and after the exercise in order to reinforce successes and identify obstacles to problem solving.

35. Teach about Coping Package (35)

A. The client was taught a variety of techniques to help manage anxiety symptoms.

B. The client was taught calming strategies, such as relaxation and breathing techniques.

C. The client was taught cognitive techniques, such as thought-stopping, positive self-talk, and attention-focusing skills (e.g., distraction from urges, staying focused, behavioral goals of abstinence).

D. The client has used his/her coping package techniques to help reduce his/her anxiety symptoms; this program was reinforced.

E. The client has not used the coping package for managing anxiety symptoms and was redirected to do so.

36. Teach Social and Communication Skills (36)

A. The client was taught general social and communication skills.

B. Instruction, modeling and role-playing were used to help build the client's general social and communicational skills.

C. The client's increased social skills were reinforced.

D. Despite attempts at increasing the subject's social and communication skills, he/she still has significant deficits in this area, and was provided with remedial treatment in this area.

37. Assign Information on Social and Communication Skills (37)

A. The client was assigned to read about general social and/or communication skills in books or treatment manuals on building social skills.

B. The client was assigned to read *Your Perfect Right* (Alberti and Emmons).

C. The client was assigned to read *Conversationally Speaking* (Garner).

D. The client has read the assigned information on social and communication skills, and key points were reviewed.

E. The client has not read the information on social and communication skills and was redirected to do so.

38. Coordinate Externally Focused Activities (38)

A. The client was encouraged to gradually increase his/her involvement in community activities, volunteering, and other externally focused activities.

B. The client was assisted in finding specific opportunities to increase his/her external focus by becoming involved in activities.

C. The client was supported for becoming regularly involved in community activities and for reporting an increase in his/her external focus.

D. The client has not been able to focus on community activities, and his/her struggles in this area were problem solved.

39. Encourage Social Relationships (39)

A. The client was encouraged to increase his/her involvement in social relationships.

B. Verbal reinforcement was used when the client reported attempts at increasing his/her social contacts.

C. The client has not increased his/her social relationships and was redirected in this area.

40. Accompany to Social/Recreational Events (40)

A. The client was accompanied to social/recreational events in order to increase his/her involvement in community-based activities.

B. The level of contact with or support from the clinician during the outing was controlled by the client.

C. The client was reinforced for successfully negotiating the social/recreational event with close contact from the clinician.

D. The client was reinforced for successfully negotiating the social/recreational event with limited contact from the clinician.

E. The client has declined any support from the clinician during social/recreational events and was reminded of the availability of this support.

41. Educate the Family about Symptoms of Mental Illness (41)

A. The client's family, friends, and caregivers were educated about the symptoms of mental illness, with specific emphasis on the nonvolitional aspects of some symptoms.

B. The client's family members were supported for their increased understanding about the symptoms of mental illness and the nonvolitional aspects of some symptoms.

C. The client's family members, friends, and caregivers rejected the information regarding his/her symptoms of mental illness and the nonvolitional aspects of some symptoms, and they were given additional feedback in this area.

42. Teach Calm Responses to Paranoia (42)

A. The client's family, friends, and caregivers were taught to give calm, assertive responses to paranoid behaviors.

B. Modeling and role-playing techniques were used to teach to the client's family, friends, and caregivers how to give calm, assertive responses to his/her paranoid behaviors.

C. The client's family, friends, and caregivers were cautioned against issuing challenges that are too vigorous for his/her delusional beliefs.

D. The client's family, friends, and caregivers were given positive feedback regarding their calm, assertive responses to his/her paranoid behavior.

E. The client's family, friends, and caregivers tend to react too strongly to his/her pattern of delusional beliefs, causing increased stress and conflicts within the relationship; this overreaction was processed.

43. Explore Stressors that Trigger Psychosis (43)

A. The client was probed for recent stressors that may have triggered his/her most recent psychotic episode.

B. The client was provided with emotional support and feedback as he/she described the stressors that have contributed to his/her most recent psychotic episode.

C. The client's feelings regarding his/her stressors were processed.

D. The client maintained a pattern of denial and minimization regarding his/her stressors and psychosis and was provided with additional feedback in this area.

44. Teach Social Skills (44)

A. The client was taught skills to help reduce his/her stress (e.g., using assertiveness, problem-solving, or other stress reduction techniques).

B. The client was referred for training to increase his/her social skills.

C. The client was reinforced for displaying a better understanding of social skills and for using them to help decrease his/her stress level.

D. The client displayed poor social skills and was redirected to use the social skills for which he/she has been trained.

45. Reduce Threats in the Environment (45)

A. The client was assisted in identifying and implementing strategies for reducing stress in his/her environment.

B. The client was provided with feedback as he/she identified specific threats in the environment.

C. The client was assisted in reducing threats in the environment (e.g., finding a safer place to live, arranging for regular visits from the clinician, arranging for family members to call more frequently, checking his/her perceptions with others).

46. Refer to a Support Group (46)

A. The client was referred to a support group for individuals with severe and persistent mental illness.

B. The client has attended the support group for individuals with severe and persistent mental illness, and the benefits of this support group were reviewed.

C. The client reported that he/she has not experienced any positive benefit from the use of a support group but was encouraged to continue to attend.

D. The client has not used the support group for individuals with severe and persistent mental illness and was redirected to do so.

PARENTING

CLIENT PRESENTATION

1. Symptoms Affect Interactions with the Child (1)*

A. The client's severe and persistent mental illness symptoms often affect his/her interactions with his/her child.

B. The client's child often appears to be confused by the client's erratic behavior due to his/her severe and persistent mental illness symptoms.

C. As treatment has progressed, the client's severe and persistent mental illness symptoms have improved.

2. Loss of Custody (2)

A. The client's child is at risk of being removed from his/her custody due to safety concerns or his/her inability to care for the child.

B. The client has lost custody of his/her child due to safety concerns or inability to care for the child.

C. The client has decompensated due to the increased stress and emotional response related to losing custody of his/her child.

D. The client has become more focused and more open to treatment subsequent to losing custody of his/her child.

E. As the client has stabilized in treatment, he/she has pursued regaining custody of his/her child.

3. Lack of Interest (3)

A. The client described a pattern of very limited or only superficial interest in the child's activities.

B. The client displayed a pattern of limited interest in his/her child's activities.

C. The client's severe and persistent mental illness has caused a decreased level of involvement in the child's activities.

D. The client has taken steps to become more involved in his/her child's activities.

4. Difficulty Coping with Parenting (4)

A. The client described a sense of being overwhelmed by the day-to-day stressors of parenting.

B. The client reported a lack of coping skills for the day-to-day stressors of parenting.

C. As the client's severe and persistent mental illness has stabilized, he/she reports an increased ability to function with day-to-day stressors.

5. Disagreement with Significant Other (5)

A. The client described a pattern of disagreement with his/her partner regarding child rearing practices.

---

* The numbers in parentheses correlate to the number of the Behavioral Definition statement in the companion chapter with the same title in *The Severe and Persistent Mental Illness Treatment Planner,* 2nd ed. (Berghuis and Jongsma) by John Wiley & Sons, 2008.

B. The client described that his/her severe and persistent mental illness symptoms have exacerbated his/her relationship conflicts.

C. The client described a pattern of increasing relationship stress due to disagreements regarding child rearing practices.

D. The client reported a decrease in his/her level of relationship stress.

6. Extended Family Involvement (6)

A. Members of the client's extended family have expressed concern about the welfare of his/her child.

B. Members of the client's extended family have taken responsibility for his/her child.

C. Support and assistance have been provided by the client's extended family to assist him/her in maintaining involvement in his/her child.

D. As the client has stabilized, his/her extended family has decreased their involvement in his/her parenting.

7. Child's Manipulation (7)

A. The client described a pattern of ineffectiveness in his/her parenting style due to his/her severe and persistent mental illness symptoms.

B. The client's child has often taken advantage of the client's pattern of ineffective parenting.

C. As the client's severe and persistent mental illness has stabilized, he/she reports an increased pattern of effectiveness in his/her parenting skills.

D. Through the client's increased parenting effectiveness and other natural supports, his/her child has been unable to take advantage of him/her.

8. Shame, Embarrassment, and Confusion (8)

A. The client's child described feeling shame and embarrassment due to the client's mental illness symptoms.

B. The client's child is often confused about his/her parent's mental illness symptoms.

C. As treatment has progressed, the client's child has displayed increased understanding and acceptance of the client's mental illness.

INTERVENTIONS IMPLEMENTED

1. Explore Parenting Concerns (1)*

A. The client's history of parenting concerns was explored.

B. The client was provided with positive feedback for being open and honest regarding his/her history of parenting concerns.

C. The client tended to minimize his/her parenting difficulties, and this was reflected to him/her.

2. Create a Family Genogram (2)

A. The client's description of family members, patterns of interactions, rules, and secrets was translated into a graphic genogram.

* The numbers in parentheses correlate to the number of the Therapeutic Intervention statement in the companion chapter with the same title in *The Severe and Persistent Mental Illness Treatment Planner,* 2nd ed. (Berghuis and Jongsma) by John Wiley & Sons, 2008.

B. A family session was conducted in which a genogram was developed that was complete, denoting family members, patterns of interaction, rules, and secrets.

C. The dysfunctional communication patterns between family members were highlighted.

D. Family members were supported as they acknowledged the lack of healthy communication that permeates the extended family.

E. The client displayed an increased understanding of his/her family's pattern of unhealthy communication and was encouraged for this progress.

F. The client failed to develop insight into family interactions and was given tentative interpretations of these patterns.

3. Develop a Time line of Parenting and Illness (3)

A. The client was assisted in developing a time line of important events regarding parenting (e.g., births, relationships beginning and/or ending, loss or return of custody/visitation).

B. The client's parenting time line was compared with milestones related to his/her illness (e.g., onset of symptoms, hospitalizations).

C. The interaction between the client's mental illness symptoms and parenting struggles was processed with him/her.

D. The client was supported for the insight of identifying a pattern of increased stress related to his/her parenting that correlates with increases in his/her symptom pattern.

E. The client denied any connection between his/her mental illness symptoms and parenting concerns and was encouraged to keep this connection in mind.

4. Review Current Parenting Concerns (4)

A. The client was asked to review current concerns and successes regarding parenting, including the child's challenging behaviors, the approach taken with the child, and legal issues.

B. The client's partner was requested to provide input regarding current parenting concerns.

C. The client was reminded to focus on the successes and positive traits of the child.

D. The client was supported and encouraged as he/she gave an accurate portrayal of his/her current parenting concerns.

E. The client tended to minimize and deny his/her current parenting concerns and was provided with confrontation in this area.

F. The client tended to be quite negative about the child and was reminded to balance this with more positive feedback.

5. Psychological Testing (5)

A. A psychological evaluation was conducted to determine the extent of the client's ability to bond with the child.

B. The client approached the psychological testing in an honest, straightforward manner and was cooperative with any requests presented to him/her.

C. The client was uncooperative and resistant to engage during the evaluation process and was advised to use this testing to discover more about himself/herself.

D. The results of the psychological evaluation were reviewed with the client.

6. Educate about Mental Illness (6)

A. The client was educated about the expected or common symptoms of his/her mental illness that may negatively impact his/her ability to function in the parent role.

B. As the client's symptoms of mental illness were discussed, he/she displayed an understanding of how these symptoms may affect his/her functioning as a parent.

C. The client struggled to identify how symptoms of his/her mental illness may negatively impact his/her parenting and was given additional feedback in this area.

7. Assign Reading on Mental Illness (7)

A. The client and his/her family were referred to books that provide information regarding the etiology, symptoms, and treatment of severe and persistent mental illness.

B. *Schizophrenia: The Facts* by Tsuang and Faraone and *Bipolar Disorder: A Guide for Patients and Families* by Mondimore were recommended to the client and his/her family.

C. The client and his/her family have read books regarding the etiology, symptoms, and treatment of mental illness, and this information was reviewed within the session.

D. The client and his/her family have not read information regarding the etiology, symptoms, and treatment of severe and persistent mental illness and were redirected to do so.

8. Discuss Mental Illness Effect on Parenting (8)

A. The effect of the client's personal experience of severe and persistent mental illness was reviewed to identify how these symptoms have affected his/her ability to parent effectively.

B. The client was praised for his/her openness and insight regarding how his/her mental illness symptoms have affected his/her parenting.

C. As the client has gained insight into his/her pattern of parenting, he/she has become more effective, and this was reviewed within the session.

D. The client has minimized and denied any effect of his/her severe and persistent mental illness symptoms on his/her ability to parent effectively and was provided with contrary feedback.

9. Refer to a Physician (9)

A. The client was referred to a physician for an evaluation for a prescription of psychotropic medications.

B. The client was reinforced for following through on a referral to a physician for an assessment for a prescription of psychotropic medications, but none were prescribed.

C. The client has been prescribed psychotropic medications.

D. The client declined evaluation by a physician for a prescription of psychotropic medications and was redirected to cooperate with this referral.

10. Educate about and Monitor Psychotropic Medications (10)

A. The client was taught about the indications for and the expected benefits of psychotropic medications.

B. As the client's psychotropic medications were reviewed, he/she displayed an understanding about the indications for and expected benefits of the medications.

C. The client was monitored for compliance with, effectiveness of, and side effects from his/her psychotropic medication regimen.

D. The client was provided with positive feedback about his/her regular use of psychotropic medications.

E. Concerns about the client's medication effectiveness and side effects were communicated to the physician.

F. Although the client was monitored for medication side effects, he/she reported no concerns in this area.

G. The client displayed a lack of understanding of the indications for and expected benefits of psychotropic medications and was provided with additional information and feedback regarding his/her medications.

11. Obtain Day Care (11)

A. The client was assisted in obtaining day care services for his/her children during his/her appointment for mental illness treatment.

B. The client was reinforced for obtaining regular day care services to assist with the supervision of his/her children during his/her appointments and becoming more regular in attending appointments.

C. The client has not obtained day care services for the times when he/she is at appointments for his/her mental illness treatment and was redirected in this area.

12. Review Side Effects of Medications (12)

A. The possible side effects related to the client's medications were reviewed with the client.

B. The client identified significant side effects, and these were reported to the medical staff.

C. Possible side effects of the client's medications were reviewed, but he/she denied experiencing any side effects.

13. Refer to a Parenting Class (13)

A. The client was referred to a parenting class to teach him/her new skills for parenting.

B. The client has attended the parenting class, and his/her implementation of new parenting skills was reviewed.

C. The client has not attended the parenting class and was redirected to do so.

14. Assign Parenting Books (14)

A. The client was assigned to read material that provides guidance on effective parenting methods.

B. The client was assigned to read *1-2-3 Magic: Effective Discipline for Children 2–12,* Second Edition, by Phelan; *Parenting Teens with Love and Logic: Preparing Adolescents for Responsible Adulthood* by Cline and Fay; or *Positive Parenting from A to Z* by Joslin.

C. The client has read the assigned parenting material, and this information was processed.

D. The client has not read the assigned parenting material and was redirected to do so.

15. Practice Parenting Skills (15)

A. Role-playing, modeling, and behavioral rehearsal were used to help the client practice implementation of new parenting skills.

B. The client was reinforced for his/her display of understanding regarding new parenting skills.

C. The client failed to display understanding of new parenting skills and was provided with remedial information in this area.

16. Focus the Couple on a Parenting Plan (16)

A. A conjoint session was arranged to help the client and his/her partner to develop mutually acceptable plans for parenting of the child.

B. The conjoint session was focused on the types of parenting approaches to be used with the child.

C. The client and his/her partner have identified specific approaches to be used with the child and were encouraged for this plan.

D. The client and his/her partner were reinforced for using parenting techniques in a similar manner.

E. The client and his/her partner have been unable to agree on a mutually acceptable plan for parenting the child and were encouraged to continue to focus on this area.

17. Regularly Review Parenting Plans (17)

A. The client and his/her partner were encouraged to regularly review their parenting plan.

B. Conjoint sessions were scheduled to focus on the review of the parenting plan.

C. The client was assisted in making appropriate adjustments to his/her parenting plan.

D. The client and his/her significant other have not reviewed the parenting plan and were encouraged to do so.

18. Explore Mental Illness Effects on Parenting (18)

A. Situations in which the client's mental illness symptoms may affect interactions with the child were explored.

B. The client identified specific situations in which his/her mental illness symptoms may affect interactions with the child and was provided with positive support and encouragement in this area.

C. The client seemed to be denying the effect of his/her mental illness symptoms on interaction with the child and was confronted about this denial.

19. Develop Contingency Plans (19)

A. The client and his/her partner were assisted in developing contingency plans for areas in which the client's mental illness symptoms may affect interactions with the child (e.g., removing the car keys when the client becomes manic).

B. The client and his/her partner were supported for developing a contingency plan for situations in which the client's mental illness symptoms may affect interaction with the child.

C. The client and his/her partner were reinforced for their regular use of contingency plans.

D. The client and his/her partner have not developed or used contingency plans and were redirected in this area.

20. Develop Emergency Child Care List (20)

A. The client and his/her partner were directed to develop a listing of family members and other individuals who can provide short-term supervision to the child when the client is feeling overwhelmed by his/her parenting responsibilities.

B. The client and his/her partner were reinforced for developing a list of support network members who are willing to provide short-term supervision to the client's child.

C. The client was supported for regularly using members of his/her support network to supervise the child when the client is feeling overwhelmed by his/her parenting responsibilities.

D. The client has not listed or used family members and other individuals who can provide short-term supervision for the child and was reminded of this resource.

21. Coordinate Child Care during Acute Phases (21)

A. The assistance of the extended family was enlisted in order to provide supervision and parenting to the child during acute stages of the client's mental illness.

B. The client was reassured and reinforced regarding the longer-term supervision of the child provided by members of the extended family.

C. The client has not agreed to have the child supervised by extended family members during his/her acute stages of mental illness and was strongly encouraged to do so.

22. Coordinate Respite Services (22)

A. The client was directed to funding resources for obtaining respite services.

B. Respite services were coordinated for the client in order to provide short- or long-term periods of relief from the additional stress of parenting.

C. The client was encouraged to use respite funds and services in order to obtain relief from the stress of parenting.

D. The client was reinforced for his/her use of respite services in order to improve the overall relationship with the child.

E. The client has not used the respite services and was encouraged to do so.

23. Suggest One-to-One Time (23)

A. The client was urged to set specific times to spend alone with each child.

B. The client was encouraged to treat his/her one-to-one time with each child as a priority while still being flexible enough to reschedule if his/her mental illness symptoms are more acute.

C. The client's use of one-to-one time with his/her child was reviewed.

D. The client was supported for using good judgment in rescheduling one-to-one time when his/her mental illness symptoms were more acute.

E. The client has not appropriately used one-to-one time with each child and was provided with feedback in this area.

24. Teach Relaxation Techniques (24)

A. The client was taught deep muscle relaxation and deep breathing techniques as ways to reduce muscle tension.

B. *The Relaxation and Stress Reduction Workbook* (Davis, Eshelman, and McKay) was used to provide the client with examples of techniques to help himself/herself relax.

C. The client was reinforced for implementing the relaxation techniques.

D. The client has not implemented the relaxation techniques presented to him/her and continues to feel quite stressed; use of relaxation procedures was again encouraged.

25. Brainstorm Diversionary Activities (25)

A. The client was assisted in brainstorming diversionary activities that can relieve parenting stress (e.g., going for a walk, calling a friend, or engaging in a hobby).

B. The client identified a variety of diversionary activities that would appeal to him/her and was encouraged to use these.

C. The client was provided with positive feedback as he/she has regularly used diversionary activities to relieve parenting stress.

D. The client has not used diversionary activities to relieve parenting stress and was encouraged to do so.

26. Coordinate Conjoint Sessions with the Child (26)

A. Conjoint sessions were coordinated for the client's child to ask questions about the client's mental illness symptoms.

B. The client was assisted in responding to the child's questions at an age-appropriate level.

C. The child was provided with additional information regarding his/her questions about the client's mental illness symptoms.

27. Provide Written Information to the Child (27)

A. The child was provided with age-appropriate written information about his/her parent's mental illness.

B. The child was provided with information from *When Parents Have Problems: A Book for Teens and Older Children with an Abusive, Alcoholic or Mentally Ill Parent* by Miller.

C. The child has read the information about his/her parent's mental illness, and this material was reviewed.

D. The child has not read the information about his/her parent's mental illness and was encouraged to do so.

28. Coach about Talking for the Child's Understanding (28)

A. The client was coached about how to talk about his/her mental illness concerns in a manner in which the child can understand.

B. The client was provided with examples of how to talk to the child in an age-appropriate manner about his/her mental illness symptoms.

C. The client's talks with the child about his/her mental illness symptoms were reviewed, and he/she was provided with feedback in this area.

D. The client has not discussed his/her mental illness concerns with his/her child and was encouraged to do so.

29. Explore the Child's Feelings (29)

A. The client's child's feelings regarding his/her parent's mental illness were explored.

B. Specific incidents of when the client's symptoms have had a painful impact on the child's life were identified.

C. The child was provided with support and encouragement regarding his/her emotional response to his/her parent's mental illness.

D. The child tends to minimize his/her emotions and painful experiences and was encouraged to talk about these emotions as he/she feels capable.

30. Reinforce Acceptance of the Child's Emotions (30)

A. The client was focused on the need to accept, without judgment, the feelings of his/her child.

B. Reassurance was provided to the client that his/her child's feelings are not a personal attack on the client.

C. The client was reinforced for his/her willingness to accept the child's emotions.

D. The client has not been willing to accept his/her child's emotions and was provided with feedback in this area.

31. Refer to a Support Group for Children (31)

A. The client and his/her child were referred to a multifamily support group for family members of an individual with a mental illness.

B. The client's child was referred to an age-appropriate support group for family members of an individual with a mental illness.

C. The client's child reported being helped by attending a support group for children with a mentally ill family member, and this attendance was reinforced.

D. The client's child has not attended a support group and was encouraged to do so.

32. Identify the Child's Accommodations (32)

A. The client and the child were assisted in identifying mild accommodations that can be made to increase functioning in the relationship.

B. The client and his/her child were reinforced for implementing mild accommodations to increase functioning in the relationship.

C. The client and his/her child identified accommodations that were inappropriate for a child to make for the parent and were provided with feedback in this area.

33. Brainstorm Responses to Teasing (33)

A. The client's child was assisted in brainstorming about how to respond to teasing or other interference from peers related to the parent's mental illness symptoms.

B. The client's child was supported for his/her appropriate response to teasing or other interference from peers due to the parent's mental illness symptoms.

C. The client's child has often responded in inappropriate ways to teasing and other interference from peers and was provided with feedback in this area.

34. Define Inability to Parent (34)

A. The client's assistance was enlisted in developing a description of the level of decompensation at which he/she would see himself/herself as temporarily unable to function as a parent.

B. The client was encouraged to commit to temporarily relinquishing responsibility as a parent when he/she decompensates to a critical level.

C. The client has agreed to temporarily relinquish his/her role as a parent when he/she decompensates and was encouraged for planning ahead in this manner.

D. The client has temporarily given up his/her parenting role due to decompensation and was supported for this difficult decision.

E. The client has refused to temporarily give up his/her parenting role when decompensating and was encouraged to review this decision.

35. Teach about Child Protection Guidelines (35)

A. The client was assisted in understanding the general guidelines under which the court or child protection agency will operate.

B. The client was reinforced for displaying an understanding of the general guidelines under which the court or child protective agency will operate (whether he/she agrees with these guidelines or not).

C. The client failed to display an understanding of the general guidelines under which the court or child protection agency will operate and was provided with remedial information in this area.

36. Assist in Custody/Child Protection Case (36)

A. The client was assisted in understanding the multiple, intricate steps that occur during a custody or child protection case.

B. The client was supported for displaying an increased understanding of the intricate steps that occur during a custody or child protection case.

C. Court hearings were attended to provide emotional support to the client.

D. The client displayed a poor understanding of the steps that are occurring in his/her custody or child protection case and was provided with additional feedback in this area.

37. Refer to an Attorney (37)

A. The client was referred to an attorney.

B. The client has followed up on the referral to an attorney, and the benefits of this were processed with the client.

C. The client has not contacted an attorney and was encouraged to do so.

38. Explore a Working Relationship with the Former Spouse (38)

A. The degree of cooperative parenting that occurs with the client's former spouse was explored.

B. Emphasis was placed on the need for the relationship with the client's former spouse to be a working relationship, focusing on the mutual job of raising their child.

C. The client was encouraged to find friendship and other emotional needs outside of the relationship with his/her former spouse when this confounds working together in the best interests of their children.

D. The client was supported for displaying a healthier relationship with his/her former spouse by emphasizing the needs of their child.

E. The client continues to have an unhealthy, dysfunctional relationship with his/her spouse and was provided with additional feedback in this area.

39. Keep the Estranged Spouse Informed (39)

A. A proper authorization to release information was obtained to allow information to be provided to the client's estranged spouse.

B. The client's estranged spouse was informed of the client's general level of functioning as it relates to his/her ability to care for the child.

C. As a result of increased information, the client's estranged spouse has been more cooperative in assisting the client with maximizing his/her contact and care for their child, and this was reviewed within the session.

D. The client has declined to allow information to be provided to his/her estranged spouse, and this decision was honored.

E. Information was provided to the client's estranged spouse, but the information has been used against the client without care as to how it relates to his/her ability to care for the child.

40. Discourage Major Decisions during Acute Illness (40)

A. The client was discouraged from making long-term, major life decisions during the acute phase of his/her illness.

B. The client was reinforced for agreeing to refrain from making any long-term, major life decisions during the acute phase of his/her illness.

C. The client continues to make life-changing decisions during the acute phase of his/her mental illness and was cautioned against this.

41. Weigh the Pros and Cons of Giving Up Custody (41)

A. The client was assisted in identifying the pros and cons of giving up custody of his/her child.

B. Empathic listening was provided to the client regarding his/her choice about giving up custody of his/her child without endorsing one choice or another.

C. The severe pain that is involved in giving up custody of his/her child was acknowledged.

D. The client has declined to make any decisions related to his/her child custody rights and was provided with feedback in this area.

42. Refer for Grief Counseling (42)

A. The client was referred for grief counseling due to his/her decision to give up custody of his/her child.

B. The client was supported for following through on the grief counseling.

C. The client has not followed through on the referral for grief counseling and was redirected to do so.

43. Review the Decision to Have Children (43)

A. The client and his/her intimate partner were focused on the pros and cons of the choice to attempt to have children.

B. The client and his/her intimate partner have reviewed the pros and cons of the choice to have children and have decided to proceed with having children; they were provided with feedback in this area.

C. The client and his/her intimate partner were supported for reviewing the pros and cons regarding having children and deciding not to have children.

POSTTRAUMATIC STRESS DISORDER (PTSD)

CLIENT PRESENTATION

1. Exposure to Death/Injury to Others (1)*

A. The client has a history of having been exposed to the death or serious injury of others that resulted in feelings of intense fear, helplessness, or horror.

B. The client's severe emotional response to fear has somewhat diminished.

C. The client can now recall being a witness to the traumatic incident without experiencing the intense emotional response of fear, helplessness, or horror.

2. Exposure to Threatened Death/Injury to Self (1)

A. The client has been a victim of a threat of death or serious injury to himself/herself that has resulted in an intense emotional response of fear, helplessness, or horror.

B. The client's intense emotional response to the traumatic event has somewhat diminished.

C. The client can now recall the traumatic event of being threatened with death or serious injury without an intense emotional response.

3. Intrusive Thoughts (2)

A. The client described experiencing intrusive, distressing thoughts or images that recall the traumatic event and its associated intense emotional response.

B. The client reported experiencing less difficulty with intrusive, distressing thoughts of the traumatic event.

C. The client reported no longer experiencing intrusive, distressing thoughts of the traumatic event.

4. Disturbing Dreams (3)

A. The client described disturbing dreams that he/she experiences and are associated with the traumatic event.

B. The frequency and intensity of the disturbing dreams associated with the traumatic event have decreased.

C. The client reported no longer experiencing disturbing dreams associated with the traumatic event.

5. Flashbacks (4)

A. The client reported experiencing illusions about or flashbacks to the traumatic event.

B. The frequency and intensity of the client's flashback experiences have diminished.

C. The client reported no longer experiencing flashbacks to the traumatic event.

6. Distressful Reminders (5)

A. The client experienced intense distress when exposed to reminders of the traumatic event.

---

* The numbers in parentheses correlate to the number of the Behavioral Definition statement in the companion chapter with the same title in *The Severe and Persistent Mental Illness Treatment Planner,* 2nd ed. (Berghuis and Jongsma) by John Wiley & Sons, 2008.

B. The client reported having been exposed to some reminders of the traumatic event without experiencing overwhelming distress.

7. Physiological Reactivity (6)

A. The client experiences physiological reactivity associated with fear and anger when he/she is exposed to the internal or external cues that symbolize the traumatic event.

B. The client's physiological reactivity has diminished when he/she is exposed to internal or external cues of the traumatic event.

C. The client reported no longer experiencing physiological reactivity when exposed to internal or external cues of the traumatic event.

8. Thought/Feeling/Conversation Avoidance (7)

A. The client described trying to avoid thinking, feeling, or talking about the traumatic event because of the associated negative emotional response.

B. The client is making less effort to avoid thoughts, feelings, or conversations about the traumatic event.

C. The client reported that he/she is now able to talk or think about the traumatic event without feeling overwhelmed with negative emotions.

9. Place/People Avoidance (8)

A. The client reported a pattern of avoidance of activity, places, or people associated with the traumatic event because he/she is fearful of the negative emotions that may be triggered.

B. The client is able to tolerate contact with people, places, or activities associated with the traumatic event without feeling overwhelmed.

10. Blocked Recall (9)

A. The client stated that he/she has an inability to recall some important aspect of the traumatic event.

B. The client's amnesia regarding some important aspects of the traumatic event has begun to lessen.

C. The client can now recall almost all of the important aspects of the traumatic event, as his/her amnesia has terminated.

11. Lack of Interest (10)

A. The client has developed a lack of interest and a pattern of lack of participation in activities that had previously been rewarding and pleasurable.

B. The client has begun to show some interest in participation in previously rewarding activities.

C. The client is not showing a normal interest in participation in rewarding activities.

12. Detachment (11)

A. The client described feeling a sense of detachment from others.

B. The client reported regaining a sense of attachment in participation with others.

C. The client reported that he/she no longer feels alienated from others and is able to participate in social and intimate interactions.

13. Blunted Emotions (12)

A. The client reported an inability to experience the full range of emotions, including love.

B. The client reported beginning to be in touch with his/her feelings again.

C. The client is able to experience the full range of emotions.

14. Pessimistic/Fatalistic (13)

A. Since the traumatic event occurred, the client has had a pessimistic and fatalistic attitude regarding the future.

B. The client is beginning to experience a somewhat hopeful attitude regarding the future.

C. The client's pessimistic, fatalistic attitude regarding the future has terminated, and he/she has begun to make plans and talk about the future with a more hopeful attitude.

15. Sleep Disturbance (14)

A. Since the traumatic event occurred, the client has experienced a desire to sleep much more than normal.

B. Since the traumatic event occurred, the client has found it very difficult to initiate and maintain sleep.

C. Since the traumatic event occurred, the client has had a fear of sleeping.

D. The client's sleep disturbance has terminated, and he/she has returned to a normal sleep pattern.

16. Irritability (15)

A. The client described a pattern of irritability that was not present before the traumatic event occurred.

B. The client reported incidents of becoming angry and losing his/her temper easily, resulting in explosive outbursts.

C. The client's irritability has diminished somewhat, and the intensity of the explosive outbursts has lessened.

D. The client reported no recent incidents of explosive, angry outbursts.

17. Lack of Concentration (16)

A. The client described a pattern of lack of concentration that began with the exposure to the traumatic event.

B. The client reported that he/she is now able to focus more clearly on cognitive processing.

C. The client's ability to concentrate has returned to normal levels.

18. Hypervigilance (17)

A. The client described a pattern of hypervigilance.

B. The client's hypervigilant pattern has diminished.

C. The client reported no longer experiencing hypervigilance.

19. Exaggerated Startle Response (18)

A. The client described having experienced an exaggerated startle response.

B. The client's exaggerated startle response has diminished.

C. The client no longer experiences an exaggerated startle response.

20. Depression (19)

A. The client described experiencing sad affect, lack of energy, social withdrawal, and guilt feelings as part of a depressive reaction.

B. The client's depression symptoms have diminished considerably.

C. The client reported that he/she is no longer experiencing symptoms of depression.

21. Alcohol/Drug Abuse (20)

A. Since the traumatic experience, the client has engaged in a pattern of alcohol and/or drug abuse as a maladaptive coping mechanism.

B. The client's alcohol and/or drug abuse has diminished as he/she has worked through the traumatic event.

C. The client reported no longer engaging in any alcohol or drug abuse.

22. Suicidal Thoughts (21)

A. The client reported experiencing suicidal thoughts since the onset of PTSD.

B. The client's suicidal thoughts have become less intense and less frequent.

C. The client reported no longer experiencing any suicidal thoughts.

23. Interpersonal Conflict (22)

A. The client described a pattern of interpersonal conflict, especially in regard to intimate relationships.

B. As the client has worked through his/her reaction to the traumatic event, there has been less conflict within personal relationships.

C. The client's partner reported that he/she is irritable, withdrawn, and preoccupied with the traumatic event.

D. The client and his/her partner reported increased communication and satisfaction with the interpersonal relationship.

24. Violent Threat/Behavior (23)

A. The client described having engaged in violent verbal threats since experiencing the traumatic event.

B. The client's irritability has been magnified into physically violent behavior.

C. As the client has worked through the emotions associated with the traumatic event, his/her verbal and physical violence has diminished.

D. The client reported having no recent experiences with verbal or physical violence or threats of violence.

25. Employment Conflicts (24)

A. The client has been unable to maintain employment due to authority/coworker conflict or anxiety symptoms.

B. As the client has worked through the feelings associated with the traumatic event, he/she has been more reliable and responsible within the employment setting.

C. The client has resumed his/her employment duties and attendance in a consistent and reliable manner.

26. Symptoms for One Month or More (25)

A. The client stated that his/her symptoms of PTSD have been present for more than a month.

B. The client's symptoms that have been present for more than a month have diminished.

C. The client no longer experiences PTSD symptoms.

INTERVENTIONS IMPLEMENTED

1. Develop Trust (1)*

A. Today's clinical contact focused on building the level of trust with the client through consistent eye contact, active listening, unconditional positive regard, and warm acceptance.

B. Empathy and support were provided for the client's expression of thoughts and feelings during today's clinical contact.

C. The client was provided with support and feedback as he/she described his/her maladaptive pattern of anxiety.

D. As the client has remained mistrustful and reluctant to share his/her underlying thoughts and feelings, he/she was provided with additional reassurance.

E. The client verbally recognized that he/she has difficulty establishing trust because he/she has often felt let down by others in the past, and he/she was accepted for this insight.

2. Assess Nature of PTSD Symptoms (2)

A. The client was asked about the frequency, intensity, duration, and history of his/her PTSD symptoms, fear, and avoidance.

B. *The Anxiety Disorder's Interview Schedule for DSM-IV* (DiNardo, Brown, and Barlow) was used to assess the client's PTSD symptoms.

C. The assessment of the client's PTSD symptoms indicated that his/her symptoms are extreme and severely interfere with his/her life.

D. The assessment of the client's PTSD symptoms indicate that these symptoms are moderate and occasionally interfere with his/her functioning.

E. The results of the assessment of the client's PTSD symptoms indicate that these symptoms are mild and rarely interfere with his/her daily functioning.

F. The results of the assessment of the client's PTSD symptoms were reviewed with the client.

3. Refer/Conduct Psychological Testing (3)

A. Psychological testing was administered to assess for the presence and strength of the PTSD symptoms.

B. The psychological testing confirmed the presence of significant PTSD symptoms.

C. The psychological testing confirmed mild PTSD symptoms.

D. The psychological testing revealed that there are no significant PTSD symptoms present.

E. The results of the psychological testing were presented to the client.

4. Assess Stimuli (4)

A. Specific stimuli that may precipitate the client's fears and avoidance were reviewed.

B. Specific thoughts and possible delusions were reviewed as to how they contribute to the client's fears and avoidance.

C. Specific situations that have precipitated the client's fears and avoidance were reviewed.

---

* The numbers in parentheses correlate to the number of the Therapeutic Intervention statement in the companion chapter with the same title in *The Severe and Persistent Mental Illness Treatment Planner,* 2nd ed. (Berghuis and Jongsma) by John Wiley & Sons, 2008.

D. Upon the review of the stimuli, thoughts and situations that precipitated the client's fears and avoidance, he/she has been able to decrease his/her level of fear and avoidance.

5. Differentiate Anxiety Symptoms (5)

A. The client was assisted in differentiating anxiety symptoms that are a direct affect of his/her severe and persistent mental illness, as opposed to a separate diagnosis of an anxiety disorder.

B. The client was provided with feedback regarding his/her differentiation of symptoms that are related to his/her severe and persistent mental illness, as opposed to a separate diagnosis.

C. The client has identified a specific anxiety disorder, which is freestanding from his/her severe and persistent mental illness, and this was reviewed within the session.

D. The client has been unsuccessful in identifying ways in which his/her anxiety symptoms are related to his/her mental illness or a separate anxiety disorder.

6. Acknowledge Anxiety Related to Delusional Experiences (6)

A. It was acknowledged that both real and delusional experiences could cause anxiety.

B. The client was provided with support regarding his/her anxieties and worries, which are related to both the real experiences and delusional experiences.

C. The client described a decreased pattern of anxiety due to the support provided to him/her.

7. Identify with Recovery from Trauma (7)

A. The client was provided with a description of Posttraumatic Stress Disorder.

B. Information from *Overcoming Posttraumatic Stress Disorder* (Smyth) was used to help describe symptoms.

C. The client was assisted in identify how he/she may recover from trauma.

8. Explore Facts of Traumatic Event (8)

A. The client was gently encouraged to tell the entire story of the traumatic event.

B. The client was given the opportunity to share what he/she recalls about the traumatic event.

C. Today's therapy session explored the sequence of events before, during, and after the traumatic event.

9. Assess Depression (9)

A. The depth of the client's depression and his/her suicide potential were assessed.

B. Since the client has significant depression and verbalizes suicidal urges, steps were taken to provide more intense treatment and constant supervision.

C. The client's depression was not noted to be particularly serious, and he/she has denied any current suicidal ideation.

10. Assess Chemical Dependence (10)

A. The client was asked to describe his/her use of alcohol and/or drugs as a means of escape from negative emotions.

B. The client was supported as he/she acknowledged that he/she has abused alcohol and/or drugs as a means of coping with the negative consequences associated with the traumatic event.

C. The client was quite defensive about giving information regarding his/her substance abuse history and minimized any such behavior; this was reflected to him/her and he/she was urged to be more open.

11. Request Substance Use Information from Support System (11)

A. The client's family and peers were asked to provide additional information regarding the client's substance use history.

B. The treatment staff that have worked closely with the client were asked to provide an objective review of the client's substance abuse history.

C. Auxiliary information about this client's substance use pattern was consistent with the client's own description.

D. Auxiliary information collected about the client's substance use was not consistent with the client's description of his/her own substance use.

12. Administer Objective Assessment of Substance Use (12)

A. The client was administered an objective assessment of his/her substance use.

B. The Alcohol Severity Index was administered to the client.

C. The findings of the objective assessment of the client's alcohol use were reviewed with the client.

13. Teach Contributing Factors to Substance Abuse (13)

A. The client was taught the familial, emotional, and social factors that have contributed to the development of his/her chemical dependence.

B. The client was supported as he/she verbalized an understanding of the factors contributing to his/her chemical dependence and acknowledged it as a problem.

C. The client's denial led to a refusal to acknowledge his/her chemical dependence and any factors that have contributed to it; this was reflected to him/her.

14. Refer to Chemical Dependence Treatment (14)

A. The client was referred for chemical dependence treatment.

B. The client consented to chemical dependence treatment referral, as he/she has acknowledged it as a significant problem.

C. The client refused to accept a referral for chemical dependence treatment and continued to deny that substance abuse is a problem.

D. The client was reinforced for following through on obtaining chemical dependence treatment.

E. The client's treatment focus was switched to his/her chemical dependence problem.

15. Refer for Medication Evaluation (15)

A. The client was referred for a medication evaluation to help stabilize his/her moods and decrease the intensity of his/her feelings.

B. The client was reinforced as he/she agreed to follow through with the medication evaluation.

C. The client was strongly opposed to being placed on medication to help stabilize his/her moods and reduce emotional distress; his/her objections were processed.

16. Monitor Effects of Medication (16)

A. The client's response to the medication was discussed in today's therapy session.

B. The client reported that the medication has helped to stabilize his/her moods and decrease the intensity of his/her feelings; he/she was directed to share this information with the prescribing clinician.

C. The client reports little to no improvement in his/her moods or anger control since being placed on the medication; he/she was directed to share this information with the prescribing clinician.

D. The client was reinforced for consistently taking the medication as prescribed.

E. The client has failed to comply with taking the medication as prescribed; he/she was encouraged to take the medication as prescribed.

17. Discuss PTSD Symptoms (17)

A. A discussion was held about how PTSD results from exposure to trauma and results in intrusive recollections, unwarranted fears, anxiety, and a vulnerability to other negative emotions.

B. The client was provided with specific examples of how PTSD symptoms occur and affect individuals.

C. The client displayed a clear understanding of the dynamics of PTSD and was provided with positive feedback.

D. The client has struggled to understand the dynamics of PTSD and was provided with remedial feedback in this area.

18. Assign Reading on Anxiety (18)

A. The client was assigned to read psychoeducational chapters of books or treatment manuals on PTSD.

B. The client was assigned information from *Finding Life Beyond Trauma* (Follette and Pistorello).

C. The client has read the assigned information on PTSD, and key points were reviewed.

D. The client has not read the assigned information on PTSD and was redirected to do so.

19. Discuss Treatment Rationale (19)

A. The client was taught about the overall rationale behind treatment of PTSD.

B. The client was assisted in identifying the appropriate goals for PTSD treatment.

C. The client was taught about coping skills, cognitive restructuring, and exposure techniques.

D. The client was taught about techniques that will help to build confidence, desensitize and overcome fears, and see oneself, others, and the world in a less fearful and/or depressing manner.

E. The client was reinforced for his/her clear understanding of the rationale for treatment of PTSD.

F. The client struggled to understand the rationale behind the treatment for PTSD and was provided with additional feedback in this area.

20. Assign Written Information on PTSD (20)

A. The client was assigned to read about stress inoculation, cognitive restructuring, and/or exposure-based therapy in chapters of books or treatment manuals on PTSD.

B. The client was assigned specific chapters from *Reclaiming Your Life After Rape* (Rothbaum and Foa).

C. The client was assigned specific chapters from *Feeling Good: The New Mood Therapy* (Burns).

D. The client has read the assigned information on PTSD; key concepts were reviewed.

E. The client has not read the assigned information on PTSD and was redirected to do so.

21. Teach Stress Inoculation Training (21)

A. The client was taught strategies from stress inoculation training, such as relaxation, breathing, covert modeling, and role-play.

B. The client was taught stress inoculation techniques for managing fears until a sense of mastery is evident from *A Clinical Handbook for Treating PTSD* (Meichenbaum).

C. The client was assisted in practicing stress inoculation training techniques.

D. The client displayed a clear understanding of the use of stress inoculation training.

E. The client has not displayed a clear understanding of the stress inoculation training techniques and was provided with additional feedback in this area.

22. Assess Anger Control (22)

A. A history of the client's anger control problems was taken in today's therapy session.

B. Active listening was used as the client shared instances in which poor control of his/her anger resulted in verbal threats of violence, actual harm or injury to others, or destruction of property.

C. The client identified events or situations that frequently trigger a loss of control of his/her anger and was helped to see his/her patterns.

D. The client was asked to identify the common targets of his/her anger to help gain greater insight into the factors contributing to his/her lack of control.

E. Today's therapy session helped the client realize how his/her anger control problems are often associated with underlying, painful emotions about the traumatic event.

F. The client was quite guarded about his/her anger control problems and was urged to be more open in this area.

23. Teach Anger Management Techniques (23)

A. The client was taught mediational and self-control strategies to help improve his/her anger control.

B. The client was taught guided imagery and relaxation techniques to help improve his/her anger control.

C. Role-playing and modeling techniques were used to demonstrate effective ways to control anger.

D. The client was strongly encouraged to express his/her anger through controlled, respectful verbalizations and healthy physical outlets.

E. A reward system was designed to reinforce the client for demonstrating good anger control.

24. Encourage Physical Exercise (24)

A. The client was assisted in developing a physical exercise routine as a means of coping with stress and developing an improved sense of well-being.

B. The client was reinforced for following through on implementing a regular exercise regimen as a stress release technique.

C. The client has failed to consistently implement a physical exercise routine and was encouraged to do so.

25. Recommend Exercising Your Way to Better Mental Health (25)

A. The book *Exercising Your Way to Better Mental Health* (Leith) was recommended to the client as a means of encouraging physical exercise.

B. The client has followed through with reading the book on exercise and mental health; the key points of this material were reviewed.

C. The client was assisted in implementing a consistent exercise regimen.

D. The client has not followed through with reading the book on exercise nor has he/she implemented a regular physical exercise regimen.

26. Monitor Sleep Patterns (26)

A. The client was encouraged to keep a record of how much sleep he/she gets every night.

B. The client was trained in the use of relaxation techniques to help induce sleep.

C. The client was trained in the use of positive imagery to help induce sleep.

D. The client was referred for a medication evaluation to determine whether medication is needed to help him/her sleep.

27. Identify Distorted Thoughts (27)

A. The client was assisted in identifying the distorted schemas and related automatic thoughts that mediate PTSD responses.

B. The client was taught the role of distorted thinking in precipitating emotional responses.

C. The client was reinforced as he/she verbalized an understanding of the cognitive beliefs and messages that mediate his/her PTSD responses.

D. The client was assisted in replacing distorted messages with positive, realistic cognitions.

E. The client failed to identify his/her distorted thoughts and cognitions and was provided with tentative examples in this area.

28. Read about Cognitive Restructuring of Fears (28)

A. The client was assigned to read about cognitive restructuring of fears or worries in books or treatment manuals.

B. *Overcoming Post-Traumatic Stress Disorder* (Smyth) was assigned to the client to help teach about cognitive restructuring.

C. Key components of cognitive restructuring and exposure therapy were reviewed.

D. The client and parents have not done the assigned reading on cognitive restructuring and were redirected to do so.

29. Assign Self-Talk Homework (29)

A. The client was assigned homework exercises in which he/she identifies fearful self-talk and creates reality-based alternatives.

B. The "Negative Thoughts Trigger Negative Feelings" exercise from the *Adult Psychotherapy Homework Planner,* 2nd ed. (Jongsma) was used to help the client develop healthy self-talk.

C. The client was directed to do homework exercises about self-talk and reality-based alternatives as described in *Overcoming Post-Traumatic Stress Disorder* (Smyth).

D. The client has completed his/her homework related to self-talk and creating reality-based alternatives; he/she was provided with positive reinforcement for his/her success in this area.

E. The client has completed his/her homework related to self-talk and creating reality-based alternatives; he/she was provided with corrective feedback for his/her failure to identify and replace self-talk with reality-based alternatives.

F. The client has not attempted his/her homework related to fearful self-talk and reality-based alternatives and was redirected to do so.

30. Construct Anxiety Stimuli Hierarchy (30)

A. The client was assisted in constructing a hierarchy of anxiety-producing situations associated with two or three spheres of worry.

B. It was difficult for the client to develop a hierarchy of stimulus situations, as the causes of his/her anxiety remain quite vague; he/she was assisted in completing the hierarchy.

C. The client was successful at creating a focused hierarchy of specific stimulus situations that provoke anxiety in a gradually increasing manner; this hierarchy was reviewed.

31. Assign Homework on Exposures (31)

A. The client was assigned homework exercises to perform exposure to feared stimuli and record his/her experience.

B. The client was assigned situational exposures homework from *Posttraumatic Distress Disorder* (Resick and Calhoun).

C. The client's use of exposure techniques was reviewed and reinforced.

D. The client has struggled in his/her implementation of exposure techniques and was provided with corrective feedback.

E. The client has not attempted to use the exposure techniques and was redirected to do so.

32. Use Imaginal Exposure (32)

A. The client was asked to describe a traumatic experience at an increasing, but client-chosen, level of detail.

B. The client was asked to continue to describe his/her traumatic experience at his/her own chosen level of detail until the associated anxiety reduces and stabilizes.

C. The client was provided with recordings of the session and was asked to listen to it between sessions.

D. The client was directed to do imaginal exposures as described in *Posttraumatic Distress Disorder* (Resick and Calhoun).

E. The client was reinforced for his/her progress in imaginal exposure.

F. The client was assisted in problem-solving obstacles to his/her imaginal exposure.

33. Assign Reading Material on Exposure (33)

A. The client was assigned to read about exposure in books or treatment manuals on PTSD.

B. The client was assigned to read information from *Reclaiming Your Life After Rape* (Rothbaum and Foa).

C. The client was assigned to read information from *Overcoming Post-Traumatic Stress Disorder* (Smyth).

D. The client has read the information on exposure techniques, and key points were reviewed.

E. The client has not read the information on exposure techniques and was redirected to do so.

34. Teach Thought Stopping (34)

A. The client was taught a thought-stopping technique.

B. The client was taught to internally voice the word STOP immediately upon noticing unwanted trauma or otherwise negative unwanted thoughts.

C. The client was taught to imagine something representing the concept of stopping (e.g., a stop sign or stoplight) immediately upon noticing unwanted trauma or otherwise negative unwanted thoughts.

D. The client was assisted in reviewing his/her use of thought-stopping techniques and was provided with positive feedback for his/her appropriate use of this technique.

E. Redirection was provided, as the client has not learned to use the thought-stopping technique.

35. Teach Self-Dialogue Procedure (35)

A. The client was taught self-dialogue procedures as described in *Posttraumatic Distress Disorder* (Resick and Calhoun).

B. The client was taught self-dialogue techniques to learn to recognize maladaptive self-talk, challenge its bias, cope with engendered feelings, overcome avoidance, and reinforce accomplishments.

C. The client was reinforced for his/her use of self-dialogue procedures.

D. The client has found significant obstacles to using self-dialogue procedures and was assisted in problem-solving these concerns.

36. Employ EMDR Techniques (36)

A. The client was trained in the use of the eye movement desensitization and reprocessing (EMDR) technique to reduce his/her emotional reactivity to the traumatic event.

B. The client reported that the EMDR technique has been helpful in reducing his/her emotional reactivity to the traumatic event.

C. The client reported partial success with the use of the EMDR technique to reduce emotional distress.

D. The client reported little to no improvement with the use of the EMDR technique to decrease his/her emotional reactivity to the traumatic event.

37. Discuss Lapse versus Relapse (37)

A. The client was assisted in differentiating between a lapse and a relapse.

B. A lapse was associated with the initial and reversible return of symptoms, fear, or urges to avoid.

C. A relapse was associated with the decision to return to fearful and avoidant patterns.

D. The client was reinforced for his/her ability to respond to a lapse without relapsing.

38. Identify and Rehearse Response to Lapse Situations (38)

A. The client was asked to identify the future situations or circumstances in which lapses could occur.

B. The client was asked to rehearse the management of his/her potential lapse situations.

C. The client was reinforced as he/she identified and rehearsed how to cope with potential lapse situations.

39. Encourage Use of Therapy Strategies (39)

A. The client was encouraged to routinely use strategies used in therapy.

B. The client was urged to use cognitive restructuring, social skill, and exposure techniques while building social interactions and relationships.

C. The client was reinforced for his/her regular use of therapy techniques within social interactions and relationships.

D. The client was unable to identify many situations in which he/she has used therapy techniques to help build social interactions and social relationships and was redirected to seek these situations out.

40. Develop a Coping Card (40)

A. The client was provided with a coping card on which specific coping strategies were listed.

B. The client was assisted in developing his/her coping card in order to list his/her helpful coping strategies.

C. The client was encouraged to use his/her coping card when struggling with anxiety producing situations.

41. Conduct Family/Conjoint Session (41)

A. A conjoint session was held to facilitate healing the hurt that the client's PTSD symptoms have caused to others.

B. The client was supported while apologizing to significant others for the irritability, withdrawal, and angry outbursts that are part of his/her PTSD symptom pattern.

C. Support was provided as the client's significant others verbalized the negative impact that the client's PTSD symptoms have had on their lives.

D. Significant others indicated support for the client and accepted apologies for previous hurts that his/her behavior caused; the benefits of this progress were highlighted.

42. Refer for Group Therapy (42)

A. The client was referred for group therapy to help him/her share and work through his/her feelings about the trauma with other individuals who have experienced traumatic incidents.

B. The client was given the directive to self-disclose at least once during the group therapy session about his/her traumatic experience.

C. It was emphasized to the client that his/her involvement in group therapy has helped him/her realize that he/she is not alone in experiencing painful emotions surrounding a traumatic event.

D. It was reflected to the client that his/her active participation in group therapy has helped him/her share and work through many of his/her emotions pertaining to the traumatic event.

E. The client has not made productive use of the group therapy sessions and has been reluctant to share his/her feelings about the traumatic event; he/she was encouraged to use this helpful technique.

43. Reinforce Reality-Based Cognitions (43)

A. The client was taught positive, reality-based self-talk to replace his/her distorted cognitive messages.

B. The client was reinforced for implementing positive, reality-based cognitive messages that enhance self-confidence and increase adaptive action.

C. The client has begun to verbalize hopeful and positive statements regarding the future and was reinforced for doing so.

PSYCHOSIS

CLIENT PRESENTATION

1. Bizarre Thought Content (1)*
A. The client demonstrated delusional thought content.
B. The client has experienced persecutory delusions.
C. The client's delusional thoughts have diminished in frequency and intensity.
D. The client no longer experiences delusional thoughts.

2. Illogical Thought/Speech (2)
A. The client's speech and thought patterns are incoherent and illogical.
B. The client demonstrated loose association of ideas and vague speech.
C. The client's illogical thought and speech have become less frequent.
D. The client no longer gives evidence of illogical forms of thought and speech.

3. Perception Disturbance (3)
A. The client has experienced auditory hallucinations.
B. The client has experienced visual hallucinations.
C. The client's hallucinations have diminished in frequency.
D. The client reported no longer experiencing hallucinations.

4. Disorganized Behavior (4)
A. The client's behavior was characterized by disorganization, confusion, and severe lack of goal direction.
B. The client displayed impulsiveness or repetitive behaviors that appear to be disjunct from reality.
C. The client's behavior has become more organized and goal directed.

5. Paranoia (5)
A. The client displayed paranoid thoughts and reactions, including extreme distrust, fear, and apprehension.
B. The client's level of distrust of others is so pervasive and obsessive that his/her daily functioning is disrupted.
C. The client is unable to fulfill job and family responsibilities because of his/her preoccupation with issues of distrust and paranoia.
D. The client's level of trust is growing, and he/she displays decreased paranoid thoughts and reactions and is more able to perform daily duties and responsibilities.

* The numbers in parentheses correlate to the number of the Behavioral Definition statement in the companion chapter with the same title in *The Severe and Persistent Mental Illness Treatment Planner*, 2nd ed. (Berghuis and Jongsma) by John Wiley & Sons, 2008.

6. Psychomotor Abnormalities (6)

A. The client demonstrated a marked decrease in reactivity to his/her environment.

B. The client demonstrated various catatonic patterns (e.g., stupor, rigidity, posturing, negativism, and excitement).

C. The client gave evidence of unusual mannerisms or grimacing.

D. The client's psychomotor abnormalities have diminished, and his/her pattern of relating has become more typical and less alienating.

7. Agitation (7)

A. The client displayed a high degree of irritability and unpredictability in his/her actions.

B. The client displayed agitation through anger outbursts and impulsive physical acting out.

C. The client is difficult to approach due to his/her extreme agitation.

D. As treatment has progressed, the client has decreased his/her level of agitation and is less irritable, angry, unpredictable, or impulsive.

8. Bizarre Dress/Grooming (8)

A. The client has not given adequate attention to his/her personal grooming.

B. The client presents in unusual clothing and bizarre manner of dress due to his/her diminished contact with reality.

C. As the client's psychosis has stabilized, he/she has become more normalized in his/her dress and grooming.

9. Disturbed Affect (9)

A. The client presented with blunted affect.

B. The client gave evidence of a lack of affect.

C. At times the client's affect was inappropriate for the context of the situation.

D. The client's affect has become more appropriate and energized.

10. Relationship Withdrawal (10)

A. The client has been withdrawn from involvement with the external world and preoccupied with egocentric ideas and fantasies.

B. The client has shown a slight improvement in his/her ability to demonstrate relationship skills.

C. The client has shown an interest in relating to others in a more appropriate manner.

INTERVENTIONS IMPLEMENTED

1. Approach in a Calm Manner (1)*

A. Due to the client's acute psychotic symptoms, he/she was approached in a calm, confident, open, direct yet soothing manner.

B. Body language when approaching the client focused on a slow approach, facing toward the client, and speaking slowly and clearly.

---

* The numbers in parentheses correlate to the number of the Therapeutic Intervention statement in the companion chapter with the same title in *The Severe and Persistent Mental Illness Treatment Planner,* 2nd ed. (Berghuis and Jongsma) by John Wiley & Sons, 2008.

C. As the client has been approached in a calmer manner, his/her psychotic agitation has decreased.

D. The client continues to display increased agitation, despite the use of calm, open, and soothing mannerisms.

2. Identify History of Psychosis (2)

A. The client was asked to identify his/her history of hallucinations, delusions, or other psychotic symptoms.

B. The client was provided with positive feedback as he/she was clearly able to identify his/her pattern of psychotic symptoms.

C. The client denied any pattern of psychotic symptoms and was provided with contrary feedback in this area.

3. Identify Current Psychotic Symptoms (3)

A. The client was asked about his/her current pattern of psychotic symptoms.

B. The client was reinforced for displaying understanding of his/her current pattern of psychotic symptoms.

C. The client denied any current psychotic symptoms and was provided with contrary feedback in this area.

4. Refer for Psychological Testing (4)

A. The client was referred for psychological testing to evaluate the depth of his/her psychosis.

B. The client was compliant with the testing, which indicated a significant pattern of psychotic symptoms.

C. The psychological test results indicate only mild psychotic symptoms, and this was reviewed.

D. The psychological testing results indicate that the client's psychosis has significantly abated, and this was reviewed.

E. The client was not compliant with the psychological testing and was redirected to this referral.

5. Obtain a History from the Family (5)

A. The client's family members were asked to provide information about his/her history of psychotic behaviors.

B. The client's family members provided information about his/her history of psychotic behaviors, and this was processed with him/her.

6. Refer to a Physician (6)

A. The client was referred to a physician for an evaluation for a prescription of psychotropic medications.

B. The client was reinforced for following through on a referral to a physician for an assessment for a prescription of psychotropic medications, but none were prescribed.

C. The client has been prescribed psychotropic medications.

D. The client declined evaluation by a physician for a prescription of psychotropic medications and was redirected to cooperate with this referral.

7. Refer to a Supervised Environment (7)

A. Because the client was judged to be uncontrollably harmful to himself/herself, arrangements were made for psychiatric hospitalization.

B. Due to concerns about the client's inability to manage himself/herself within a less restrictive setting, he/she was referred to a crisis residential facility.

C. The client was supported for cooperating voluntarily with admission to a more supervised environment.

D. The client refused to voluntarily admit himself/herself to a more supervised environment; therefore, civil commitment procedures were initiated.

8. Arrange for a Stable Setting (8)

A. Arrangements were made for the client to remain in a stable, supervised setting.

B. The client has been able to decrease his/her psychotic symptoms as he/she has remained in a stable, supervised setting, and the benefits of this were reviewed with him/her.

C. Despite remaining in a stable, supervised setting, the client has continued to decompensate and he/she was admitted to a more intensive treatment setting.

9. Coordinate Mobile Crisis Response Services (9)

A. Arrangements were made for mobile crisis response services for the client, including a physical exam, psychiatric evaluation, medication access, and triage to inpatient care.

B. The client was sought out in his/her home environment for the mobile crisis response services.

C. Mobile crisis response services have assisted the client in becoming stabilized.

D. The client continues to decompensate despite the use of mobile crisis response services, and a more structured placement was arranged.

10. Assess Suicidal Ideation (10)

A. The client was asked to describe the frequency and intensity of his/her suicidal ideation, the details of any existing suicide plan, the history of any previous suicide attempts, and any family history of depression or suicide.

B. The client was encouraged to be forthright regarding the current strength of his/her suicidal feelings and the ability to control such suicidal urges.

C. The client was monitored on an ongoing basis for his/her suicide potential.

D. Precautionary steps were taken to keep the client from committing suicide, including more direct supervision or placement in a locked, monitored environment.

11. Remove Potentially Hazardous Materials (11)

A. Significant others were encouraged to remove firearms and other potentially lethal means of suicide from the client's easy access.

B. With the client's permission, potentially hazardous materials were removed and stored until he/she has become more stable.

C. The client declined to allow hazardous materials to be removed, and he/she was provided with feedback about this decision and the additional steps that may be taken to assure his/her safety.

12. Develop a Short-Term Crisis Plan (12)

A. A short-term round-the-clock crisis plan was developed.

B. It was determined that components of the client's short-term round-the-clock crisis plan must include multiple caregivers, psychiatric involvement, and/or crisis assistance in order to maintain him/her within the community.

C. As the crisis plan has been implemented, the client has been able to remain within the community as he/she stabilizes from his/her period of psychosis.

D. The client continues to decompensate and is not safe to maintain within the community, despite the use of the crisis plan, and arrangements for a more restrictive setting were initiated.

13. Coordinate Access to Professional Consultation (13)

A. The client and his/her caregivers were told how to access round-the-clock professional consultation.

B. The client was supported for using the 24-hour, professionally staffed crisis line to help decrease his/her agitation and psychosis.

C. The client's caregivers were reinforced for accessing professional consultation on an as-needed basis to help determine how best to cope with his/her difficult behaviors in this less restrictive setting.

D. The client and his/her caregivers have not used the available professional consultation and were encouraged to do so.

14. Provide Cues to Focus on Reality (14)

A. The client was provided with visual and verbal cues to increase his/her focus on reality.

B. The date, time, and place were written in a clearly visible area to help anchor the client in reality.

C. Verbal interactions with the client focused on the here and now.

15. Use a Wristband (15)

A. A wristband was placed on the client's arm with the date, place, and his/her name written clearly.

B. The client was reinforced for being more reality-focused with the use of the wristband.

C. The client continues with illogical and unrealistic psychotic thoughts, despite implementing visual cues with the client (e.g., a wristband on the arm).

16. Focus on Concrete Events (16)

A. Conversations with the client focused on real events in basic, concrete terms.

B. As the client displayed his/her psychotic process, he/she was consistently refocused onto actual, current events described in basic, concrete terms.

C. As the client has been focused onto more concrete information, he/she has decreased his/her bizarre or irrational comments in favor of more reality-based thoughts.

D. The client continues to experience psychotic process, despite others focusing on real events in basic, concrete terms.

17. Reinforce a Focus on Reality (17)

A. The client was provided with positive reinforcement as he/she displayed an appropriate focus on reality.

B. As the client became more reality-focused, he/she was gradually returned to a less restrictive environment and decreased supervision.

C. The client has relapsed into more delusional thought and other psychotic processes, despite being reinforced for his/her appropriate focus on reality.

18. Investigate Sleep-Inducing Medications with the Physician (18)

A. The client's treating physician was consulted regarding the need for sleep-inducing medications to provide the client and his/her caregivers time to regroup relative to this current psychotic episode.

B. The treating physician has prescribed sleep-inducing medications that have helped the client to sleep, which has resulted in a more reality-based orientation.

C. Caregivers were supported for providing intensive support to the client subsequent to his/her being induced to sleep.

D. The treating physician has declined to use sleep-inducing medication.

19. Educate about Psychotropic Medications (19)

A. The client was taught about the indications for and the expected benefits of psychotropic medications.

B. As the client's psychotropic medications were reviewed, he/she displayed an understanding about the indications for and expected benefits of the medications.

C. The client displayed a lack of understanding of the indications for and expected benefits of psychotropic medications and was provided with additional information and feedback regarding his/her medications.

20. Monitor Medications (20)

A. The client was monitored for compliance with his/her psychotropic medication regimen.

B. The client was provided with positive feedback about his/her regular use of psychotropic medications.

C. The client was monitored for the effectiveness and side effects of his/her prescribed medications.

D. Concerns about the client's medication effectiveness and side effects were communicated to the physician.

E. Although the client was monitored for medication side effects, he/she reported no concerns in this area.

21. Review Side Effects of Medications (21)

A. The possible side effects related to the client's medications were reviewed with the client.

B. The client identified significant side effects, and these were reported to the medical staff.

C. Possible side effects of the client's medications were reviewed, but he/she denied experiencing any side effects.

22. Assess Tardive Symptoms (22)

A. Arrangements were made for an assessment of the client's tardive symptoms.

B. Objective measurement of the client's tardive symptoms was performed by qualified personnel using a specific instrument [e.g., the Abnormal Involuntary Movement Scale (AIMS)].

C. The client displayed no evidence of tardive symptoms, and this was reflected to him/her.

D. The client displayed both subjective and objective evidence of tardive symptoms, and this was reported to the physician who prescribed the client's psychotropic medications.

23. Educate the Family about Symptoms of Mental Illness (23)

A. The client's family, friends, and caregivers were educated about the symptoms of mental illness, with specific emphasis on the nonvolitional aspects of some symptoms.

B. The client's family members, friends, and caregivers were supported for their increased understanding about the symptoms of mental illness and the nonvolitional aspects of some symptoms.

C. The client's family members, friends, and caregivers rejected the information regarding his/her symptoms of mental illness and the nonvolitional aspects of some symptoms and were given additional feedback in this area.

24. Role-Play Response to Anger Outbursts (24)

A. Specific responses to the client's anger outbursts were role-played with his/her family members.

B. The client's family, friends, and caregivers were advised to focus on providing short, specific directions and to avoid arguing about reality.

C. The client's family, friends, and caregivers were reinforced for their understanding of assertive, safe, direct responses to his/her anger outbursts.

D. The client's family, friends, and caregivers remain confused about how to respond directly to his/her anger outbursts in an assertive, safe manner; further direction was provided to them.

25. Refer to Family Psychoeducational Program (25)

A. The family was referred to a psychoeducational program to help demonstrate techniques to cope with the client's psychotic behaviors.

B. The client was referred to a multigroup family psychoeducational program to help learn and share about techniques to cope with the client's psychotic behaviors.

C. The family was engaged in the psychoeducational program and has identified ways in which they have learned to cope with the client's psychotic behaviors.

D. The client's family has not engaged in the psychoeducational program and was redirected to do so.

26. Identify Psychosis Triggers (26)

A. The client was requested to identify specific behaviors, situations, and feelings that occurred prior to decompensation or psychotic episodes.

B. The client identified specific behaviors, situations, and feelings that occurred prior to his/her decompensation, and these triggers were processed.

C. The client was unable to identify specific behaviors, situations, and feelings that have occurred prior to decompensation and was given suggestions in these areas.

27. Identify Symptoms Maintenance Cycles (27)

A. The client was assisted in identifying emotional reactions that tend to maintain his/her symptoms.

B. The client was assisted in identifying how the effects of his/her psychotic symptoms may exacerbate those symptoms.

C. Examples were used to identify the self-reinforcing nature of some psychotic symptoms (e.g., withdrawal leading to isolation and loneliness; paranoid accusations leading to negative actions of others that falsely support the delusion).

D. The client was reinforced for his/her insight into the effects of his/her psychosis.

E. The client has not understood or accepted the effects of his/her psychotic symptoms, and was provided with remedial assistance in this area.

28. Assess Adaptive and Maladaptive Strategies (28)

A. The client was assessed for his/her adaptive and maladaptive strategies for coping with his/her psychotic symptoms.

B. Inquiries were made regarding how the client uses deficit strategies to cope with his/her psychotic symptoms.

C. The client was provided with feedback about his/her use of maladaptive and adaptive strategies for coping with his/her psychotic symptoms.

29. Use Cognitive-Behavioral Strategies (29)

A. Cognitive-behavioral strategies were used to help the client learn coping and compensation strategies for managing his/her psychotic symptoms.

B. The client was referred for cognitive-behavioral therapy to help the coping compensation strategies for managing his/her psychotic symptoms.

C. The client was asked to provide examples of the cognitive-behavioral strategies that he/she has learned in order to cope with his/her psychotic symptoms.

D. The client was reinforced for his/her use of cognitive-behavioral strategies.

E. The client has not used cognitive-behavioral strategies to cope with his/her psychotic symptoms and was redirect to do so.

30. Desensitize Fearfulness of Hallucinations (30)

A. The client was encouraged to talk about his/her hallucinations, their frequency, intensity, and meaning, in order to desensitize his/her level of fear.

B. "What Do You Hear and See?" from the *Adult Psychotherapy Homework Planner,* 2nd ed. (Jongsma) was used to help the client talk about his/her hallucinations.

C. As the client talked about his/her hallucinations, he/she was provided with support, encouragement, and empathy.

D. The client was reinforced for reporting a decreased sense of fear related to his/her hallucinations, now seeing them as simply a symptom.

E. The client continues to exhibit significant fear related to his/her hallucinations and was provided with additional support in this area.

31. Teach Coping and Compensation Strategies (31)

A. The client was taught coping and compensations strategies for managing his/her psychotic symptoms.

B. The client was taught self-calming techniques and attention switching/narrowing techniques to help manage his/her psychotic symptoms.

C. The client was taught healthy internal cognition techniques, such as realistic self-talk or realistic attribution of the source of the symptom in order to help manage his/her psychotic symptoms.

D. The client was taught to increase adaptive personal and social activity to help manage his/her psychotic symptoms.

E. The client was reinforced for his/her use of coping and compensation strategies.

F. The client has not used the coping and compensation strategies and was redirected to do so.

32. Teach/Refer for Communication and Social Skills (32)

A. The client was referred for an assertiveness-training group that will educate and facilitate assertiveness skills and other adaptive communication techniques.

B. Role-playing, modeling, and behavioral rehearsal were used to train the client in assertiveness skills, communication, and social skills.

C. The client has demonstrated a clearer understanding of important social skills and was provided with positive feedback in this area.

D. The client could not demonstrate a clear understanding of important social and communication skills and was provided with additional feedback in this area.

33. Practice New Skills In Session and Out (33)

A. The client was asked to practice new skills in reality testing, changing his/her maladaptive beliefs and managing his/her symptoms within the session.

B. The client was provided with homework assignments between sessions that focus on practicing his/her new skills, reality testing, changing maladaptive beliefs, and managing his/her symptoms.

C. The client was helped to process his/her maintenance exercises.

D. The client has not completed his/her maintenance exercises and was redirected to do so.

34. Identify Emotional Indicators of Stress (34)

A. The client was requested to identify three emotional indicators of stress and how they affect his/her functioning.

B. The client identified three emotional indicators of stress (e.g., anxiousness, uncertainty, and anger) as well as how they affect his/her functioning, and these indicators were processed.

C. The client failed to identify indicators of stress and how they affect his/her functioning and was provided with feedback in this area.

35. Identify Physical Indicators of Stress (35)

A. The client was requested to identify three physical indicators of stress and how they affect his/her functioning.

B. The client identified three physical indicators of stress (e.g., tense muscles, headaches, psychomotor agitation) and how they affect his/her functioning, and these indicators were processed.

C. The client failed to identify physical indicators of stress and was provided with additional feedback in this area.

36. Teach Stress Management Strategies (36)

A. The client was taught stress management strategies to help him/her decrease his/her overall subjective level of stress.

B. The client was taught relaxation techniques to help him/her manage his/her level of stress.

C. The client was taught positive self-talk, problem-solving, and communication skills to help him/her decrease his/her level of stress.

D. The client was taught lifestyle management considerations that may help to decrease his/her level of stress.

E. The client has implemented many stress management techniques, and the benefits of these techniques were reviewed and reinforced.

F. The client has not utilized many stress management techniques and was redirected to do so.

37. Refer to an Activity Therapist (37)

A. The client was referred to an activity therapist for recommendations regarding physical fitness activities that are available to help reduce his/her stress level.

B. The client was referred to community physical fitness resources (e.g., health clubs and other recreational programs).

C. The client has been actively participating in community physical fitness programs and was reinforced for this.

D. The client has declined involvement in community physical fitness programs and was redirected to do so.

38. Identify Decompensation (38)

A. The client was assisted in identifying symptoms that indicate that he/she is decompensating.

B. The client identified several symptoms of his/her decompensation, and these were reviewed.

C. The client has failed to identify symptoms of his/her decompensation and was provided with additional feedback in this area.

39. Train Support Network about Decompensation Indicators (39)

A. The client's support network was trained about the indicators of decompensation.

B. The client's support network was focused on when to take appropriate action to get professional services for him/her.

C. The client's support network has displayed an understanding of his/her decompensation indicators and the appropriate time to obtain professional services for him/her and was encouraged to use this information.

D. Members of the client's support network have displayed a poor understanding of decompensation and when to obtain professional services for him/her and were provided with additional feedback in this area.

40. Encourage Discontinuation of Substance Use (40)

A. The client was encouraged to decrease or to discontinue his/her substance use, including drugs, alcohol, nicotine, and caffeine.

B. The client was reinforced for decreasing his/her substance use.

C. The client was reinforced for discontinuing his/her substance use.

D. The client continues to use a variety of substances and was refocused on the need to discontinue his/her substance use.

41. Refer for Substance Abuse Treatment (41)

A. The client was evaluated regarding his/her use of substances, the severity of his/her substance abuse, and treatment needs/options.

B. The client was referred to a substance abuse program knowledgeable in the treatment of both substance abuse and severe and persistent mental illness.

C. The client was compliant with the substance abuse evaluation, and the results of the evaluation were discussed with him/her, resulting in admission to a substance abuse program.

D. The client declined to participate in the substance abuse evaluation or treatment and was encouraged to do so.

42. Teach Coping Skills to Caregivers (42)

A. Caregivers for the client were taught problem-solving and assertiveness skills, as well as respite care options to assist in meeting their own needs when they feel overly stressed by his/her psychosis.

B. Caregivers for the client have appropriately used problem-solving and assertiveness skills, as well as respite care to help meet their own needs when they feel overly stressed by his/her psychosis and were encouraged for this as a positive way to care for him/her.

C. Caregivers for the client have not used coping skills to help meet their own needs when they feel overly stressed by his/her psychosis and were redirected in this area.

43. Encourage Emotions Regarding Mental Illness (43)

A. The client was encouraged to express his/her feelings related to the acceptance of his/her mental illness.

B. The client was provided with positive support and empathy as he/she expressed his/her emotions related to his/her mental illness.

C. As the client has expressed his/her feelings, he/she reports a greater acceptance of his/her mental illness, and this was processed.

D. The client tends to deny and minimize his/her feelings related to the acceptance of his/her mental illness and was provided with additional feedback in this area.

44. Explain Psychosis (44)

A. The client was provided with information related to the psychotic process, it's biochemical component, and its confusing effect on rational thought.

B. The client's questions regarding his/her psychotic process were answered.

C. As the client has gained a greater understanding of his/her psychotic process, he/she has been observed to be more at ease with his/her pattern of symptoms.

D. The client failed to understand the nature of his/her psychotic process and was provided with additional feedback in this area.

45. Refer to a Support Group (45)

A. The client was referred to a support group for individuals with severe and persistent mental illness.

B. The client has attended the support group for individuals with severe and persistent mental illness, and the benefits of this support group were reviewed.

C. The client reported that he/she has not experienced any positive benefit from the use of a support group but was encouraged to continue to attend.

D. The client has not used the support group for individuals with severe and persistent mental illness and was redirected to do so.

RECREATIONAL DEFICITS

CLIENT PRESENTATION

1. Lack of Involvement (1)*

A. The client described a history of limited involvement in recreational activities.

B. The client displayed a pattern of limited involvement in recreational activities.

C. The client has become more involved in his/her chosen recreational activities.

D. As treatment has progressed, the client has significantly increased his/her involvement in recreational activities.

2. Lack of Interest (2)

A. The client displayed a lack of interest in leisure activities.

B. The client's involvement in leisure activity options has declined.

C. The client regularly declines any involvement in leisure activities due to his/her deflated mood.

D. As the client has stabilized, he/she displayed increased interest in leisure activities.

3. Limited Knowledge/Experience (3)

A. The client displayed a limited knowledge of recreational opportunities that are available to him/her.

B. The client described a pattern of inexperience in recreational activities.

C. As the client has experienced and learned about recreational opportunities, he/she has increased his/her desire for involvement in recreational activities.

4. Embarrassment (4)

A. The client described that he/she is often embarrassed about his/her presentation and therefore declines involvement in recreational activities.

B. The client displayed signs of embarrassment (e.g., shyness, anxiousness, and a lack of involvement in recreational activities).

C. As the client has become more self-assured, he/she reports decreased embarrassment in recreational activities.

5. Frustration/Agitation (4)

A. The client often becomes frustrated or agitated when involved in recreational activities.

B. The client expressed feelings of frustration and sees this as a barrier to his/her involvement in recreational activities.

C. As the client has learned anger control techniques, his/her pattern of frustration and agitation in recreational activities has significantly decreased.

---

* The numbers in parentheses correlate to the number of the Behavioral Definition statement in the companion chapter with the same title in *The Severe and Persistent Mental Illness Treatment Planner,* 2nd ed. (Berghuis and Jongsma) by John Wiley & Sons, 2008.

6. Symptoms Disrupt Recreational Activities (5)

A. The client described that his/her mental illness symptoms often disrupt involvement in recreational activity.

B. The client's poor reality orientation makes it difficult for him/her to appropriately interact with others in recreational activities.

C. The client finds it difficult to maintain recreational interest due to his/her widely varying moods.

D. As the client has stabilized his/her mental illness symptoms, he/she has become more capable of involvement in recreational activities.

7. Discrimination (6)

A. The client described a pattern of discrimination due to his/her mental illness symptoms, which prohibits involvement in community activities.

B. The client has often been barred from involvement in community activities due to his/her bizarre behavior or other symptoms of his/her mental illness.

C. The client is often discouraged from involvement in community activities by those who have organized the activities.

D. As advocacy has been provided for and by the client, discrimination regarding his/her involvement in community activities has declined.

8. Negative Medication Effects (7)

A. The client reports decreased coordination due to his/her medications, which decreases his/her ability to be involved in some recreational activities (e.g., sports).

B. The client's medications are known to have negative side effects, which will decrease his/her ability to perform in some recreational activities.

C. The client has replaced those activities that are affected by his/her medication with other activities not affected by the medication.

9. Lack of Invitations (8)

A. The client described that he/she is rarely invited to recreational activities due to limited social contact.

B. The client has rarely been invited to recreational activities due to his/her poor social skills.

C. The client rarely reciprocates invitations to recreational activities.

D. As the client has learned increased social skills and stabilized his/her mental illness symptoms, he/she reports increased social contacts.

10. Lack of Funds (9)

A. The client described that he/she is often unable to pay for recreational activities.

B. The client is often unable to obtain transportation to recreational activities.

C. As the client's severe and persistent mental illness symptoms have stabilized, he/she reports increased ability to procure funds for transportation and involvement in recreational activities.

INTERVENTIONS IMPLEMENTED

1. Request a History of Recreational Involvement (1)*

A. The client was requested to relate his/her history or pattern of recreational involvement.

B. The client was assisted in developing an understanding of his/her pattern of recreational deficiencies.

C. The client displayed an increased understanding of his/her syndrome of recreational problems and how they relate to his/her severe and persistent mental illness symptoms and was provided with positive feedback about this insight.

D. The client has a very limited understanding of his/her pattern of recreational problems and was provided with additional feedback in this area.

2. Develop a Graphic Display (2)

A. A graphic time line display was used to help the client chart his/her pattern of recreational difficulties.

B. The client identified his/her pattern of recreational involvement, struggle, failure, and the effects of these problems and was assisted in charting them on a time line.

C. The client displayed a greater understanding of his/her pattern of decreased recreational involvement and was given support and feedback in this area.

D. The client failed to understand his/her pattern of recreational struggles and was redirected in this area.

3. Educate about Mental Illness (3)

A. The client was educated about the expected or common symptoms of his/her mental illness that may negatively impact his/her recreational enjoyment.

B. As the client's symptoms of mental illness were discussed, he/she displayed an understanding of how these symptoms may affect his/her level of involvement in recreational activities.

C. The client struggled to identify how symptoms of his/her mental illness may negatively impact his/her recreational activities and was given additional feedback in this area.

4. Connect Mental Illness and Social/Recreational Problems (4)

A. The client was assisted in making the connection between his/her mental illness symptoms and social/recreational problems.

B. The client was reinforced for displaying an understanding of how his/her mental illness symptoms affect his/her social/recreational problems.

C. The client has failed to make the connection between his/her mental illness symptoms and social/recreational problems and was provided with additional information in this area.

5. Identify Inexperience (5)

A. The client was asked to identify the recreational areas in which he/she has had little experience due to his/her severe and persistent mental illness.

---

* The numbers in parentheses correlate to the number of the Therapeutic Intervention statement in the companion chapter with the same title in *The Severe and Persistent Mental Illness Treatment Planner,* 2nd ed. (Berghuis and Jongsma) by John Wiley & Sons, 2008.

B. The client was assisted in identifying recreational areas in which he/she has had little experience due to severe and persistent mental illness.

C. The client received positive feedback as he/she identified areas in which he/she has experienced limited involvement.

D. The client has failed to identify recreation areas in which he/she has had little experience and was redirected to review this area.

6. Refer to a Physician (6)

A. The client was referred to a physician for an evaluation for a prescription of psychotropic medications.

B. The client was reinforced for following through on a referral to a physician for an assessment for a prescription of psychotropic medications, but none were prescribed.

C. The client has been prescribed psychotropic medications.

D. The client declined evaluation by a physician for a prescription of psychotropic medications and was redirected to cooperate with this referral.

7. Educate about Psychotropic Medications (7)

A. The client was taught about the indications for and the expected benefits of psychotropic medications.

B. As the client's psychotropic medications were reviewed, he/she displayed an understanding about the indications for and expected benefits of the medications.

C. The client displayed a lack of understanding of the indications for and expected benefits of psychotropic medications and was provided with additional information and feedback regarding his/her medications.

8. Monitor Medications (8)

A. The client was monitored for compliance with his/her psychotropic medication regimen.

B. The client was provided with positive feedback about his/her regular use of psychotropic medications.

C. The possible side effects related to the client's medications were reviewed with the client.

D. The client was monitored for the effectiveness and side effects of his/her prescribed medications.

E. Concerns about the client's medication effectiveness and side effects were communicated to the physician.

F. Although the client was monitored for medication side effects, he/she reported no concerns in this area.

9. Acknowledge/Consult about Medication Effects (9)

A. The manner in which the side effects of the medications may inhibit the client's involvement in some recreational activities was acknowledged.

B. The client endorsed examples in which his/her medications have inhibited his/her involvement in recreational activities (e.g., slowed reaction time, decreased motor dexterity), and this was processed.

C. The client's physician was consulted regarding the possible change in the client's medication regimen to decrease side effects that inhibit involvement in recreational activities.

D. The client's medications have been adjusted in order to increase his/her involvement in recreational activities.

E. The client's medications have not been able to be adjusted in order to increase his/her involvement in recreational activities.

10. Refer to an Activity Therapist (10)

A. The client was referred to an activity therapist for recommendations regarding current interests and abilities relative to recreational activities that are available in the community.

B. The results of the activity therapist's review of the client's interests and aptitudes were examined with him/her.

C. The client was referred to community activities and other recreational programs.

D. The client was reinforced for actively participating in community programs.

E. The client has declined involvement in community programs and was urged to consider this as he/she is able.

11. Contract for Interest Development (11)

A. An agreement was made with the client to have him/her pursue a short-term involvement with a variety of activities.

B. Emphasis was placed on the need for the client to explore several different activity areas to develop interests.

C. The client was supported for committing to involvement in a variety of short-term activities in order to develop recreational interests.

D. The client has declined involvement in short-term recreational activities and was redirected in this area.

12. Develop a Schedule (12)

A. An activity schedule for the client was developed that samples a broad range of types of activities, settings, length of time, level of involvement, cultural needs, and social contact.

B. The client was provided with positive feedback regarding his/her participation in the schedule of activities.

C. The client has not complied with his/her schedule of activities to help sample a broad range of activities and was redirected to do so.

13. Review a Sample of Activities (13)

A. The client's involvement in a sample of activities was reviewed on a regular basis.

B. The client provided feedback about his/her involvement in activities, and this was processed.

C. The client was requested to identify his/her preferences regarding the activities that he/she has experienced.

D. The client has identified specific preferences, and these were accepted and processed.

E. The client has not used the sampling of activities and was redirected to do so.

14. Explore Social Reactions (14)

A. The client's reactions to difficult social situations in the past were explored.

B. The client was assisted in identifying specific emotions regarding his/her previous difficult social experiences.

C. The client has identified difficult social experiences and the emotions that he/she has experienced relative to these social problems, and these experiences were processed.

D. The client found it difficult to identify problematic social experiences and the emotions relative to these experiences and was provided with support and encouragement in this area.

15. Acknowledge Emotions (15)

A. The emotions that the client may be experiencing, including fear, embarrassment, and uncertainty, were acknowledged.

B. The effect of the client's emotions on limiting his/her willingness to be involved in new activities was acknowledged.

C. As the client has worked through his/her emotions, he/she is more interested in recreational activities, and this was processed.

D. The client tends to deny any feelings related to his/her involvement in activities and was provided with feedback in this area.

16. Request an Inventory of Community Activities (16)

A. The client was requested to develop an inventory of activities that are available in the community.

B. The client was directed to review information from the local newspaper, telephone book, or magazines.

C. The client was reinforced for developing an inventory of activities that are available in the community.

D. The client has not developed his/her inventory of activities available in the community and was redirected to do so.

17. Obtain Additional Resources Regarding Available Activities (17)

A. Additional resources were obtained for the client's review regarding the recreational activities that are available in the community (e.g., brochures from a local tourism board, current events calendar).

B. Additional resources regarding recreational activities were reviewed with the client.

C. The client has identified additional interests, and these were processed.

18. Develop Income Sources (18)

A. The client was assisted in obtaining, completing, and filing forms for Social Security Disability benefits or other public aid.

B. The client was assisted in identifying ways to increase income through obtaining employment.

C. The client has obtained regular income, and he/she is now able to afford the use of resources within the community and was provided with positive feedback for this progress.

D. The client has not developed any regular sources of income and was redirected to do so.

19. Access Available Funding or Sponsors (19)

A. The client was assisted in seeking access to funds that are available for assisting people with disabilities in their recreational pursuits.

B. The benefits of the use of funds for recreational activities were reviewed.

C. Community recreational businesses were contacted to sponsor the client's involvement in recreational activities (e.g., free tickets or supplies).

D. The client has increased his/her involvement in recreational activities through the use of materials or other support from recreational businesses in the community, and the benefits of this were processed.

E. The client has not accessed funds from the agency or from sponsors/community organizations for assisting people with disabilities and was redirected to do so.

F. The client has not used available resources from recreational businesses in the community and was redirected to do so.

20. Coordinate Ride Sharing and Public Transportation (20)

A. Transportation to recreational events was coordinated through ride sharing with other clients or community members.

B. The client was reinforced for increasing his/her involvement in recreational events through the use of ride sharing and public transportation.

C. The client was assisted in identifying community-based transportation resources for his/her use in getting to recreational activities.

D. The client was assisted in scheduling community-based transportation resources for his/her use in recreational activities.

E. The client has not taken advantage of ride sharing with other clients or community members or the use of public transportation in order to attend recreational events and was redirected to do so.

21. Refer to an Activity Therapist (21)

A. The client was referred to an activity therapist for recommendations regarding basic skills necessary for involvement in recreational activities.

B. The client was taught specific skills useful in leisure or recreational activities (e.g., how to bowl or play bridge).

C. The client was reinforced for displaying increased knowledge and ability in leisure and recreational activities.

D. The client has declined to learn more or be involved in community recreational activities and was redirected to do so.

22. Increase Socialization Online (22)

A. The client was provided with access to online services in order to increase his/her social contact in a safer setting.

B. The client has identified an increased comfort level regarding social contact through his/her online social involvement, and this was processed.

C. The client appears to be less social since accessing online services and was redirected in this area.

D. The client has not used online services as a way to increase social contact in a safer setting and was redirected in this area.

23. Incorporate Meals as a Training Incentive (23)

A. During recreational skills training, cooking and meal preparation were incorporated as an added incentive for the completion of each training session.

B. The client was supported for being more regular in his/her completion of training sessions through the use of cooking and meal preparation as an added incentive, and the benefits of this were reviewed with him/her.

C. The client has not been regularly involved in recreational skills training, despite added incentives, and was redirected to increase his/her involvement.

24. Refer to a Support Group (24)

A. The client was referred to a support group for individuals with severe and persistent mental illness.

B. The client has attended the support group for individuals with severe and persistent mental illness, and the benefits of this support group were reviewed.

C. The client reported that he/she has not experienced any positive benefit from the use of a support group, but was encouraged to continue to attend.

D. The client has not used the support group for individuals with severe and persistent mental illness, and was redirected to do so.

25. Refer for Individual Therapy (25)

A. The client was referred for individual therapy to a therapist who specializes in the treatment of the severely and persistently mentally ill and social skill development.

B. The client was referred to a therapist who specializes in the treatment of the severely and persistently mentally ill for group therapy focused on social skill development.

C. The client has followed up on the referral to therapy to develop social skills, and this treatment was reviewed.

D. The client has not followed up on the referral to therapy to develop social skills and was encouraged to make this contact.

26. Teach/Practice Social Skills (26)

A. Role-playing, behavioral rehearsal, and role reversal techniques were used to help the client understand the use of social skills.

B. Social skills were modeled to the client (e.g., assertiveness, clear communication, handling anger).

C. The client was encouraged to use the modeled social skills on a regular basis.

D. The client was provided with feedback regarding his/her use of social skills.

E. The client has not regularly used the social skills on which he/she has been educated and was provided with remedial information in this area.

27. Train Caregivers/Staff Members on Incidental Learning (27)

A. The caregivers/staff members for the client were trained in the use of incidental learning techniques (e.g., teaching the client social and recreational skills during the course of everyday activities).

B. The caregivers/staff members have regularly used incidental learning techniques to assist the client in learning social and recreational skills, and the benefits of this teaching were reviewed with the caregivers/staff members and the client.

C. The client's increased functioning regarding social and recreational skills was processed.

D. The ongoing use of the incidental learning techniques by the caregivers/staff members was monitored to avoid "program drift."

E. Positive feedback was provided to the caregivers/staff members regarding their regular continued use of incidental learning techniques.

F. The caregivers/staff members have not used the incidental learning techniques and were redirected to do so.

28. List Interesting Activities (28)

A. The client was provided with a list of recreational activities in which he/she has indicated some interest.

B. The client was urged to use his/her list of interesting recreational activities to initiate activity during free times.

C. The client received positive feedback regarding his/her use of his/her list of recreational activities.

D. The client has not used his/her list of recreational activities in order to initiate activity during his/her free time and was redirected to do so.

29. Chart Involvement in Activities (29)

A. A chart was provided to the client and his/her caretakers to monitor and track his/her involvement in various recreational activities.

B. The chart of the client's involvement in recreational activities was reviewed.

C. The chart of the client's involvement in recreational activities indicated an increased pattern of involvement, and this was reflected to the client.

D. The client was verbally reinforced for his/her involvement in recreational activities.

E. The client was reinforced for identifying the positive effects of his/her increased involvement in recreational activities.

F. The chart of the client's involvement in recreational activities has indicated a limited amount of involvement in recreational activities, and this was reflected to him/her.

G. The client denied any positive effect of his/her involvement in recreational activities, and contrary evidence was presented to him/her.

30. Shadow at Recreational Activities (30)

A. As the client attended his/her chosen recreational activities, he/she was shadowed in order to provide support and direction.

B. To decrease stigma and increase independent functioning, the client was allowed to determine how closely the clinician was involved as the client was shadowed at his/her selected activity.

C. As a result of the support and encouragement provided by the shadowing clinician, the client has been able to increase his/her involvement and comfort level at his/her chosen activities.

D. The client declined to have the clinician shadow him/her at the chosen activities, and he/she was accepted for this position.

31. Solicit Volunteers to Accompany the Client (31)

A. Volunteers were solicited from the client's family and peers to attend recreational activities with him/her.

B. The family members and peers have volunteered to attend recreational activities with the client, and he/she described an increased comfort level.

C. The client continues to feel uncomfortable, despite the use of family members and peers to accompany the client to recreational activities, and was provided with additional support in this area.

32. Refer for a Complete Physical (32)

A. The client was referred to a physician for a complete physical examination to determine his/her ability to participate in physical activities.

B. The client has completed the physical examination, and the physician has identified that he/she is able to participate in physical activities.

C. The client has completed the physical examination, and specific limitations were identified regarding his/her ability to participate in physical activities, and these were reviewed with him/her.

D. The client has not submitted himself/herself for the physical examination and was redirected to do so.

33. Coordinate Exercising with Others (33)

A. The client's physical exercise involvement with others who have similar interests was coordinated.

B. The client was assisted in locating and attending physical exercise with other individuals with severe and persistent mental illness.

C. The client was assisted in locating and attending physical exercise with the nondisabled population.

D. The client was reinforced for increasing his/her physical exercise involvement with others.

E. The client does not take advantage of physical exercise involvement with others and was redirected in this area.

34. Advise Nondisabled Peers on Coping with Mental Illness (34)

A. An appropriate authorization to release confidential information was obtained in order to meet with the client's nondisabled peers.

B. The client's nondisabled peers were provided with information about how best to cope with their friend's severe and persistent mental illness symptoms.

C. The client's involvement in social relationships has increased as his/her nondisabled peers have developed better coping skills for his/her severe and persistent mental illness symptoms.

35. Review Social Experiences Regularly (35)

A. The client's successes and difficulties in social settings were reviewed.

B. The client identified a variety of successes and difficulties in social settings and was provided with support and feedback in this area.

C. A specific time to reassess these concerns was identified with the client.

36. Teach Relaxation Techniques (36)

A. The client was taught deep muscle relaxation and deep breathing techniques as ways to reduce muscle tension when feelings of stress are experienced.

B. *The Relaxation and Stress Reduction Workbook* (Davis, Eshelman, and McKay) was used to provide the client with examples of techniques to help himself/herself relax.

C. The client was reinforced for implementing the relaxation techniques and reporting decreased reactivity when experiencing stress.

D. The client has not implemented the relaxation techniques presented to him/her and continues to feel quite stressed; use of relaxation procedures was again encouraged.

37. Coordinate Respite Services (37)

A. Access to funds was coordinated in order to obtain respite services.

B. Respite services were coordinated for the client in order to provide short-term periods of relief from parenting in order to engage in recreational activities.

C. The client was encouraged to use respite funds and services in order to spend quality time alone with each child in their identified recreational pursuits.

D. The client was encouraged for his/her use of respite services in order to be involved in recreational activities and improve the overall relationship with the child.

E. The client has not used the respite services and was encouraged to do so.

38. Incorporate Recreation in Other Programming (38)

A. A recreational component was incorporated into the client's day program.

B. A recreational component was incorporated into the client's supported employment program.

C. A recreational component was incorporated into other programming for the client.

D. The client was reinforced for increasing his/her recreational involvement through incorporating this into other types of programming.

E. The client continues to struggle with his/her recreational involvement, despite the use of recreational activities in other types of programming.

39. Review Risks of Manipulation/Abuse (39)

A. The possible situations in which an individual with severe and persistent mental illness might be manipulated or abused were reviewed.

B. The client was provided with positive feedback regarding his/her understanding of situations in which he/she might be manipulated or abused while participating in recreational activities.

C. The client was reminded of the support system that he/she has and is able to use if uncertain about the treatment from others.

D. The client was supported for contacting members of his/her support system that can help keep him/her from being manipulated or abused.

E. The client continues to be at risk for being manipulated or abused, despite support, and further remediation of these concerns was implemented.

40. Emphasize Nonsubstance-Oriented Activities (40)

A. The need for developing social and recreational activities that are not related to the use of mood-altering substances was reviewed.

B. The client was assisted in developing recreational activities that are not related to the use of mood-altering substances.

C. As a result of the client's increased involvement in recreational activities, his/her use of mood-altering substances has decreased, and he/she was provided with positive feedback in this area.

SELF-DETERMINATION DEFICITS

CLIENT PRESENTATION

1. Lack of Choices (1)*

A. The client identified a lack of involvement in making the choices related to his/her daily life, school, residence, or vocation.

B. Others often take away from the client the responsibility for making choices.

C. As self-determination techniques have been used, the client has experienced an increase in his/her freedom to choose in his/her daily life, school, residence, or vocational situation.

2. Limited Decision-Making Experience (2)

A. The client described that he/she has often not been allowed to make important decisions for himself/herself.

B. The client has limited experience with using decision-making techniques.

C. As self-determination techniques have been used, the client has increased his/her experience in making decisions.

D. As the client has made more of his/her own decisions, he/she reported increased satisfaction and function.

3. Poor Planning for Transitions (3)

A. The client often fails to plan for his/her near or distant future.

B. The client often experiences difficult transitions regarding relationships, residence, vocational, or financial concerns due to his/her pattern of poor planning.

C. The client has often abdicated his/her responsibility for planning and expected others to complete this for him/her.

D. As the client has become more focused on taking responsibility for his/her own future, his/her planning has increased.

E. The client described better transitions in his/her relationships and financial, residential, or vocational situations due to his/her implementation of positive planning.

4. Decreased Responsibilities (4)

A. The client described a pattern of decreased responsibility due to his/her mental illness.

B. Others often take responsibility for the client's needs due to his/her mental illness.

C. The client often fails to take responsibility for those areas in which he/she is capable due to his/her mental illness and others' tendency to take responsibility for him/her.

D. As the client has taken responsibility for his/her own needs, others have decreased taking responsibility for him/her.

---

* The numbers in parentheses correlate to the number of the Behavioral Definition statement in the companion chapter with the same title in *The Severe and Persistent Mental Illness Treatment Planner,* 2nd ed. (Berghuis and Jongsma) by John Wiley & Sons, 2008.

5. Decreased Opportunities (4)

A. The client described decreased opportunities due to his/her mental illness.

B. The client has often been prohibited from age-appropriate activities or other opportunities due to his/her mental illness.

C. As the client has taken responsibility for his/her own needs, he/she has been more assertive in obtaining opportunities appropriate to his/her age and station, in spite of his/her mental illness, and he/she has reported increased satisfaction.

6. Agencies Limiting Freedom of Choice (5)

A. The client described involvement in agencies that have consistently dictated the options/services that are available.

B. The client has often been denied the assistance he/she desires due to agencies dictating the options/services that are available.

C. As the client has been more responsible for determining his/her own needs and services, his/her choice of services has expanded.

D. The client reports increased satisfaction with the services that he/she selects.

7. Lack of Independent Living Skills (6)

A. The client displayed limited knowledge and lack of skills necessary for living in an independent setting.

B. The client has been dependent on others for basic needs, limiting his/her ability to obtain independent living skills.

C. As the client has obtained skills for living independently, he/she has become more independent and has increased his/her level of functioning.

8. Vocational/Residential Failures (7)

A. The client described a pattern of vocational placement failures due to a lack of appropriate decision-making skills and an inability to adjust to changing situations.

B. The client described a pattern of residential placement failures due to a lack of appropriate decision-making skills and an inability to adjust to changing situations.

C. The client has begun to use appropriate decision-making skills to assist him/her in adjusting to changing situations.

D. As treatment has progressed, the client displayed increased success in vocational and residential placements.

9. Lack of Assertiveness (8)

A. The client displayed a lack of assertiveness.

B. The client described that he/she has decreased his/her assertiveness due to his/her caregivers' pattern of overprotecting him/her.

C. As the client takes more responsibility for his/her own needs, he/she has increased in assertiveness.

10. Poor Decision Making and Problem Solving (8)

A. The client described a pattern of poor decision making and poor problem solving.

B. The client is often overprotected by his/her caregiver, resulting in limited opportunities to solve problems and make decisions.

C. As the client has become more involved in determining and meeting his/her own needs, he/she has had increased experience in problem solving and decision making.

D. The client displays an increased ability regarding solving problems and making decisions.

11. Choice Limited by Treatment Agency Structure (9)

A. The agency providing treatment to the client has limited his/her choice of services.

B. The agency providing treatment to the client has limited his/her choice regarding which provider provides services to him/her.

C. Agency structure tends to limit the client's choices.

D. As the client has been allowed to have greater choice regarding his/her services and providers, he/she has been more motivated in treatment.

12. Limited Knowledge Regarding Self-Determination (10)

A. The client, family, caregivers, and clinical staff lack knowledge or training in the concepts of self-determination.

B. As the client, family, caregivers, and clinical staff have gained knowledge in the concepts of self-determination, the client has been given more responsibility for his/her own needs and choices.

C. As the client, family, caregivers, and clinical staff have used self-determination techniques, the client has experienced increased functioning.

INTERVENTIONS IMPLEMENTED

1. Assess Understanding of Self-Determination (1)*

A. The client's understanding of the concept of self-determination or person-centered planning was assessed.

B. The client displayed a partial understanding of the concept of self-determination and person-centered planning and was provided with additional information in this area.

C. The client was reinforced for displaying a complete understanding of the concepts related to self-determination and person-centered planning.

D. The client described very little understanding of the concepts of self-determination or person-centered planning and was provided with remedial information in this area.

2. Identify Examples of Self-Determination (2)

A. The client was assisted in identifying examples of self-determination in his/her own life, as well as in the lives of others.

B. The client's caregivers were assisted in identifying examples of self-determination in their own lives, as well as in the lives of others.

C. Personal examples of how the clinician experiences self-determination were provided.

D. Additional information was provided in areas in which the client and caregivers have limited knowledge or experiences regarding self-determination.

---

* The numbers in parentheses correlate to the number of the Therapeutic Intervention statement in the companion chapter with the same title in *The Severe and Persistent Mental Illness Treatment Planner,* 2nd ed. (Berghuis and Jongsma) by John Wiley & Sons, 2008.

3. Invite to Training (3)

A. The client and his/her caregivers were invited to agency trainings on person-centered planning and self-determination.

B. The client and his/her caregivers have attended agency training on person-centered planning and self-determination, and the key points of this training were processed.

C. The client and his/her caregivers have not attended agency training on person-centered planning and self-determination and were redirected to do so.

4. Encourage Discussion (4)

A. The client and his/her caregivers were encouraged to discuss the use of self-determination principles relative to his/her treatment, dreams, and desires.

B. Caregivers have discussed self-determination principles with the client, and their expectations in this area were reviewed.

C. The client and his/her caregivers have not discussed the use of self-determination principles and were redirected to do so.

5. Assess Strengths and Weaknesses Regarding Self-Determination (5)

A. The client was assessed for his/her strengths and weaknesses in the area of self-determination.

B. Specific areas (e.g., the client's autonomy, self-regulation, psychological empowerment, and self-realization) were identified as strengths or weaknesses.

C. Based on the assessment of the client's strengths and weaknesses in self-determination, a plan to promote his/her involvement in his/her future goals with the support of his/her family was developed.

D. The findings of the client's self-determination assessment were shared with him/her and his/her caregivers.

E. The client's strengths related to self-determination were emphasized.

6. Facilitate Agenda Development (6)

A. The client's development of an agenda for a person-centered planning meeting was facilitated.

B. The client was provided with examples of goals that he/she might like to achieve, but emphasis was placed on his/her input regarding goal areas.

C. As the client has been provided with support in developing his/her agenda for the person-centered planning meeting, he/she has become more directive, and this was processed with him/her.

7. Assist with Invitations (7)

A. The client was assisted with inviting all of the individuals whom he/she would like to have present during the person-centered planning meeting.

B. The client was provided with minimal direction related to the clinicians, family members, peers, advocates, friends, and others that he/she chooses to invite to the person-centered planning meeting.

C. The client was allowed to choose how the members of his/her person-centered planning meeting were invited and where the meeting is held.

D. A review was conducted with the client of those people whom he/she would prefer not to have at his/her person-centered planning meeting.

E. The procedures were developed that the client wishes to use if those whom he/she would prefer not to have at the meeting indicate an interest in coming.

F. The implications of not inviting specific individuals were reviewed.

8. Request Facilitator Choice (8)

A. The client was requested to choose a facilitator for his/her person-centered planning meeting.

B. Emphasis was placed on the idea that the client's facilitator does not have to be a clinical person.

C. The client's request for a certain facilitator was honored.

9. Identify Off-Limits Topics (9)

A. The client was encouraged to identify any off-limits topics (e.g., topics that he/she does not wish to be brought up at the person-centered planning meeting).

B. The client identified off-limits topics, and this was accepted.

C. The client was prompted to identify a setting in which he/she would be willing to discuss the off-limits topics.

D. The client was reinforced for his/her willingness to review the off-limits topics in an alternative setting.

E. The client has not been willing to review the off-limits topics in an alternative setting and was redirected to make sure that he/she covers these important areas.

10. Review Current Issues (10)

A. The client was assisted in articulating his/her current concerns related to relationships, preferences, dreams, hopes and fears, community choices, and issues related to home, career, and health.

B. The client was supported as he/she identified a variety of issues and concerns in many different areas of his/her life.

C. The client has failed to address many areas in his/her life in preparation for the person-centered planning meeting and was redirected to review these areas.

11. Identify Barriers and Supports (11)

A. The client was asked to identify barriers that interfere with his/her stated desires.

B. The client was supported as he/she identified a variety of barriers that interfere with his/her stated desires.

C. The client was assisted in identifying supports that are needed to attain future goals and dreams.

D. The client has struggled to identify barriers and/or supports and was provided with additional feedback in this area.

12. Identify Areas for Improvement (12)

A. The client was requested to identify areas in which he/she would like to improve (e.g., living situation, work setting, relationships).

B. The client was reinforced for identifying areas in which he/she would like to improve.

C. The client has not identified areas in which he/she would like to improve and was redirected to do so.

13. Conduct Person-Centered Planning Meeting (13)

A. The person-centered planning meeting was held, led by the client's chosen facilitator.

B. Participants in the person-centered planning meeting were requested to direct their comments to the client.

C. When comments were directed to the clinician or the facilitator, he/she consistently redirected those comments to the client.

D. Participants in the person-centered planning meeting were reinforced for consistently directing their comments to the client.

E. Participants in the person-centered planning meeting were encouraged to focus on the client and his/her desires and needs.

F. Participants in the person-centered planning meeting did not focus on the client and his/her stated desires and needs, and they were redirected to do so.

14. Ask Client's and Others' Opinion (14)

A. The client was asked to answer first, then the rest of the participants were asked, "Who is ___?"

B. The client was asked to answer first, then the rest of the participants were asked, "What are ___'s strengths and problems?"

C. The client was asked to answer first, then the rest of the participants were asked, "What supports, accommodations, or barriers exist?"

D. The client was asked to answer first, then the rest of the participants were asked, "What shall we put in the action plan for goals/objectives?"

15. List, Prioritize, and Coordinate Goals (15)

A. The client was assisted in making a list of his/her short- and long-term goals.

B. The client was requested to identify his/her favorite three goals.

C. Continuity was ensured between the client's short- and long-term goals.

D. The client's goals were written in a behaviorally observable and attainable manner.

E. The client failed to identify and prioritize his/her goals and was provided with additional feedback in this area.

16. Develop Conditions to Realize Goals (16)

A. The client was assisted in identifying and creating conditions that will facilitate the realization of his/her goals and desires.

B. Creative solutions were identified for breaking the existing barriers to identified goals.

C. As the client has identified and created conditions to facilitate the realization of his/her goals, he/she has experienced increased functioning, and this was reviewed.

D. The client continues to struggle to develop conditions that will help him/her to realize his/her goals and desires and was provided with additional feedback.

17. Explore Participation in Activities (17)

A. The client's desire to participate in a wide range of possible activities was explored.

B. The client was encouraged to participate in activities that promote community integration (e.g., social contacts, independent living, volunteer or work placement, service groups, church or recreational involvement).

C. The client was reinforced for participating in a wide range of possible activities, and developing self-determination skills.

D. The client continues to be quite limited in his/her involvement in community activities and was provided with additional assistance in this area.

18. Arrange Brainstorming and Commitment to Goals (18)

A. The significant people in the client's life were encouraged to brainstorm regarding creative options to expand his/her personal choices.

B. The significant people in the client's life were asked to commit to assist him/her in attaining the identified goals.

C. As a result of brainstorming, a variety of creative options was identified and processed.

D. As a result of the assistance given by the significant people in the client's life, he/she has increased his/her involvement in chosen activities.

E. Very few creative options were identified for helping the client attain his/her identified goals, and the significant people in his/her life were encouraged to think more creatively.

19. Assess the Potential for Adverse Choices (19)

A. The client's potential for making adverse choices was assessed.

B. The risk of the client's choices was determined by talking with the client, his/her family, and professionals, as well as by direct observation.

C. Those choices that have a low potential for resulting in physical and/or mental harm were identified and processed with the client.

D. Those choices that have a high potential for resulting in physical and/or mental harm were identified and processed with the client.

20. Weigh Risks against Rights (20)

A. The risk-of-harm level regarding the client's choices was weighed against his/her right to make his/her own choices.

B. A variety of factors was used to help weigh risks versus rights (e.g., the likelihood of short- or long-term harm, physical or psychological harm, direct or indirect harm, and predictable or unpredictable harm to the client or others).

C. The weight of the risk of harm versus the client's right to make his/her own choices was used to determine the degree of freedom of choice that is best suited for the client.

D. The client was urged to identify his/her desired level of freedom of choice when factoring in his/her risk of harm and right to make own choices.

E. Total independence with unrestricted choice was identified as a healthy option for the client.

F. Limited independence with restricted options available from which to choose was identified as the best level of freedom for the client.

21. Remind about Service Choice (21)

A. The client was reminded that he/she has a choice about the services to be provided, who provides them, and where he/she receives these services.

B. The client's guardian was reminded about the choice of services provided, who provides these services, and where the client receives the services.

C. The client's choice of services, service providers, and locations was processed.

D. The client's guardian was provided with feedback regarding the client's choice of services, service providers, and locations.

22. Develop a Provider Network (22)

A. A network of providers was developed from which the client can choose to identify from whom he/she would like to receive services.

B. The client's guardian was provided with a list of providers from which to choose someone to provide service to the client.

C. Specific providers have been identified, and additional feedback was given regarding the choices of providers.

23. Select Services within Financial Boundaries (23)

A. The costs of all the services that are currently being provided to the client were identified.

B. The client was provided with the cost of each individual service/provider that is available and appropriate for meeting his/her needs.

C. The client or guardian was allowed to choose whatever services and providers they see fit within their financial resources.

D. The client or guardian was provided with feedback regarding the choices of services and providers within the financial resource pool.

24. Focus on Customer Service (24)

A. Service providers were focused on the need to provide customer service.

B. An emphasis was placed on the concept that the client has a choice of providers available.

C. Providers were encouraged to adopt a "We need them!" philosophy rather than "They need us."

25. Identify Decision-Making Experience (25)

A. The client was assisted in identifying actual examples from his/her life when he/she has used decision-making skills.

B. The specific situations in which the client has used decision-making skills (e.g., gathering information, weighing pros and cons, consulting with others) were reviewed with him/her.

C. The client was unable to identify specific situations in which he/she has used decision-making skills and was provided with additional feedback in this area.

26. Teach Assertive Self-Advocacy (26)

A. The client was taught techniques for assertive self-advocacy.

B. The client was taught specific self-advocacy techniques from *The Self-Advocacy Manual for Consumers* by the Michigan Protection and Advocacy Service, Inc., or *The Self-Advocacy Workbook* by Gardner.

C. The client was provided with self-advocacy and leadership practice opportunities (e.g., with counselors, personal care support personnel, and residential supervisors).

27. Teach about Passiveness, Assertiveness, and Aggressiveness (27)

A. The client was taught about the difference between passive, assertive, and aggressive behaviors.

B. Assertive, aggressive, and passive responses to the same situation were modeled to the client, and he/she was requested to identify the most effective style.

C. The client was reinforced for identifying an assertive style for dealing with a problem situation.

D. The client has not identified the most assertive manner in which to respond to situations and was provided with additional feedback in this area.

28. Teach Problem-Solving and Logging Skills (28)

A. The client was taught problem-solving techniques via didactics, role-playing, and modeling.

B. Specific problem-solving techniques were taught to the client as found in *Thinking It Through: Teaching a Problem-Solving Strategy for Community Living* by Foxx and Bittle.

C. The client was reinforced as he/she displayed significant skills related to problem-solving techniques.

D. The client was encouraged to keep a journal of his/her conflicts and problem solutions.

E. The client's problem-solving journal entries were reviewed with him/her.

F. The client displays poor problem-solving techniques and was provided with additional information in this area.

G. The client has failed to keep a problem-solving journal and was redirected to do so.

29. Identify Preferences (29)

A. The client's responses to various activities and situations were assessed in order to understand his/her preferences better.

B. The client's approach, verbalizations, gestures, and affect were reviewed to best understand his/her preferences.

C. The client was provided with feedback regarding his/her preferences based on his/her responses to various activities.

30. Provide Choice Opportunities (30)

A. The client was provided with opportunities to choose in all areas in his/her life (e.g., leisure, shopping, mealtime, lifestyle, or employment).

B. The client was supported as he/she has made more independent choices.

C. The client has not made independent choices, despite attempts to provide these opportunities to him/her and was provided with additional direction in this area

D. The importance of the client being able to express his/her own choices and preferences and to have them honored was stressed with the family, caregivers, and support staff.

E. Family, caregivers, and support staff were reinforced as they endorsed the importance of the client being able to express his/her own choices and preferences and to have them honored.

F. Family, caregivers, and support staff have not allowed the client to express his/her own choices and preferences and were redirected to do so.

31. Generalize Self-Determination Skills (31)

A. The client was provided with learning opportunities for self-determination skills.

B. The client was assisted in generalizing his/her self-determination skills by processing his/her self-determination learning opportunities to a range of other situations.

C. As the client has learned self-determination skills, he/she was supported for generalizing them into other areas.

D. The client has failed to generalize self-determination skills from one area to another and was provided with remedial information in this area.

32. Review Goal-Oriented Decisions (32)

A. The client was assisted in reviewing his/her decisions and evaluating the compatibility of the decisions with the identified goals.

B. The client was supported as he/she identified his/her behavior as being consistent with his/her identified goals.

C. The client does not see his/her behavior as being consistent with his/her identified goals and was assisted in changing these behaviors as needed.

33. Develop Reinforcers (33)

A. The reinforcers that the client desires were identified.

B. The client was focused on establishing his/her reinforcers as an attainable contingent of the occurrence of his/her own predetermined target behavior.

C. The client was reinforced for using positive reinforcers to increase the frequency of his/her target behaviors.

D. The client has not maintained the use of positive reinforcers and was redirected in this area.

34. Teach Social Skills (34)

A. The client was taught social skills through didactic presentations and role playing.

B. Specific social skills (e.g., basic conversational skills, self-assertion, honesty, truthfulness, and how to handle negative comments) were reviewed and role-played.

C. The client was reinforced as he/she displayed mastery of the social skills that have been taught.

D. The client has failed to learn and implement the social skills and was provided with additional encouragement in this area.

35. Arrange Social Skills Practice (35)

A. Arrangements were made for the client to use social skills that he/she has identified as desirable.

B. The client's practice of social skills has improved his/her functioning, and this was reflected to him/her.

C. The client was urged to take risks to participate in social situations with people who have disabilities and with those who do not.

D. The client was reinforced for his/her increased attempts at participating in social situations.

E. The client tends to limit his/her social involvement with other people who have disabilities and was urged to expand this involvement to those who do not have a disability.

F. The client has not practiced social skills and was redirected to do so.

36. Advise Nondisabled Peers on Coping with Mental Illness (36)

A. An appropriate authorization to release confidential information was obtained in order to meet with the client's nondisabled peers.

B. The client's nondisabled peers were provided with information about how best to cope with their friend's severe and persistent mental illness symptoms.

C. The client's nondisabled peers were reinforced for implementing better coping skills for the client's severe and persistent mental illness symptoms.

37. Teach about Community Resources (37)

A. The client was provided with information about the availability and use of community resources.

B. The client was taught skills necessary for accessing entertainment, services, and other resources within the community.

C. As the client has increased his/her community access, he/she was reinforced for reporting a greater sense of self-determination.

D. The client was reinforced for displaying an increased understanding of the availability and use of community resources.

E. The client has not developed an increased understanding of the use of community resources and was provided with additional information in this area.

38. Assist in Obtaining Employment (38)

A. The client was assisted in obtaining employment.

B. The client was referred to a supported employment program.

C. The client was assisted with preparation of a resume, job application, and other needs for obtaining employment.

D. The client has not obtained employment and was provided with additional support in this area.

39. Prompt Support Network to Plan for Self-Determination (39)

A. The client's caregivers were encouraged to identify a plan of supporting lifelong learning opportunities and experiences for him/her.

B. The client's support network was assisted in identifying specific steps to promote his/her decision-making, problem-solving, goal-setting, and goal-attainment skills.

C. Caregivers were supported in their attempts to develop self-awareness and knowledge for the client within the home setting.

D. The client's caregivers have not supported ongoing steps toward self-determination and were provided with redirection in this area.

40. Demonstrate Opportunities for Identifying Preferences (40)

A. The many opportunities throughout the day that the client can use for exerting choices and preferences were demonstrated to the family.

B. Opportunities for the client to exert his/her personal preference (e.g., meal choices, scheduling for the day, clothing choices) were identified with the family.

C. The client's support network was encouraged to foster independence by helping him/her only when needed.

D. The client's family was reinforced for encouraging and supporting him/her to exert his/her choices and preferences while he/she maximizes his/her abilities and independence.

E. The client's family has not allowed him/her to exert his/her choices and preferences and was redirected to do so.

41. Emphasize Freedom (41)

A. An emphasis was placed on the client's freedom to make choices (even harmful choices) as a freedom that most people value.

B. The client's family and support network were encouraged to allow him/her to assume responsibility for his/her own actions and the natural consequences of these actions.

C. The family was reinforced for allowing the client to take responsibility for his/her own actions and to experience the natural consequences.

D. The client's family and support system have not allowed him/her to assume the responsibility for his/her actions, and this was reviewed.

SEXUALITY CONCERNS

CLIENT PRESENTATION

1. Sexual Victimization (1)*

A. The client recalled a history of being victimized in a sexual manner due to the vulnerability that is caused by his/her severe and persistent mental illness symptoms.

B. The client recalled specific memories of being sexually victimized.

C. The client has experienced a variety of secondary symptoms due to his/her sexual victimization.

D. As the client has stabilized his/her severe and persistent mental illness symptoms, he/she is less vulnerable to sexual victimization.

2. Bizarre Sexual Thoughts (2)

A. The client's hallucinations, delusions, and other severe and persistent mental illness symptoms have caused him/her to experience bizarre sexual thoughts.

B. The client's hallucinations and delusions contain strong sexual themes.

C. The client's support system has become alienated due to his/her expression of bizarre sexual thoughts.

D. As the client has become more stable in regard to his/her hallucinations and delusions, his/her bizarre sexual thoughts have decreased as well.

3. High Risk for STDs (3)

A. The client has reported engaging in high-risk behavior for sexually transmitted diseases (STDs).

B. The client appears to lack an understanding about sexual behavior that puts him/her at a higher risk for STDs.

C. As the client has gained understanding about safer sexual behavior, his/her risk for STDs has decreased.

4. Impulsive Sexual Acting Out (4)

A. The client reported a behavior pattern that reflected a lack of normal inhibition and an increase in sexual impulsivity, without regard for potentially painful consequences.

B. The client's impulsivity has been reflected in sexual acting out.

C. The client has gained more control over his/her impulses and has returned to a normal level of inhibition and sexual propriety.

5. Hypersexuality (4)

A. The client described a pervasive pattern of promiscuity and an increased focus on sexual matters.

---

* The numbers in parentheses correlate to the number of the Behavioral Definition statement in the companion chapter with the same title in *The Severe and Persistent Mental Illness Treatment Planner,* 2nd ed. (Berghuis and Jongsma) by John Wiley & Sons, 2008.

B. The client has a pattern of seduction and sexualization of relationships.

C. The client acknowledged that he/she has developed an unhealthy sexualization of relationships.

D. The client has terminated his/her pattern of sexual promiscuity and seduction.

6. Sexual Dysfunction (5)

A. The client described a consistently very low desire for or pleasurable anticipation of sexual activity.

B. The client has experienced a recurrent lack of the usual physiological response of sexual excitement and arousal.

C. The client reported a persistent delay in or absence of orgasm after achieving arousal, in spite of sensitive sexual pleasuring by a caring partner.

D. The client's sexual dysfunction appears to be due to the side effects of long-term psychotropic medication use.

E. The client's sexual dysfunction has been ameliorated, and he/she reports increased pleasure and enjoyment in sexual activity.

7. Medical Problems Due to STDs (6)

A. The client has a medical condition related to an STD that requires a physician's care.

B. The client reported that he/she has tested positive for the human immunodeficiency virus (HIV).

C. The client's HIV status has resulted in the development of acquired immunodeficiency syndrome (AIDS).

D. As the client has received medical treatment for his/her STD, he/she reports better health functioning.

8. Inadequate Prenatal Care (7)

A. The client reported that she is pregnant.

B. The client has received inadequate prenatal care due to her homelessness, confusion, or other effects of severe mental illness.

C. As the client has stabilized her mental illness condition, she has accessed more appropriate prenatal care.

9. Conflicts in Romantic Relationships (8)

A. The client described conflicts in his/her sexual or romantic relationships due to his/her bizarre behavior or other severe mental illness symptoms.

B. The client described a pattern of multiple lost romantic relationships due to his/her severe mental illness symptoms.

C. As the client has stabilized his/her bizarre behavior and other severe mental illness symptoms, his/her romantic relationship has improved as well.

INTERVENTIONS IMPLEMENTED

1. Explore Sexual History (1)*

A. The client's history of sexual abuse and vulnerability to sexual victimization was explored.

B. The client's pattern of sexual dysfunction and deviant sexual practices was explored.

C. The client was supported during his/her open and honest description of his/her history of sexuality concerns.

D. The client appeared to be rather defensive and withholding regarding his/her history regarding sexuality concerns and was urged to be more open in this area.

2. Inquire in a Tentative, Open Manner (2)

A. Inquiries regarding the client's sexuality issues were presented to him/her in a tentative, open manner, due to the highly personal and sensitive nature of such issues.

B. The client was focused on the voluntary nature of working on sexuality issues and that he/she will have the power to control how quickly or intensely these issues are addressed.

C. As the client has felt more in control over how intensely the sexuality issues are worked on, he/she has been more capable of addressing these issues, and this was reflected to him/her.

D. The client was reinforced for openly discussing matters of a sexual nature.

E. Despite inquiries into sexuality issues being presented in a tentative, open manner, the client was very cautious and withholding regarding these issues; he/she was urged to address these issues as he/she is able.

3. Identify History of Sexuality Concerns (3)

A. The client was requested to provide specific information regarding his/her history of sexual difficulties, dysfunction, or confusion.

B. The client's specific information regarding his/her history of sexual difficulties, dysfunction, or confusion was reviewed.

C. The client has not provided more specific information regarding his/her sexuality concerns and was redirected to do so.

4. Obtain Additional Sources of Information (4)

A. A written consent to release information was obtained in order to procure additional information about the client's sexuality concerns from outside sources.

B. Specific information was obtained from the client's spouse, partner, or other family members regarding the client's sexuality concerns.

C. The additional information regarding sexuality issues obtained from the client's spouse, partner, or other family members was reviewed with the client.

D. The client's choice not to have others provide information regarding his/her sexuality concerns was respected.

* The numbers in parentheses correlate to the number of the Therapeutic Intervention statement in the companion chapter with the same title in *The Severe and Persistent Mental Illness Treatment Planner*, 2nd ed. (Berghuis and Jongsma) by John Wiley & Sons, 2008.

5. Prepare a Time line of Sexual Involvement (5)

A. A graphic time line display was used to help the client chart his/her sexual history.

B. The client noted patterns of sexual behavior, sexual abuse history, and other sexual history concerns, which were graphically displayed on a time line.

C. The client was provided with support as he/she developed a greater understanding of his/her pattern of sexuality concerns.

D. The client failed to gain insight into his/her pattern of sexuality concerns and was redirected in this area.

6. Focus on Reality (6)

A. The client was encouraged to check out his/her beliefs regarding others by verifying his/her conclusions with others directly.

B. The client was encouraged to identify respected individuals with whom he/she can check the reality of his/her delusional or paranoid thoughts.

C. The client is beginning to verbalize a sense of trust in significant others, and this was processed within the session.

D. The client has followed through on checking out his/her distrustful beliefs and has found that others do not share them; he/she was assisted in reexamining and processing his/her unreasonable beliefs.

E. The client has attempted to use reality testing but has become more agitated when his/her beliefs are not supported, so he/she was encouraged to temporarily suspend this type of self-analysis.

7. Define Sexual Abuse (7)

A. The client was provided with a definition of sexual abuse.

B. The definition of sexual abuse was compared with the client's experience, and this was processed.

8. Explore Sexual Abuse History (8)

A. The client was encouraged to tell the entire story of the sexual abuse, giving as many details as he/she felt comfortable with providing.

B. The client was supported and encouraged as he/she appeared overwhelmed with feelings of sadness and shame due to talking about his/her childhood sexual abuse.

C. The client was supported as he/she spoke of the childhood sexual abuse without becoming emotionally overwhelmed.

9. Review Common Effects of Sexual Abuse (9)

A. Common emotional, self-esteem, and relationship effects of sexual abuse were reviewed with the client.

B. It was noted that the client displayed understanding of the effects of sexual abuse but did not identify with any of these concerns.

C. The client was supported as he/she identified emotional, self-esteem, and relationship effects that he/she has experienced due to his/her sexual abuse.

10. Assign Reading Regarding Sexual Abuse (10)

A. The client was assigned to read information to assist in processing his/her feelings related to the sexual abuse.

B. The client was assigned specific readings from *The Courage to Heal: A Guide for Women Survivors of Sexual Abuse* by Bass and Davis or *Reach for the Rainbow: Advanced Healing for Survivors of Sexual Abuse* by Finney.

C. The client was directed to complete assignments from the *Courage to Heal Workbook: for Men and Women Survivors of Sexual Abuse* (Davis); his/her assignments were processed.

D. The client has read the assigned material regarding sexual abuse healing, and his/her reaction to this information was processed.

E. The client has not read the assigned material regarding the sexual abuse and was redirected to do so.

11. Refer for Psychotherapy (11)

A. The client was referred for individual psychotherapy to a therapist who specializes in the treatment of sexuality issues and severe mental illness.

B. The client has followed up on the referral for psychotherapy, and this treatment was reviewed.

C. The client has not followed up on the referral to psychotherapy and was encouraged to make this contact.

12. Inquire/Report about Current Abuse (12)

A. The client was asked whether he/she is currently experiencing any sexual assault or abuse.

B. Specific situations and individuals were identified as possible current sexual assault or abuse risks and were processed with the client.

C. The client identified specific sexual abuse/victimization that is currently occurring for him/her, and immediate steps were taken to protect him/her.

D. Current sexual victimization was reported to the police and/or adult protective services agency in accordance with agency guidelines and local legal requirements.

E. Based on agency guidelines and local legal requirements, no report was necessary regarding current sexual victimization

F. The client denied any specific risk factors or specific situations for sexual assault or abuse but was urged to remain vigilant about such risks.

G. The client was informed of the report made to the police and/or adult protective services agency.

13. Advocate for Supports to End Abuse (13)

A. Advocacy was provided for the client in order to assist him/her with obtaining the needed support that will remove him/her from an abusive situation (e.g., domestic violence shelter, protection order).

B. The client has obtained the needed support and has used it to change his/her situation to end the abuse.

C. The client has not been able to obtain the needed support to remove himself/herself from an abusive situation and was provided with additional advocacy and direction.

14. Stabilize Financial/Residential Needs (14)

A. The client was assisted in meeting financial and residential needs in order to decrease the likelihood of having to be dependent on a sexually or physically abusive partner.

B. As the client's financial and residential needs have been met, he/she has become more independent, and the benefits of this were reviewed.

C. As the client has become more independent, he/she has been able to terminate involvement with the sexually or physically abusive partner, and he/she was supported for this.

D. The client continues to experience unmet financial and residential needs, which has continued his/her dependence on a sexually or physically abusive partner, and he/she was provided with additional encouragement to end this pattern.

15. Educate about Self-Defense (15)

A. The client was taught self-defense strategies to make him/her less vulnerable to abuse.

B. The client was provided with specific techniques for self-defense, as described in *Self-Defense: Steps to Success* by Nelson.

C. The client was provided with positive feedback as he/she displayed increased understanding of self-defense strategies.

D. The client has not learned self-defense strategies and was provided with additional encouragement to do so.

16. Review Sexually Inappropriate Behavior (16)

A. The client was provided with feedback about his/her sexually inappropriate behavior.

B. The client was provided with feedback about the illegality of his/her sexually inappropriate behavior.

C. The client was reinforced for terminating his/her sexually inappropriate behavior.

D. The client continues to display sexually inappropriate behavior and was confronted more directly about these concerns.

E. The client was referred to group therapy for sexual offenders.

F. The client's experience in the sexual offender treatment group was processed.

G. The client has not attended the sexual offender treatment group and was redirected to do so.

17. Educate about Human Sexuality (17)

A. The client was provided with educational materials on human sexuality.

B. The client was referred to books on human sexuality: *All about Sex: A Family Resource on Sex and Sexuality* by Moglia and Knowles and *Sexual Health: Questions You Have, Answers You Need* by Reitano and Ebel.

C. The client has reviewed the information on human sexuality, and this was processed with him/her.

D. The client has not reviewed the information on human sexuality and was redirected to do so.

18. Refer to a Sex Education Group (18)

A. The client was referred to a sex education group.

B. The client was referred to a sex education group based on *Positive Partnerships: A Sexuality Education Curriculum for Persons with Serious Mental Illness* by Caldwell and Reynolds.

C. The client has attended the sex education group, and the information learned was processed.

D. The client has not attended the sex education group and was redirected to do so.

19. Refer to a Physician (19)

A. The client was referred to a physician for an evaluation for a prescription of psychotropic medications.

B. The client was reinforced for following through on a referral to a physician for an assessment for a prescription of psychotropic medications, but none were prescribed.

C. The client has been prescribed psychotropic medications.

D. The client declined evaluation by a physician for a prescription of psychotropic medication and was redirected to cooperate with this referral.

20. Educate about and Monitor Psychotropic Medications (20)

A. The client was taught about the indications for and the expected benefits of psychotropic medications.

B. As the client's psychotropic medications were reviewed, he/she displayed an understanding about the indications for and expected benefits of the medications.

C. The client displayed a lack of understanding of the indications for and expected benefits of psychotropic medications and was provided with additional information and feedback regarding his/her medications.

D. The client was monitored for compliance with his/her psychotropic medication regimen.

E. The client was provided with positive feedback about his/her regular use of psychotropic medications.

F. The client was monitored for the effectiveness and side effects of his/her prescribed medications; concerns about the client's medication effectiveness and side effects were communicated to the physician.

G. Although the client was monitored for medication side effects, he/she reported no concerns in this area.

21. Advocate for Medications that Reduce Extrapyramidal Side Effects (EPSs) (21)

A. Advocacy was provided for the client to his/her prescribing physician regarding the use of medications that reduce the likelihood of extrapyramidal side effects (EPSs).

B. The client's prescribing physician has agreed to adjust medications to reduce EPSs, and this was told to the client.

C. The client's prescribing physician has indicated that the client's medications cannot be adjusted to further decrease the likelihood of EPSs, and this was told to him/her.

22. Assist in Increasing ADLs (22)

A. The client was encouraged to increase performance on his/her activities of daily living (ADLs).

B. The client was reinforced for his/her improvement in personal appearance as a result of his/her increased focus on ADLs.

C. The client was supported as he/she reported an enhanced self-image as a result of his/her improved ADLs and personal appearance.

D. The client has not improved his/her performance on ADLs and was encouraged to do so.

23. Refer to a Support Group (23)

A. The client was referred to a support group for individuals with severe and persistent mental illness.

B. The client has attended the support group for individuals with severe and persistent mental illness, and the benefits of this support group were reviewed.

C. The client reported that he/she has not experienced any positive benefit from the use of a support group but was encouraged to continue to attend.

D. The client has not used the support group for individuals with severe and persistent mental illness and was redirected to do so.

24. Teach Social Skills (24)

A. The client was taught social skills that could be applied to a range of intimate relationships.

B. The client was reinforced for using social skills to improve his/her intimate relationships.

C. The client has not used social skills to increase his/her involvement in intimate relationships and was redirected to do so.

25. Educate the Partner Regarding Mental Illness (25)

A. The client's partner was educated about the client's mental illness.

B. The client's partner was assisted in identifying how the client's mental illness symptoms impact on their intimacy and their relationship.

C. The client's partner was reinforced for demonstrating more understanding of the client's mental illness symptoms and the impact on their intimacy.

D. The client's partner has difficulty understanding the client's mental illness symptoms and accepting the impact on their pattern of intimacy and was given additional feedback in this area.

26. Resolve Family Needs (26)

A. The client's partner was assisted in resolving family needs that are not directly related to the client's mental illness symptoms.

B. Tension levels within the client's relationship have decreased as family needs have been met.

27. Engage Partner in Treatment (27)

A. The client's partner was encouraged to take an active role in the client's treatment (e.g., attend treatment meetings, provide feedback to the clinicians, or manage medications) as allowed by the client/partner.

B. The client's partner has been active in the client's treatment, and the benefits of this were reviewed.

C. The client's partner has not been active in the client's treatment, despite encouragement, and was encouraged to increase that role in his/her treatment.

D. The client has not allowed his/her partner to be very active in his/her treatment and was asked to consider this resource.

28. Refer for Marital Therapy (28)

A. The client and his/her partner were referred for couple's therapy related to ongoing conflicts between them.

B. The client and his/her partner were reinforced for using the marital therapy to help inoculate the relationship from future troubles.

C. The client and his/her partner have attended marital therapy, found it to be productive, and were encouraged to continue.

D. The client and his/her partner have attended marital therapy, have not found it helpful, and this was problem solved.

E. The client and his/her partner have not followed through on the referral for marital therapy and were redirected to do so.

29. Review Sexual Needs and Dysfunction (29)

A. The client's typical sexual needs that may have been neglected due to his/her mental illness symptoms were reviewed.

B. The client was supported as he/she acknowledged his/her own typical sexual needs that he/she has neglected due to his/her mental illness symptoms.

C. The client was supported as he/she acknowledged his/her partner's sexual needs that have been neglected due to his/her mental illness symptoms.

D. The client denied any pattern of sexual needs that have been neglected due to his/her mental illness symptoms and was provided with feedback in this area.

E. The client was asked about sexual dysfunction symptoms.

F. The client identified specific sexual dysfunction symptoms and was provided with information about how to address these problems.

G. The client denied any sexual dysfunction symptoms, and this was accepted.

30. Review Side Effects of Medications (30)

A. The client was taught about the sexual side effects of prescribed medications so that he/she can make an informed decision about whether to use them.

B. The client's decision against using medications due to their sexual side effects was processed.

C. The client is aware of the sexual side effects of the medications but was supported in his/her decision to use them despite these problems.

D. As the client continues to have a poor understanding of side effects of his/her medications, he/she was provided with additional information.

E. The client identified significant side effects, and these were reported to the medical staff.

F. Possible side effects of the client's medications were reviewed, but he/she denied experiencing any side effects.

31. Refer for a Physical Evaluation of Sexual Dysfunction (31)

A. The client was referred to a physician for a complete physical to rule out any organic basis for his/her sexual dysfunction.

B. The client was reinforced for cooperating with the referral for a physical evaluation to rule out any organic basis for his/her sexual dysfunction.

C. The client's physical did identify medical conditions or medications that may have a harmful effect on his/her sexual functioning, and this finding was processed.

D. An evaluation by a physician found no organic basis for the client's sexual dysfunction, and this conclusion was processed.

E. The client was supported in following up on the recommendations from the medical evaluation.

F. The client has been following up on the recommendations from the medical evaluation, and he/she was encouraged for this.

G. The client has not regularly followed up on his/her medical evaluation recommendations and was redirected to do so.

32. Review Sexual Dysfunction with a Physician (32)

A. The client's sexual dysfunction concerns were reviewed with his/her prescribing physician.

B. The physician was urged to consider the sexual dysfunction concerns in the choice for the client's medication regimen.

C. The client's physician has modified the client's medication regimen to minimize the impact on sexual libido and sexual functioning, and the impact of this was reviewed.

D. The client's physician has indicated an unwillingness to further modify the client's medications to minimize the impact on sexual libido and sexual functioning, and this was told to him/her.

33. Monitor for Decompensation (33)

A. The client was carefully assessed for decompensation.

B. The client's sexual dysfunction was interpreted as a precursor or a signal for a potential decompensation crisis.

C. The client needs further intervention as he/she appears to be decompensating.

D. The client does not appear to be otherwise decompensating, and this was reflected to him/her.

34. Educate about STDs (34)

A. The client was educated about STDs and how to avoid them.

B. The client was referred to read *Sexually Transmitted Diseases: A Physician Tells You What You Need to Know* by Marr.

C. The client has reviewed the assigned material on STDs, and key points were processed.

D. The client was supported for implementing safer sex practices.

E. The client has not read the assigned material on STDs and was redirected to do so.

F. The client does not display an accurate understanding of STDs and how to avoid them and was provided with remedial feedback in this area.

35. Refer for or Provide Free Condoms (35)

A. The client was provided with free condoms.

B. The client was referred to an agency that provides free condoms.

C. The client was taught about the proper and timely use of condoms to decrease his/her risk for STDs.

D. The client was reinforced for reporting regular use of condoms to decrease his/her risk of STDs.

E. The client has not regularly used condoms and was redirected to do so.

36. Refer for an STD Test and Treatment, If Needed (36)

A. The client was referred to a public health facility or to a physician to be tested for HIV/AIDS or other STDs.

B. The client has complied with the request to be tested for STDs, and the negative outcome of this test was reflected to him/her.

C. The client has complied with the request to be tested for STDs, has been found to have an STD, and the implications of this were discussed.

D. The client was supported in making arrangements for following up on his/her treatment for STDs.

E. The client's follow-up on the recommendations for his/her STD was reviewed.

F. The client was reinforced for following up on the recommendations for treatment for STDs.

G. The client has not complied with the request to be evaluated for STDs or treatment recommendations and was redirected to do so.

37. Refer to an HIV-Positive Support Group (37)

A. The client has tested positive for HIV and was referred to an appropriate support group.

B. The client has attended the support group for individuals who are HIV-positive, and the benefits of this support group were reviewed.

C. The client reported that he/she has not experienced any positive benefit from the use of a support group but was encouraged to continue to attend.

D. The client has not used the HIV-positive support group and was redirected to do so.

38. Review Motivations for Parenthood (38)

A. The possible motivations for the client's interest in parenthood (e.g., a redefinition of his/her self-concept from "mentally ill individual" to "parent" or a greater desire to maintain his/her psychological health) were reviewed.

B. The client's specific motivations for parenthood related to his/her mental illness were reviewed.

C. The client denied any specific motivations related to parenthood and was redirected to review this area.

39. Focus on Parenthood Stressors (39)

A. The client was focused on stressors that are related to parenthood (e.g., financial burdens, increased responsibilities) and how these may exacerbate his/her mental illness symptoms.

B. The client displayed an adequate understanding of the stressors related to parenthood, and the effects of these stressors on his/her mental illness symptoms were processed.

C. The client displayed a poor understanding of the stressors related to parenthood, or how these may exacerbate his/her mental illness symptoms, and was provided with additional feedback in this area.

40. Teach about Birth Control (40)

A. The client was taught about the correct and effective use of condoms, birth control pills, and other contraceptives.

B. The client was praised as he/she displayed an adequate understanding of the use of contraceptives.

C. The client was reinforced for his/her report of regularly using contraceptives.

D. The client displayed a poor understanding of the use of contraceptives and was provided with remedial information in this area.

41. Refer for Long-Lasting Birth Control (41)

A. The client was referred for birth control measures that are less likely to fail due to human error (i.e., Depo-Provera shots).

B. The client was reinforced for following through on the procurement of longer-lasting birth control measures.

C. The client has declined to use longer-lasting birth control measures, and his/her decision was accepted.

42. Provide Options Regarding Pregnancy (42)

A. The client was provided with information regarding options that are available for reacting to a pregnancy (e.g., abortion, release for adoption, keeping the baby).

B. The client was assisted in processing the effects of each option available regarding reacting to the pregnancy.

C. The client has made a specific decision about how to react to the pregnancy and was provided with support and/or feedback in this area.

D. The client is vacillating regarding options for reacting to the pregnancy and was provided with additional feedback in this area.

43. Emphasize Discontinuing Substances Due to Pregnancy (43)

A. The client was taught about the need for discontinuing alcohol or street drug use if it is possible that she is pregnant.

B. The client was taught about the effects of alcohol and street drug use during a pregnancy.

C. The client has been provided with positive feedback regarding her discontinuation of substances due to her possible pregnancy.

D. The client was provided with additional assistance and support, as she has struggled to discontinue substances during the pregnancy.

E. The client was referred to a substance abuse treatment program to assist in discontinuing her substance use due to the pregnancy.

F. The client's physician was immediately informed when the client suspected that she might be pregnant.

G. The client's physician's recommendations regarding a possible pregnancy were reviewed with the client.

44. Identify Atypical Sexual Behaviors (44)

A. The client was assisted in identifying atypical sexual behavior that is related to psychosis, mania, or other severe and persistent mental illness symptoms.

B. The client's atypical sexual behavior related to mental illness symptoms was compared with his/her typical sexual behavior or sexual orientation.

C. The client identified his/her pattern of atypical sexual behavior related to mental illness symptoms.

D. The client has developed a response plan that he/she would prefer to be implemented if his/her mental illness symptoms cause atypical sexual behavior.

45. Validate the Experience of Stigmatization/Discrimination (45)

A. Inquiries were made regarding the client's experience of stigmatization or discrimination due to being mentally ill *and* gay/lesbian.

B. The client's stigmatization and discrimination experience due to his/her sexual orientation was processed.

C. The client denies any stigmatization or discrimination related to his/her sexual orientation, and this was accepted.

D. It was acknowledged that family and societal issues regarding sexual orientation may cause increased stress.

E. The effects of increased stress on the client's symptoms were reviewed.

F. The client's worth was affirmed regardless of his/her sexual identity.

46. Refer to a Support Group for Sexual Orientation/Mental Illness Concerns (46)

A. The client was referred to a support group for those who are struggling with sexual orientation issues and severe and persistent mental illness concerns.

B. The client has attended the support group for individuals with sexual orientation issues and severe and persistent mental illness, and the benefits of this support group were reviewed.

C. The client reported that he/she has not experienced any positive benefit from the use of a support group, but he/she was encouraged to continue to attend.

D. The client has not used the support group for individuals with sexual orientation issues and severe and persistent mental illness and was redirected to do so.

SOCIAL ANXIETY

CLIENT PRESENTATION

1. Social Anxiety/Shyness (1)*

A. The client described a pattern of social anxiety and shyness that presents itself in almost any interpersonal situation.

B. The client's social anxiety presents itself whenever he/she has to interact with people whom he/she does not know or must interact in a group situation.

C. The client's social anxiety has diminished, and he/she is more confident in social situations.

D. The client has begun to overcome his/her shyness and can initiate social contact with some degree of comfort and confidence.

E. The client reported that he/she no longer experiences feelings of social anxiety or shyness when having to interact with new people or group situations.

2. Disapproval/Hypersensitivity (2)

A. The client described a pattern of hypersensitivity to the criticism or disapproval of others.

B. The client's insecurity and lack of confidence has resulted in an extreme sensitivity to any hint of disapproval from others.

C. The client has acknowledged that his/her sensitivity to criticism or disapproval is extreme and has begun to take steps to overcome it.

D. The client reported increased tolerance for incidents of criticism or disapproval.

3. Social Isolation (3)

A. The client has no close friends or confidants outside of first-degree relatives.

B. The client's social anxiety has prevented him/her from building and maintaining a social network of friends and acquaintances.

C. The client has begun to reach out socially and to respond favorably to the overtures of others.

D. The client reported enjoying contact with friends and sharing personal information with them.

4. Social Avoidance (4)

A. The client reported a pattern of avoiding situations that require a degree of interpersonal contact.

B. The client's social anxiety has caused him/her to avoid social situations within work, family, and neighborhood settings.

C. The client has shown some willingness to interact socially as he/she has overcome some of the social anxiety that was formerly present.

D. The client indicated that he/she feels free now to interact socially and does not go out of his/her way to avoid such situations.

---

* The numbers in parentheses correlate to the number of the Behavioral Definition statement in the companion chapter with the same title in *The Severe and Persistent Mental Illness Treatment Planner,* 2nd ed. (Berghuis and Jongsma) by John Wiley & Sons, 2008.

5. Fear of Social Mistakes (5)

A. The client reported resisting involvement in social situations because of a fear of saying or doing something foolish or embarrassing in front of others.

B. The client has been reluctant to involve himself/herself in social situations because he/she is fearful of his/her social anxiety becoming apparent to others.

C. The client has become more confident of his/her social skills and has begun to interact with more comfort.

D. The client reported being able to interact socially without showing signs of social anxiety that would embarrass him/her.

6. Performance Anxiety (6)

A. The client reported experiencing debilitating performance anxiety when expected to participate in required social performance demands.

B. The client described himself/herself as unable to function when expected to complete typical social performance demands.

C. The client avoids required social performance demands.

D. As treatment has progressed, the client has become more at ease with typical social performance demands.

E. The client reports no struggles with performance anxiety.

7. Physiological Anxiety Symptoms (7)

A. The client has an increased heart rate and experiences sweating, dry mouth, muscle tension, and shakiness in most social situations.

B. As the client has learned new social skills and developed more confidence in himself/herself, the intensity and frequency of physiological anxiety symptoms has diminished.

C. The client reported engaging in social activities without experiencing any physiological anxiety symptoms.

INTERVENTIONS IMPLEMENTED

1. Build Rapport (1)*

A. Consistent eye contact, active listening, unconditional positive regard, and warm acceptance were used to build rapport with the client.

B. The client began to express feelings more freely as rapport and trust levels increased.

C. The client has continued to experience difficulty being open and direct in his/her expression of painful feelings; he/she was encouraged to be more open as he/she feels safer.

2. Assess Nature of Social Discomfort Symptoms (2)

A. The client was asked about the frequency, intensity, duration, and history of his/her social discomfort symptoms, fear, and avoidance.

---

* The numbers in parentheses correlate to the number of the Therapeutic Intervention statement in the companion chapter with the same title in *The Severe and Persistent Mental Illness Treatment Planner*, 2nd ed. (Berghuis and Jongsma) by John Wiley & Sons, 2008.

B. *The Anxiety Disorder's Interview Schedule for DSM-IV* (DiNardo, Brown, and Barlow) was used to assess the client's social discomfort symptoms.

C. The assessment of the client's social discomfort symptoms indicated that his/her symptoms are extreme and severely interfere with his/her life.

D. The assessment of the client's social discomfort symptoms indicates that these symptoms are moderate and occasionally interfere with his/her daily functioning.

E. The results of the assessment of the client's social discomfort symptoms indicate that these symptoms are mild and rarely interfere with his/her daily functioning.

F. The results of the assessment of the client's social discomfort symptoms were reviewed with the client.

3. Explore Social Discomfort Stimulus Situations (3)

A. The client was assisted in identifying specific stimulus situations that precipitate social discomfort symptoms.

B. The client was assigned "Monitoring My Panic Attack Experiences" from the *Adult Psychotherapy Homework Planner,* 2nd ed. (Jongsma).

C. The client could not identify any specific stimulus situations that produce social discomfort; he/she was helped to identify that they occur unexpectedly and without any pattern.

D. The client was helped to identify that his/her social discomfort symptoms occur when he/she is expected to perform basic social interaction expectations.

4. Administer Social Anxiety Assessment (4)

A. The client was administered a measure of social anxiety to further assess the depth and breadth of his/her social fears and avoidance.

B. The client was administered *The Social Interaction Anxiety Scale* and/or *Social Phobia Scale* (Mattick and Clarke).

C. The result of the assessment of social anxiety indicated a high level of social fears and avoidance; this was reflected to the client.

D. The result of the assessment of social anxiety indicated a medium level of social fears and avoidance; this was reflected to the client.

E. The result of the assessment of social anxiety indicated a low level of social fears and avoidance; this was reflected to the client.

F. The client declined to participate in an assessment of social anxiety; the focus of treatment was turned to this resistance.

5. Differentiate Anxiety Symptoms (5)

A. The client was assisted in differentiating anxiety symptoms that are a direct affect of his/her severe and persistent mental illness, as opposed to a separate diagnosis of an anxiety disorder.

B. The client was provided with feedback regarding his/her differentiation of symptoms that are related to his/her severe and persistent mental illness, as opposed to a separate diagnosis.

C. The client has identified a specific anxiety disorder, which is freestanding from his/her severe and persistent mental illness, and this was reviewed within the session.

D. The client has been unsuccessful in identifying ways in which his/her anxiety symptoms are related to his/her mental illness or a separate anxiety disorder; remedial feedback was provided.

6. Acknowledge Anxiety Related to Delusional Experiences (6)

A. It was acknowledged that both real and delusional experiences could cause anxiety.

B. The client was provided with support regarding his/her anxieties and worries, which are related to both the real experiences and delusional experiences.

C. The client described a decreased pattern of anxiety due to the support provided to him/her.

7. Identify Diagnostic Classification (7)

A. The client was assisted in identifying a specific diagnostic classification for his/her anxiety symptoms.

B. Utilizing a description of anxiety symptoms such as that found in Bourne's *The Anxiety and Phobia Workbook*, the client was taken through a detailed review of his/her anxiety symptoms, diagnosis, and treatment needs.

C. The client has failed to clearly understand and classify his/her anxiety symptoms and was given additional feedback in this area.

8. Refer for Medication Evaluation (8)

A. Arrangements were made for the client to have a physician evaluation for the purpose of considering psychotropic medication to alleviate social discomfort symptoms.

B. The client has followed through with seeing a physician for an evaluation of any organic causes for the anxiety and the need for psychotropic medication to control the anxiety response.

C. The client has not cooperated with the referral to a physician for a medication evaluation and was encouraged to do so.

9. Monitor Medication Compliance (9)

A. The client reported that he/she has taken the prescribed medication consistently and that it has helped to control the anxiety; this was relayed to the prescribing clinician.

B. The client reported that he/she has not take the prescribed medication consistently and was encouraged to do so.

C. The client reported taking the prescribed medication and stated that he/she has not noted any beneficial effect from it; this was reflected to the prescribing clinician.

D. The client was evaluated but was not prescribed any psychotropic medication by the physician.

10. Refer to Group Therapy (10)

A. The client was referred to a small (closed enrollment) group for social anxiety.

B. The client was enrolled in a social anxiety group as defined in *The Group Therapy Treatment Planner,* 2nd ed. (Paleg and Jongsma).

C. The client was enrolled in a social anxiety group as defined in *Social Anxiety Disorder* (Turk, Heimberg, and Hope) and *Clinical Handbook of Psychological Disorders* (Barlow).

D. The client has participated in the group therapy for social anxiety; his/her experience was reviewed and processed.

E. The client has not been involved in group therapy for social anxiety concerns and was redirected to do so.

11. Discuss Cognitive Biases (11)

A. A discussion was held regarding how social anxiety derives from cognitive biases that overestimate negative evaluation by others, undervalue the self, increase distress, and often lead to unnecessary avoidance.

B. The client was provided with examples of cognitive biases that support social anxiety symptoms.

C. The client was reinforced as he/she identified his/her own cognitive biases.

D. The client was unable to identify any cognitive biases that support his/her anxiety symptoms and was provided with tentative examples in this area.

12. Assign Information on Social Anxiety, Avoidance, and Treatment (12)

A. The client was assigned to read information on social anxiety that explains the cycle of social anxiety and avoidance and provides a rationale for treatment.

B. The client was assigned information about social anxiety, avoidance, and treatment from *Overcoming Shyness and Social Phobia* (Rapee).

C. The client was assigned information about social anxiety, avoidance, and treatment from *Overcoming Social Anxiety and Shyness* (Butler).

D. The client has read the information on social anxiety, avoidance, and treatment, and key concepts were reviewed.

E. The client has not read the assigned material on social anxiety, avoidance, and treatment and was redirected to do so.

13. Discuss Cognitive Restructuring (13)

A. A discussion was held about how cognitive restructuring and exposure serve as an arena to desensitize learned fear, build social skills and confidence, and reality test biased thoughts.

B. The client was reinforced as he/she displayed a clear understanding of the use of cognitive restructuring and exposure to desensitize learned fear, build social skills and confidence, and reality test biased thoughts.

C. The client did not display a clear understanding of the use of cognitive restructuring and exposure and was provided with remedial feedback in this area.

14. Assign Information on Cognitive Restructuring and Exposure (14)

A. The client was assigned to read about how cognitive restructuring and exposure-based therapy could be beneficial.

B. The client was assigned to read excerpts from *Managing Social Anxiety* (Hope, Heimberg, Juster, and Turk).

C. The client was assigned to read portions of *Dying of Embarrassment* (Markaway, Carmin, Pollard, and Flynn).

D. The client has read the assigned information on cognitive restructuring and exposure-based therapy techniques, and key points were reviewed.

E. The client has not read the assigned information on cognitive restructuring and exposure-based therapy techniques, and he/she was redirected to do so.

15. Teach Anxiety Management Skills (15)

A. The client was taught anxiety management skills.

B. The client was taught about staying focused on behavioral goals and riding the wave of anxiety.

C. Techniques for muscular relaxation and paced diaphragmatic breathing were taught to the client.

D. The client was reinforced for his/her clear understanding and use of anxiety management skills.

E. The client has not used his/her new anxiety management skills and was redirected to do so.

16. Assign Calming and Coping Strategy Information (16)

A. The client was assigned to read about calming and coping strategies in books or treatment manuals on social anxiety.

B. The client was assigned to read portions of *Overcoming Shyness and Social Phobia* (Rapee).

C. The client has read the assigned information on calming and coping strategies, and key points were reviewed.

D. The client has not read the information on calming and coping strategies, and he/she was redirected to do so.

17. Identify Distorted Thoughts (17)

A. The client was assisted in identifying the distorted schemas and related automatic thoughts that mediate social anxiety responses.

B. The client was taught the role of distorted thinking in precipitating emotional responses.

C. The client was reinforced as he/she verbalized an understanding of the cognitive beliefs and messages that mediate his/her anxiety responses.

D. The client was assisted in replacing distorted messages with positive, realistic cognitions.

E. The client failed to identify his/her distorted thoughts and cognitions and was provided with tentative examples in this area.

18. Assign Reading on Cognitive Restructuring (18)

A. The client was assigned to read information about cognitive restructuring in books or treatment manuals on social anxiety.

B. The client was assigned to read excerpts from *The Shyness and Social Anxiety Workbook* (Antony and Swinson).

C. The client has read the assigned information on cognitive restructuring, and key points were reviewed.

D. The client has not read the assigned information on cognitive restructuring and was redirected to do so.

19. Assign Exercises on Self-Talk (19)

A. The client was assigned homework exercises in which he/she identifies fearful self-talk and creates reality-based alternatives.

B. The client was assigned "Bad Thoughts Lead to Depressed Feelings" from the *Adolescent Psychotherapy Handbook Planner,* 2nd ed. (Jongsma, Peterson, and McInnis).

C. The client was directed to do assignments from *The Shyness and Social Anxiety Workbook* (Antony and Swinson).

D. The client was directed to complete assignments from *Overcoming Shyness and Social Phobia* (Rapee).

E. The client's replacement of fearful self-talk with reality-based alternatives was critiqued.

F. The client was reinforced for his/her successes at replacing fearful self-talk reality-based alternatives.

G. The client was provided with corrective feedback for his/her failures to replace fearful self-talk with reality-based alternatives.

H. The client has not completed his/her assignment homework regarding fearful self-talk and was redirected to do so.

20. **Construct Anxiety Stimuli Hierarchy (20)**

A. The client was assisted in constructing a hierarchy of anxiety-producing situations associated with his/her phobic fear.

B. It was difficult for the client to develop a hierarchy of stimulus situations, as the causes of his/her fear remain quite vague; he/she was assisted in completing the hierarchy.

C. The client was successful at completing a focused hierarchy of specific stimulus situations that provoke anxiety in a gradually increasing manner; this hierarchy was reviewed.

21. **Select Exposures That Are Likely to Succeed (21)**

A. Initial *in vivo* or role-played exposures were selected, with a bias toward those that have a high likelihood of being a successful experience for the client.

B. Cognitive restructuring was done within and after the exposure using behavioral strategies (e.g., modeling, rehearsal, social reinforcement).

C. *In vivo* or role-played exposures were patterned after those in "Social Anxiety Disorder" by Turk, Heimberg, and Hope in the *Clinical Handbook of Psychological Disorders* (Barlow).

D. A review was conducted with the client about his/her use of *in vivo* or role-played exposure.

E. The client was provided with positive feedback regarding his/her use of exposures.

F. The client has not used *in vivo* or role-played exposures and was redirected to do so.

22. **Assign Reading on Exposure (22)**

A. The client was assigned to read about exposure in books or treatment manuals on social anxiety.

B. The client was assigned to read excerpts from *The Shyness and Social Anxiety Workbook* (Antony and Swinson).

C. The client was assigned portions of *Overcoming Shyness and Social Phobia* (Rapee).

D. The client's information about exposure was reviewed and processed.

E. The client has not read the information on exposure and was redirected to do so.

23. **Assign Homework on Exposure (23)**

A. The client was assigned homework exercises to perform sensation exposure and record his/her experience.

B. The client was assigned "Gradually Reducing Your Phobic Fear" from the *Adult Psychotherapy Homework Planner,* 2nd ed. (Jongsma).

C. The client was assigned sensation exposure homework from *The Shyness and Social Anxiety Workbook* (Antony and Swinson).

D. The client was directed to complete assignments from *Overcoming Shyness and Social Phobia* (Rapee).

E. The client's use of sensation exposure techniques was reviewed and reinforced.

F. The client has struggled in his/her implementation of sensation exposure techniques and was provided with corrective feedback.

G. The client has not attempted to use the sensation exposure techniques and was redirected to do so.

24. Build Social and Communication Skills (24)

A. Instruction, modeling, and role-playing were used to build the client's general social and communication skills.

B. Techniques from *Social Effectiveness Therapy* (Turner, Beidel, and Cooley) were used to teach social and communication skills.

C. Positive feedback was provided to the client for his/her use of increased use of social and communication skills.

D. Despite the instruction, modeling, and role-playing about social and communication skills, the client continues to struggle with these techniques and was provided with additional feedback in this area.

25. Assign Information on Social and Communication Skills (25)

A. The client was assigned to read about general social and/or communication skills in books or treatment manuals on building social skills.

B. The client was assigned to read *Your Perfect Right* (Alberti and Emmons).

C. The client was assigned to read *Conversationally Speaking* (Garner).

D. The client has read the assigned information on social and communication skills, and key points were reviewed.

E. The client has not read the information on social and communication skills and was redirected to do so.

26. Differentiate between Lapse and Relapse (26)

A. A discussion was held with the client regarding the distinction between a lapse and a relapse.

B. A lapse was associated with an initial and reversible return of symptoms, fear, or urges to avoid.

C. A relapse was associated with the decision to return to fearful and avoidant patterns.

D. The client was provided with support and encouragement as he/she displayed an understanding of the difference between a lapse and a relapse.

E. The client struggled to understand the difference between a lapse and a relapse, and he/she was provided with remedial feedback in this area.

27. Discuss Management of Lapse Risk Situations (27)

A. The client was assisted in identifying future situations or circumstances in which lapses could occur.

B. The session focused on rehearsing the management of future situations or circumstances in which lapses could occur.

C. The client was reinforced for his/her appropriate use of lapse management skills.

D. The client was redirected in regard to his/her poor use of lapse management skills.

28. Encourage Routine Use of Strategies (28)

A. The client was instructed to routinely use the strategies that he/she has learned in therapy (e.g., cognitive restructuring, exposure).

B. The client was urged to find ways to build his/her new strategies into his/her life as much as possible.

C. The client was reinforced as he/she reported ways in which he/she has incorporated coping strategies into his/her life and routine.

D. The client was redirected about ways to incorporate his/her new strategies into his/her routine and life.

29. Develop a Coping Card (29)

A. The client was provided with a coping card on which specific coping strategies were listed.

B. The client was assisted in developing his/her coping card in order to list his/her helpful coping strategies.

C. The client was encouraged to use his/her coping card when struggling with anxiety-producing situations.

30. Explore Rejection Experiences (30)

A. The client was asked to identify childhood and adolescent experiences of social rejection and neglect that have contributed to his/her current feelings of social anxiety.

B. Active listening was provided as the client described in detail many incidences of feeling rejected by peers, which has led to social anxiety and social withdrawal.

C. The client denied any history of rejection experiences and was urged to speak about these if he/she should recall them in the future.

31. Assign Books on Shame (31)

A. The client was directed to read books on shame.

B. It was recommended to the client that he/she read *Healing the Shame That Binds You* (Bradshaw) and *Facing Shame* (Fossum and Mason).

C. The client has read the assigned books on shame and can now better identify how shame has affected his/her relating to others; key points from the reading material were reviewed.

D. As the client has overcome his/her feelings of shame, he/she was asked to initiate one social contact per day for increasing lengths of time.

E. The client has failed to follow through on reading the recommended materials on shame and was urged to do so.

32. Identify Defense Mechanisms (32)

A. The client was assisted in identifying the defense mechanisms that he/she uses to avoid close relationships.

B. The client was assisted in reducing his/her defensiveness so as to be able to build social relationships and not alienate himself/herself from others.

33. Schedule a Booster Session (33)

A. The client was scheduled for a booster session between one and three months after therapy ends.

B. The client was advised to contact the therapist if he/she needs to be seen prior to the booster session.

C. The client's booster session was held, and he/she was reinforced for his/her successful implementation of therapy techniques.

D. The client's booster session was held, and he/she was coordinated for further treatment as his/her progress has not been sustained.

SOCIAL SKILLS DEFICITS

CLIENT PRESENTATION

1. Bizarre Behavior (1)*

A. The client has demonstrated a repeated pattern of bizarre or other inappropriate social behavior.

B. The client's social behavior appears to be disorganized and causes conflict in relationships.

C. The client's bizarre behavior has diminished in frequency and intensity.

D. The client no longer displays bizarre or other inappropriate social behavior.

2. Broken/Conflicted Relationships (2)

A. The client described a history of broken or conflicted relationships.

B. The client has a history of problems in relationships due to personal deficiencies in problem solving.

C. The client has found it difficult to maintain trust in relationships.

D. The client tends to choose abusive/dysfunctional partners/friends.

E. As the client's severe and persistent mental illness symptoms have abated, his/her relationships have become more stable and healthy.

3. Social Anxiety (3)

A. The client described a pattern of social anxiety, shyness, and timidity that presents itself in almost any interpersonal situation.

B. The client's social anxiety presents itself whenever he/she has to interact with others or in group situations with people whom he/she does not know well.

C. The client's social anxiety has diminished, and he/she is more confident in social situations.

D. The client has begun to overcome his/her shyness and can initiate social contact with some degree of comfort and confidence.

E. The client reported that he/she no longer experiences feelings of social anxiety or shyness when having to interact with new people or group situations.

4. Rude/Angry (4)

A. The client presented in an angry, resentful, oppositional manner.

B. The client was often rude and demanding in his/her comments toward peers and others.

C. Anger predominated the client's mood.

D. The client's overall manner was sullen and quiet, which covered a strong mood of anger and resentfulness.

E. The client's general mood and presentation reflected a notable decrease in anger and a general increase in pleasant, polite cooperation.

---

* The numbers in parentheses correlate to the number of the Behavioral Definition statement in the companion chapter with the same title in *The Severe and Persistent Mental Illness Treatment Planner,* 2nd ed. (Berghuis and Jongsma) by John Wiley & Sons, 2008.

5. Inability to Establish and Maintain Relationships (5)

A. The client described an inability to establish, nurture, and maintain meaningful, interpersonal relationships.

B. The client's difficulty in relationships is related to his/her failure to listen, support, communicate, or negotiate differences of opinion.

C. The client often fails to work through problem situations within his/her relationships, often leading to a lost or diminished relationship.

D. As the client's severe and persistent mental illness symptoms have stabilized, he/she has learned to listen, support, communicate, and negotiate, which has helped him/her to maintain meaningful interpersonal relationships.

6. Estrangement Due to Mental Illness Symptoms (6)

A. The client's psychotic symptoms (i.e., hallucinations, delusions, bizarre behavior, manic phases) have had a significant negative effect on his/her social interactions.

B. The client tends to be estranged from others due to the negative impact of his/her psychotic symptoms.

C. Others often avoid the client due to his/her mental illness symptoms.

D. As the client has stabilized his/her mental illness symptoms, his/her social relationships have improved.

7. Loneliness (7)

A. The client has no close friends or confidants outside of first-degree relatives.

B. The client identified ongoing feelings of loneliness.

C. The client's social anxiety has prevented him/her from building and maintaining a social network of friends and acquaintances.

D. The client has begun to reach out socially and respond favorably to the overtures of others.

E. The client reported enjoying contact with friends and sharing personal information with them.

8. Poor Support Network (7)

A. The client described a lack of friends to provide support during crises.

B. The client sees all of his/her relationships as fair-weather friends.

C. The client displayed a pattern of decompensation, which is exacerbated by the lack of a social network to provide support to him/her during these crises.

D. As the client has developed better relationships, he/she has found more support and been more stable during crisis times.

9. Lack of Assertiveness (8)

A. The client has difficulty saying no to other people when he/she is presented with a request for a favor.

B. The client attempts to ingratiate himself/herself to others by being eager to meet their needs.

C. The client often fails to be assertive in the appropriate situation.

D. The client has been taken advantage of by others because he/she fears rejection if he/she refuses to comply with others' requests.

E. The client has begun to set limits in doing things for others and not complying with their requests.

10. Lack of Experience in Social Activities (9)

A. The client described that he/she has had little experience in recreational/leisure activities.

B. The client is often unsure of the social aspects of recreational/leisure activities.

C. The client's involvement in recreational/leisure activities has increased, as he/she has stabilized.

D. The client reports an increased confidence in the social aspects of recreational/leisure activities.

INTERVENTIONS IMPLEMENTED

1. List Important Relationships (1)*

A. The client was asked to prepare a list of all important relationships, including friends, family, and treatment providers.

B. The client was provided with feedback regarding his/her list of important relationships, and important additions were made.

C. The client has not completed his/her homework of preparing a list of important relationships and was redirected to do so.

2. Develop a Genogram (2)

A. The client was assisted in developing a family genogram.

B. Important relationships within the family were identified through the use of the genogram.

3. Assess Social Skills Strengths and Weaknesses (3)

A. The client's social skill strengths and weakness were assessed.

B. Information from a variety of settings was used to assess the client's social skills.

C. The client was assessed in settings that demand a variety of different types of social involvement.

D. The client's social skill strengths and weaknesses were reflected to him/her.

4. Conduct Semi-Structured Interview (4)

A. An interview was conducted with the client and a person familiar with him/her in regard to the social skills that the client displays.

B. The Social Behavior Schedule was used to conduct a semi-structured interview of social skills with a client and a person familiar with him/her.

C. The Social Adjustment Scale was used to conduct a semi-structured interview of social skills with the client and a person familiar with him/her.

D. The client participated openly in the assessment of his/her social skills, and the results of this assessment were reflected to him/her.

E. The client did not participate significantly in the assessment of his/her social skills and was redirected to do so.

---

* The numbers in parentheses correlate to the number of the Therapeutic Intervention statement in the companion chapter with the same title in *The Severe and Persistent Mental Illness Treatment Planner,* 2nd ed. (Berghuis and Jongsma) by John Wiley & Sons, 2008.

5. Differentiate Etiology of Social Skill Deficits (5)

A. An attempt was made to differentiate among the social skill deficits that the client displays in regard to the etiological factors that create the deficits.

B. Social skill deficits that were related to social anxiety were identified.

C. Social skill deficits that are symptoms of a severe persistent mental disorder were identified.

D. Social skill deficits were identified as a negative symptom of the client's schizophrenia.

E. Social skill deficits were identified as a symptom of the client's manic episode.

6. Assess Cognitive Ability (6)

A. The client was referred for an assessment of cognitive abilities and deficits relative to social skills functioning.

B. The client underwent objective psychological testing to assess his/her cognitive strengths and weaknesses.

C. The client cooperated with the psychological testing, and feedback about the results was given to him/her.

D. The psychological testing confirmed the presence of specific cognitive abilities and deficits.

E. The client was not compliant with taking the psychological evaluation and was encouraged to participate completely.

7. Educate about Mental Illness Symptoms (7)

A. The client was educated about the expected or common symptoms of his/her mental illness that may negatively impact basic social skills.

B. As the client's symptoms of mental illness were discussed, he/she displayed an understanding of how these symptoms may affect his/her social skills.

C. The client struggled to identify how symptoms of his/her mental illness may negatively impact basic social skill functioning and was given additional feedback in this area.

8. Refer to a Physician (8)

A. The client was referred to a physician for an evaluation for a prescription of psychotropic medications.

B. The client was reinforced for following through on a referral to a physician for an assessment for a prescription of psychotropic medications, but none were prescribed.

C. The client has been prescribed psychotropic medications.

D. The client declined an evaluation by a physician for a prescription of psychotropic medication and was redirected to cooperate with this referral.

9. Monitor Medications (9)

A. The client was monitored for compliance with his/her psychotropic medication regimen.

B. The client was provided with positive feedback about his/her regular use of psychotropic medications.

C. The client was monitored for the effectiveness and side effects of his/her prescribed medications.

D. Concerns about the client's medication effectiveness and side effects were communicated to the physician.

E. Although the client was monitored for medication side effects, he/she reported no concerns in this area.

10. Identify Positive Effects of the Medications (10)

A. The client was assisted in recognizing the positive impact of his/her consistent use of the psychotropic medications on social interactions.

B. The positive social effects of the client's consistent use of psychotropic medications were processed.

C. The client was unable to identify the positive impact of his/her consistent use of psychotropic medications on social interactions and was given feedback in this area.

11. Provide Rationale for Social Skills Training (11)

A. A rationale for social skills training was provided to the client to help increase his/her commitment to the social skills training.

B. An emphasis was placed on the improved social interactions that may occur from social skills training.

C. An emphasis was placed on how social skills training may decrease negative social interactions.

D. The client was reinforced for his/her increased commitment and motivation in social skills training.

E. The client has displayed indifference in regards to social skills training and was provided with additional motivation in this area.

12. Provide Social Skills Training (12)

A. The client was provided with social skills training through the use of cognitive behavioral strategies.

B. Individual social skills training was provided to the client.

C. Group social skills training was provided to the client.

D. The client was taught through education, modeling, role-play, practice, reinforcement, and generalization techniques about new social skills.

13. Assign Social and Communication Information (13)

A. The client was assigned to read about social skills.

B. The client was assigned to read about communication skills.

C. The client was assigned to read *Your Perfect Right* (Alberti and Emmons).

D. The client was assigned to read *Conversationally Speaking* (Garner).

E. The client has read the assigned information about social and communication skills and key points were reviewed.

F. The client has not read the assigned information on social and communication skills and was redirected to do so.

14. Refer for Conduct Assertiveness Training (14)

A. Education, modeling, role-playing, practice, reinforcement, and generalization skills were used to teach assertiveness skills.

B. The client was referred to an assertiveness-training workshop.

C. The client was educated in the concepts related to assertiveness skills through lectures, assignments, and role-playing within the assertiveness-training group.

D. The client has displayed increased assertiveness as a result of attending the assertiveness-training group.

E. The client has not displayed an increased understanding of assertiveness, despite the use of assertiveness training, and was provided with additional feedback in this area.

15. Teach about Body Language (15)

A. The client was asked to identify three different body language messages from preselected photographs.

B. The client was reinforced as he/she correctly identified body language messages from material (e.g., magazines, family photos).

C. The client seemed to struggle with correctly identifying body language signals and was provided with feedback in this area.

16. Teach Accurate Interpretation of Body Language (16)

A. Role-playing, modeling, and behavioral rehearsal were used to teach the client how to accurately interpret body language signals.

B. In several practice situations, the client was able to correctly identify the body language signals that were being provided to him/her.

C. The client was given additional feedback as he/she failed to correctly identify the body language signals being provided to him/her.

17. Improve Eye Contact (17)

A. The client was confronted for his/her pattern of poor eye contact.

B. The client was reinforced for his/her spontaneous use of positive eye contact with others.

C. Subsequent to observing the client in social interactions, he/she was provided with feedback regarding his/her pattern of eye contact.

D. The client continues to be quite avoidant of eye contact with others and was urged to be more cognizant of these concerns.

E. The client was reinforced for using more regular eye contact.

18. Practice Eye Contact (18)

A. Role-playing and behavioral rehearsal were used to teach the client proper eye contact during social interactions.

B. The client was provided with positive feedback regarding his/her socially appropriate use of eye contact during practice social interactions.

C. The client was provided with feedback as he/she continued to display a pattern of poor eye contact during practice social interactions.

19. Develop Topics of Interest (19)

A. The client was directed to develop a list of five topics in which he/she is interested.

B. The client was directed to identify five topics in which others seem to be interested.

C. The client's list of topics of interest was processed.

D. The client has not developed lists of interests and was redirected to do so.

20. Role-Play Inquiries about Interests (20)

A. Role-playing techniques were used to practice asking questions about others' areas of interest, modeling eye contact, noninterruptive listening, and assertiveness in the process.

B. To facilitate the client's social skills, role-playing was used with him/her initiating conversation with others.

C. The client was supported as he/she expressed more confidence in his/her social initiation ability after the role-playing experience.

D. The client was reinforced for following through on implementing the initiation of social contact and reporting a feeling of success with this experience.

E. The client has not followed through with the implementation of asking questions about others' interests and was redirected to do so.

21. Assign Skill Practice (21)

A. The client was assigned to practice the use of listening and speaking skills in three social situations.

B. The client's experience of using social skills, including his/her successes and difficulties, was reviewed.

C. The complexity of the client's social skill practice situations was gradually increased.

D. The client has not followed through on practicing listening skills and was redirected to do so.

22. Refer to a Support Group (22)

A. The client was referred to a support group for individuals with severe and persistent mental illness.

B. The client has attended the support group for individuals with severe and persistent mental illness, and the benefits of this support group were reviewed.

C. The client reported that he/she has not experienced any positive benefit from the use of a support group but was encouraged to continue to attend.

D. The client has not used the support group for individuals with severe and persistent mental illness and was redirected to do so.

23. Teach Calming and Intentional Focusing Skills (23)

A. The client was taught calming and intentional focusing skills.

B. The client was reminded to stay focused on external and behavioral goals.

C. The client was taught physiological techniques to help calm his/her social anxiety, including muscular relaxation, evenly paced diaphragmatic breathing and "riding the wave of anxiety."

D. The client was reinforced for his/her increased calm, focused management of his/her social anxiety symptoms.

E. The client has not used calming and intentional focusing skills to manage his/her social anxiety symptoms and was reminded about these helpful skills.

24. Identify Distorted Thoughts (24)

A. The client was assisted in identifying the distorted schemas and related automatic thoughts that mediate problems with social skills.

B. The client was taught the role of distorted thinking in precipitating emotional responses.

C. The client was reinforced as he/she verbalized an understanding of the cognitive beliefs and messages that mediate his/her problem with social skills.

D. The client was assisted in replacing distorted messages with positive, realistic cognitions.

E. The client failed to identify his/her distorted thoughts and cognitions and was provided with tentative examples in this area.

25. Assign Exercises on Self-Talk (25)

A. The client was assigned homework exercises in which he/she identifies fearful self-talk and creates reality-based alternatives.

B. The client's replacement of fearful self-talk with reality-based alternatives was critiqued.

C. The client was reinforced for his/her successes at replacing fearful self-talk with reality-based alternatives.

D. "Restoring Socialization Comfort" from *Adult Psychotherapy Homework Planner,* 2nd ed. (Jongsma) was used to help identify fearful self-talk and create reality-based alternatives.

E. The client was provided with corrective feedback for his/her failures to replace fearful self-talk with reality-based alternatives.

F. The client has not completed his/her assigned homework regarding fearful self-talk and was redirected to do so.

26. Monitor Thought Process (26)

A. The effect of the client's mental illness symptoms on his/her thought process was monitored.

B. The client was provided with specific feedback about the areas in which his/her mental illness symptoms are currently affecting his/her thought process.

C. The client was provided with general feedback regarding areas in which his/her mental illness symptoms may potentially affect his/her thought process.

D. The client denied that his/her symptoms had any effect on his/her thought process and was provided with additional feedback in this area.

27. Develop Support and Feedback from Others (27)

A. The client was encouraged to seek frequent reality testing to challenge his/her distorted beliefs.

B. The client was provided with positive reinforcement for others' comparing his/her cognitions with the experience of trusted caregivers, friends, and family.

C. The client has sought out emotional support from family and friends, and the benefits of this were reviewed.

D. The client was reinforced for demonstrating an increased reality orientation.

E. The client failed to use reality testing from others to challenge his/her distorted beliefs and was encouraged to do so.

28. Assign Feedback Homework (28)

A. The client was assigned the homework of gaining feedback from others in three social situations.

B. The client completed the homework of obtaining feedback from others in social situations.

C. The client was reinforced for displaying an increased understanding of his/her social presentation as a result of the review of his/her feedback from others.

D. The client has not participated in obtaining feedback from others in social situations and was redirected to do so.

29. Accept Praise Graciously (29)

A. The client was assigned to focus on situations in which others provide praise and compliments to him/her.

B. The client was urged to graciously acknowledge (without discounting) praise and compliments from others.

C. The client's identified situations in which he/she received and responded to praise and compliments from others were processed.

D. The client was unable to identify any situations in which he/she received praise and compliments from others and was urged to continue to search for these areas.

30. Role-Play Requests for Group Involvement (30)

A. Role-playing techniques were used to assist the client in practicing how to ask others to allow him/her to be included in a group activity.

B. The client was supported as he/she practiced approaching others to increase his/her involvement in activities.

C. The client failed to use socially appropriate means to assert himself/herself into others' activities, and he/she was provided with encouragement.

31. Identify Mutually Satisfying Activities (31)

A. The client was assisted in identifying mutually satisfying social activities for himself/herself and friends/family members.

B. The client was supported as he/she identified a wide variety of activities that were satisfying for both himself/herself, as well as friends/family members.

C. The client tended to identify activities in which he/she has interest, but which hold very little interest for his/her friends/family members and was provided with additional feedback in this area.

32. Encourage/Facilitate Involvement in Social/Recreational Opportunities (32)

A. The client was encouraged to be involved in community- or agency-sponsored social/ recreational opportunities.

B. The client's involvement in community- or agency-sponsored social/recreational opportunities was facilitated.

C. The client was reinforced for selecting specific social/recreational opportunities in which he/she would like to be involved (e.g., bowling, exercise groups, church groups).

D. The client was supported for increasing his/her involvement in social and recreational opportunities.

E. The client has not increased his/her involvement in social/recreational opportunities and was provided with additional encouragement in this area.

33. Reframe Discrimination (33)

A. The client was assisted in identifying instances in which he/she has experienced discrimination while trying to be more involved in the community.

B. Instances of discrimination toward the client in his/her attempts to be involved in the community were reframed as a fault of the discriminating individual or group.

C. The client's emotional pain experienced due to being discriminated against was acknowledged regardless of the fault of the discriminating person or group.

34. Identify/Process Rejection (34)

A. The client was supported as he/she identified childhood and adolescent experiences of social rejection and neglect that contributed to his/her current feelings of social anxiety.

B. A reciprocal relationship was identified between the client's experience of mental illness symptoms and the emotional pain from social rejection.

C. The client tended to avoid any emotional content related to his/her history of social interaction or rejection, and this was accepted.

35. Teach Self-Affirmation Techniques (35)

A. The client was taught positive self-affirmation techniques to increase his/her focus on positive characteristics that may draw others toward him/her.

B. The client was instructed to write from 6 to 10 positive statements about himself/herself on 3-by-5-inch cards and review them several times per day.

C. The client has used positive self-affirmation techniques to increase his/her focus on positive characteristics, and the benefits of this were reviewed.

D. The client has not used positive self-affirmation techniques and was redirected to do so.

36. Encourage Family Members' Venting (36)

A. The client's family members were encouraged to vent their feelings about his/her past behavior and symptoms.

B. The client's family members were cautioned about making disrespectful or dehumanizing remarks about him/her as they vented about his/her past behavior and symptoms.

C. As the client's family members have been able to vent their emotions regarding his/her past behavior and symptoms, they have been able to increase their support for him/her.

37. Coordinate Family Therapy (37)

A. Family therapy appointments were scheduled to allow the family to express concerns, emotions, and expectations directly to the client.

B. The family's expressions of concerns, emotions, and expectations directly to the client were processed within the family session.

C. The client was supported as he/she accepted his/her family members' feedback.

D. The client has significant difficulties accepting the feedback from his/her family and was encouraged to allow them to vent their healthy emotions.

38. Answer Family Questions (38)

A. An appropriate release of information was obtained to allow the clinician to answer the family's questions regarding the client's mental illness symptoms and abilities.

B. Specific information was provided to the family regarding the client's mental illness symptoms, as well as his/her abilities.

C. The client's family members were reinforced as they displayed an increased understanding of his/her overall level of functioning.

D. The client's family continues to have a poor understanding of his/her mental illness symptoms, abilities, and needs and were provided with remedial information in this area.

39. Refer to a Family/Caregiver Support Group (39)

A. The client's family members/caregivers were referred to a support group for those who care for the chronically mentally ill.

B. The client's family members/caregivers reported being helped by attending a support group for those who care for the chronically mentally ill, and this attendance was reinforced.

C. The client's family members/caregivers have not attended a support group and were encouraged to do so.

40. Review Relationships Damaged by Mental Illness (40)

A. The client was requested to make a list of his/her important relationships, including those that have been damaged by his/her pattern of mental illness symptoms.

B. The client's list of important relationships was reviewed, focusing on lost relationships that can be salvaged, developed, or resurrected.

C. The client's experience of the loss of these relationships was processed.

D. The client has not developed a list of lost relationships and was redirected to do so.

41. Identify Individuals Hurt in Relationships (41)

A. The client was assisted in identifying those who have been hurt in previous relationships.

B. The client was assisted in identifying those to whom he must make amends.

C. The client was assisted in identifying how to apologize to those whom he has hurt in previous relationships.

42. Coordinate Conjoint Session for Making Amends (42)

A. A conjoint session was held to assist the client in making an apology or making amends to individuals whom he/she has harmed.

B. The client was reinforced for making amends or providing apologies to those whom he/she has offended or hurt due to his/her mental illness symptoms.

C. The client has denied any need for making amends to others and was encouraged to review this area.

SPECIFIC FEARS AND AVOIDANCE

CLIENT PRESENTATION

1. Unreasonable Fear of Object/Situation (1)*

A. The client described a pattern of persistent and unreasonable phobic fear that promotes avoidance behaviors because an encounter with the phobic stimulus provokes an immediate anxiety response.

B. The client has shown a willingness to begin to encounter the phobic stimulus and endure some of the anxiety response that is precipitated.

C. The client has been able to tolerate the previously phobic stimulus without debilitating anxiety.

D. The client verbalized that he/she no longer holds fearful beliefs or experiences anxiety during an encounter with the phobic stimulus.

2. Interference with Normal Routines (2)

A. The client's avoidance of phobic stimulus situations is so severe as to interfere with normal functioning.

B. The degree of the client's distrust associated with avoidance behaviors related to phobic experiences is such that he/she is not able to function normally.

C. The client is beginning to take on normal responsibilities and function with limited distress.

D. The client has returned to normal functioning and reported that he/she is no longer troubled by avoidance behaviors and phobic fears.

3. Recognition That Fear Is Unreasonable (3)

A. The client's phobic fear has persisted in spite of the fact that he/she acknowledges that the fear is unreasonable.

B. The client has made many attempts to ignore or overcome his/her unreasonable fear, but has been unsuccessful.

4. Phobia without Panic (4)

A. The client does not display panic attacks.

B. Although the client feels anxious whenever leaving his/her constricted safety zone, he/she does not experience panic symptoms apart from the agoraphobia symptoms.

---

* The numbers in parentheses correlate to the number of the Behavioral Definition statement in the companion chapter with the same title in *The Severe and Persistent Mental Illness Treatment Planner,* 2nd ed. (Berghuis and Jongsma) by John Wiley & Sons, 2008.

INTERVENTIONS IMPLEMENTED

1. Build Trust (1)*

A. An initial trust level was established with the client through the use of unconditional positive regard.

B. Warm acceptance and active-listening techniques were utilized to establish the basis for a trusting relationship.

C. The client has formed a trust-based relationship and was urged to begin to express his/her fearful thoughts and feelings.

D. Despite the use of active listening, warm acceptance, and unconditional positive regard, the client remains hesitant to trust and to share his/her thoughts and feelings.

2. Administer Fear Survey (2)

A. An objective fear survey was administered to the client to assess the depth and breadth of his/her phobic fear, including the focus of the fear, types of avoidance, development, and disability.

B. *The Anxiety Disorder's Interview Schedule for the DSM-IV (*DiNardo, Brown, and Barlow) was used to assess the client's phobia concerns.

C. The fear survey results indicate that the client's phobic fear is extreme and severely interferes with his/her life.

D. The fear survey results indicate that the client's phobic fear is moderate and occasionally interferes with his/her daily functioning.

E. The fear survey results indicate that the client's phobic fear is mild and rarely interferes with his/her daily functioning.

F. The results of the fear survey were reviewed with the client.

3. Assess Cues (3)

A. The client was assessed in regard to the stimuli that precipitate his/her specific fears and avoidance.

B. The client was assessed in regard to the thoughts that go along with his specific fears and avoidance.

C. The client was assisted in identifying situations that seemed to precipitate his/her specific fears and avoidance.

D. The client displayed significant insight into the precursors of his/her specific fears and avoidance and was provided with support and encouragement for being open about this.

E. The client struggled to identify any stimuli, thoughts, or situations that precipitated his/her specific fears and avoidance and was provided with several possibilities in this area.

4. Administer Client-Report Measure (4)

A. A client-report measure was used to further assess the depth and breadth of the client's phobic responses.

---

* The numbers in parentheses correlate to the number of the Therapeutic Intervention statement in the companion chapter with the same title in *The Severe and Persistent Mental Illness Treatment Planner,* 2nd ed. (Berghuis and Jongsma) by John Wiley & Sons, 2008.

B. The *Measures for Specific Phobias* (Antony) was used to assess the depth and breadth of the client's phobic responses.

C. The client-report measures indicated that the client's phobic fear is extreme and severely interferes with his/her life.

D. The client-report measures indicated that the client's phobic fear is moderate and occasionally interferes with his/her life.

E. The client-report measures indicated that the client's fear is mild and rarely interferes with his/her life.

F. The client declined to complete the client-report measure and the focus of treatment was changed to this resistance.

5. Differentiate Anxiety Symptoms (5)

A. The client was assisted in differentiating anxiety symptoms that are a direct affect of his/her severe and persistent mental illness, as opposed to a separate diagnosis of an anxiety disorder.

B. The client was provided with feedback regarding his/her differentiation of symptoms that are related to his/her severe and persistent mental illness, as opposed to a separate diagnosis.

C. The client has identified a specific anxiety disorder, which is freestanding from his/her severe and persistent mental illness, and this was reviewed within the session.

D. The client has been unsuccessful in identifying ways in which his/her anxiety symptoms are related to his/her mental illness or a separate anxiety disorder.

6. Acknowledge Anxiety Related to Delusional Experiences (6)

A. It was acknowledged that both real and delusional experiences could cause anxiety.

B. The client was provided with support regarding his/her anxieties and worries, which are related to both the real experiences and delusional experiences.

C. The client described a decreased pattern of anxiety due to the support provided to him/her.

7. Identify Diagnostic Classification (7)

A. The client was assisted in identifying a specific diagnostic classification for his/her anxiety symptoms.

B. Utilizing a description of anxiety symptoms such as that found in Bourne's *The Anxiety and Phobia Workbook,* the client was taken through a detailed review of his/her anxiety symptoms, diagnosis, and treatment needs.

C. The client has failed to clearly understand and classify his/her anxiety symptoms and was given additional feedback in this area.

8. Refer to Physician (8)

A. A referral to a physician was made for the purpose of evaluating the client for a prescription of psychotropic medications.

B. The client was reinforced for following through on a referral to a physician for an assessment for a prescription of psychotropic medications, but none were prescribed.

C. The client has been prescribed psychotropic medications.

D. The client declined evaluation by a physician for a prescription of psychotropic medication and was redirected to cooperate with this referral.

9. Monitor Medications (9)

A. The client was monitored for compliance with his/her psychotropic medication regimen.

B. The client was provided with positive feedback about his/her regular use of psychotropic medication.

C. The client was monitored for the effectiveness and side effects of his/her prescribed medications.

D. Concerns about the client's medication compliance, effectiveness, and side effects were communicated to the physician.

E. Although the client was monitored for medication side effects, he/she reported no concerns in this area.

10. Normalize Phobias (10)

A. A discussion was held about how phobias are very common.

B. The client was focused on how phobias are a natural, but irrational expression of our fight or flight response.

C. It was emphasized to the client that phobias are not a sign of weakness, but cause unnecessary distress and disability.

D. The client was reinforced as he/she displayed a better understanding of the natural facets of phobias.

E. The client struggled to understand the natural aspects of phobias and was provided with remedial feedback in this area.

11. Discuss Phobic Cycle (11)

A. The client was taught about how phobic fears are maintained by a phobic cycle of unwarranted fear and avoidance that precludes positive, corrective experiences with the feared object or situation.

B. The client was taught about how treatment breaks the phobic cycle by encouraging positive, corrective experiences.

C. The client was taught information from *Mastery of Your Specific Phobia—Therapist Guide* (Craske, Antony, and Barlow) regarding the phobic cycle.

D. The client was taught about the phobic cycle from information in *Specific Phobias* (Bruce and Sanderson).

E. The client was reinforced as he/she displayed a better understanding of the phobic cycle of unwarranted fear and avoidance and how treatment breaks the cycle.

F. The client displayed a poor understanding of the phobic cycle and was provided with remedial feedback in this area.

12. Assign Reading on Specific Phobias (12)

A. The client was assigned to read psychoeducational chapters of books or treatment manuals on specific phobias.

B. The client was assigned information from *Mastery of Your Specific Phobia—Client Manual* (Antony, Craske, and Barlow).

C. The client was directed to read information about specific phobias from *The Anxiety and Phobic Workbook* (Bourne).

D. The client was assigned to read from *Living with Fear* (Marks).

E. The client has read the assigned information on phobias, and key points were reviewed.

F. The client has not read the assigned information on phobias and was redirected to do so.

13. Discuss Unrealistic Threats, Physical Fear, and Avoidance (13)

A. A discussion was held about how phobias involve perceiving unrealistic threats, bodily expressions of fear, and avoidance of what is threatening that interact to maintain the problem.

B. The client was taught about factors that interact to maintain the problem phobia from information in *Mastery of Your Specific Phobia—Therapist Guide* (Craske, Antony, and Barlow).

C. The client was taught about factors that interact to maintain the problem phobia from information in *Specific Phobias* (Bruce and Sanderson).

D. The client displayed a clear understanding of how unrealistic threats, bodily expression of fear, and avoidance combine to maintain the phobic problem; his/her insight was reinforced.

E. Despite specific information about factors that interact to maintain the problem, the client displayed a poor understanding of these issues; he/she was provided with remedial information in this area.

14. Discuss Benefits of Exposure (14)

A. A discussion was held about how exposure serves as an arena to desensitize learned fear, build confidence, and make one feel safer by building a new history of success experiences.

B. The client was taught about the benefits of exposure as described in *Mastery of Your Specific Phobia—Therapist Guide* (Craske, Antony, and Barlow).

C. The client was taught about the benefits of exposure as described in *Specific Phobias* (Bruce and Sanderson).

D. The client displayed a clear understanding of how exposure serves to desensitize learned fear, build confidence, and make one feel safer by building a new history of success experiences; his/her insight was reinforced.

E. Despite specific information about how exposure serves to desensitize learned fear, build confidence, and make one feel safer by building a new history of success experiences, the client displayed a poor understanding of these issues; he/she was provided with remedial information in this area.

15. Teach Anxiety Management Skills (15)

A. The client was taught anxiety management skills.

B. The client was taught about staying focused on behavioral goals and positive self-talk.

C. Techniques for muscular relaxation and paced diaphragmatic breathing were taught to the client.

D. The client was reinforced for his/her clear understanding and use of anxiety management skills.

E. The client has not used new anxiety management skills and was redirected to do so.

16. Assign Reading about Calming Strategies (16)

A. The client was assigned to read psychoeducational chapters of books or treatment manuals describing calming strategies.

B. The client was assigned portions of *Mastery of Your Specific Phobia—Client Manual* (Antony, Craske, and Barlow).

C. The client has read the assigned information on calming strategies, and his/her favorite strategies were reviewed.

D. The client has not read the assigned information on calming strategies, and he/she was redirected to do so.

17. Assign Calming Skills Exercises (17)

A. The client was assigned a homework exercise in which he/she practices daily calming skills.

B. The client's use of the exercises for practicing daily calming skills was closely monitored.

C. The client's success at using daily calming skills was reinforced.

D. The client was provided with corrective feedback for his/her failures at practicing daily calming skills.

18. Use (Electromygraph) EMG Biofeedback (18)

A. EMG biofeedback techniques were utilized to facilitate the client's relaxation skills.

B. The client achieved deeper levels of relaxation from the EMG biofeedback experience.

C. The client did not develop deep relaxation as a result of EMG biofeedback.

19. Teach Applied Tension Technique (19)

A. The client was taught the applied tension technique to help prevent fainting during encounters with phobic objects or situations.

B. The client was taught to tense his/her neck and upper torso muscles to curtail blood flow out of the brain to help prevent fainting during encounters with phobic objects or situations involving blood, injection, or injury.

C. The client was taught specific applied tension techniques as indicated in "Applied Tension, Exposure In Vivo, and Tension-Only in the Treatment of Blood Phobia" in *Behavior Research and Therapy* (Ost, Fellenius, and Sterner).

D. The client was provided with positive feedback for his/her use of the applied tension technique.

E. The client has struggled to appropriately use the applied tension technique and was provided with remedial feedback in this area.

20. Assign Daily Applied Tension Practice (20)

A. The client was assigned a homework exercise in which he/she practices daily use of the applied tension skills.

B. The client's daily use of the applied tension technique was reviewed.

C. The client was reinforced for his/her success at using daily applied tension skills.

D. The client was provided with corrective feedback for his/her failure to appropriately use daily applied tension skills.

21. Identify Distorted Thoughts (21)

A. The client was assisted in identifying the distorted schemas and related automatic thoughts that mediate anxiety responses.

B. The client was taught the role of distorted thinking in precipitating emotional responses.

C. The client was reinforced as he/she verbalized an understanding of the cognitive beliefs and messages that mediate his/her anxiety responses.

D. The client was assisted in replacing distorted messages with positive, realistic cognitions.

E. The client failed to identify his/her distorted thoughts and cognitions and was provided with tentative examples in this area.

22. Assign Reading about Cognitive Restructuring (22)

A. The client was assigned to read about cognitive restructuring in books or treatment manuals on Panic Disorder and Agoraphobia.

B. The client was assigned to read *Mastery of Your Specific Phobia—Client Manual* (Antony, Craske, and Barlow).

C. The client was assigned to read excerpts from *The Anxiety and Phobia Workbook* (Bourne).

D. The client has read the assigned material on cognitive restructuring, and important concepts were reviewed within the session.

E. The client has not read the assigned material on cognitive restructuring and was redirected to do so.

23. Assign Homework on Self-Talk (23)

A. The client was assigned homework exercises to identify fearful self-talk, create reality-based alternatives, and record his/her experiences.

B. The client was assigned "Journal and Replace Self-Defeating Thoughts" from the *Adult Psychotherapy Homework Planner,* 2nd ed. (Jongsma).

C. The client's use of self-talk techniques was reviewed and reinforced.

D. The client has struggled in his/her implementation of self-talk techniques and was provided with corrective feedback.

E. The client has not attempted to use the self-talk techniques and was redirected to do so.

24. Model/Rehearse Self-Talk (24)

A. Modeling and behavioral rehearsal were used to train the client in positive self-talk that reassured him/her of the ability to work through and endure anxiety symptoms without serious consequences.

B. The client has implemented positive self-talk to reassure himself/herself of the ability to endure anxiety without serious consequences; he/she was reinforced for this progress.

C. The client has not used positive self-talk to help endure anxiety and was provided with additional direction in this area.

25. Construct Anxiety Hierarchy (25)

A. The client was directed and assisted in constructing a hierarchy of anxiety-producing situations.

B. The client was successful in identifying a range of stimulus situations that produced increasingly greater amounts of anxiety, and this hierarchy was reviewed.

C. The client found it difficult to identify a range of stimulus situations that produce increasingly greater amounts of anxiety and was provided with assistance in this area.

26. **Select Initial Exposures (26)**
   A. Initial exposures were selected from the hierarchy of anxiety-producing situations, with a bias toward likelihood of being successful.
   B. A plan was developed with the client for managing the symptoms that may occur during the initial exposure.
   C. The client was assisted in rehearsing the plan for managing the exposure-related symptoms within his/her imagination.
   D. Positive feedback was provided for the client's helpful use of symptom management techniques.
   E. The client was redirected for ways to improve his/her symptom management techniques.

27. **Assign Reading about Situational Exposure (27)**
   A. The client was assigned to read about situational exposure.
   B. The client was assigned to read excerpts from *Mastery of Your Specific Phobia—Client Manual* (Antony, Craske, and Barlow).
   C. The client was assigned to read portions of *Living with Fear* (Marks).
   D. The information that the client has read regarding situational exposures was reviewed and processed within the session.
   E. The client has not read information about situational exposure and was redirected to do so.

28. **Assign Homework on Situational Exposures (28)**
   A. The client was assigned homework exercises to perform situational exposures and record his/her experience.
   B. The client was assigned "Gradually Facing a Phobic Fear" from the *Adult Psychotherapy Homework Planner,* 2nd ed. (Jongsma).
   C. The client was assigned situational exposure homework from *Mastery of Your Specific Phobia—Client Manual* (Antony, Craske, and Barlow).
   D. The client was assigned situational exposure homework from *Living with Fear* (Marks).
   E. The client's use of situational exposure techniques was reviewed and reinforced.
   F. The client has struggled in his/her implementation of situational exposure techniques and was provided with corrective feedback.
   G. The client has not attempted to use the situational exposure techniques and was redirected to do so.

29. **Differentiate between Lapse and Relapse (29)**
   A. A discussion was held with the client regarding the distinction between a lapse and a relapse.
   B. A lapse was associated with a temporary and reversible return of symptoms, fear, or urges to avoid.
   C. A relapse was associated with the decision to return to fearful and avoidant patterns.
   D. The client was provided with support and encouragement as he/she displayed an understanding of the difference between a lapse and a relapse.
   E. The client struggled to understand the difference between a lapse and a relapse, and he/she was provided with remedial feedback in this area.

30. Discuss Management of Lapse Risk Situations (30)

A. The client was assisted in identifying future situations or circumstances in which lapses could occur.

B. The session focused on rehearsing the management of future situations or circumstances in which lapses could occur.

C. The client was reinforced for his/her appropriate use of the lapse management skills.

D. The client was redirected in regard to his/her poor use of lapse management skills.

31. Encourage Routine Use of Strategies (31)

A. The client was instructed to routinely use the strategies that he/she has learned in therapy (e.g., cognitive restructuring, exposure).

B. The client was urged to find ways to build his/her new strategies into his/her life as much as possible.

C. The client was reinforced as he/she reported ways in which he/she has incorporated coping strategies into his/her life and routine.

32. Develop a Coping Card (32)

A. The client was provided with a coping card on which specific coping strategies were listed.

B. The client was assisted in developing his/her coping card in order to list his/her helpful coping strategies.

C. The client was encouraged to use his/her coping card when struggling with anxiety-producing situations.

33. Explore Secondary Gain (33)

A. Secondary gain was identified for the client's panic symptoms because of his/her tendency to escape or avoid certain situations.

B. The client denied any role for secondary gain that results from his/her modification of life to accommodate panic; he/she was provided with tentative examples.

C. The client was reinforced for accepting the role of secondary gain in promoting and maintaining the panic symptoms and encouraged to overcome this gain through living a more normal life.

34. Differentiate Current Fear from Past Pain (34)

A. The client was taught to verbalize the separate realities of the current fear and the emotionally painful experience from the past that has been evoked by the phobic stimulus.

B. The client was reinforced when he/she expressed insight into the unresolved fear from the past that is linked to his/her current phobic fear.

C. The irrational nature of the client's current phobic fear was emphasized and clarified.

D. The client's unresolved emotional issue from the past was clarified.

35. Encourage Sharing of Feelings (35)

A. The client was encouraged to share the emotionally painful experience from the past that has been evoked by the phobic stimulus.

B. The client was taught to separate the realities of the irrational feared object or situation and the painful experience from his/her past.

36. Reinforce Responsibility Acceptance (36)

A. The client was supported and reinforced for following through with work, family, and social responsibilities rather than using escape and avoidance to focus on panic symptoms.

B. The client reported performing responsibilities more consistently and being less preoccupied with panic symptoms or fear that panic symptoms might occur, his/her progress was highlighted.

37. List Expectations for Improvement (37)

A. The client was asked to list several ways that his/her life will become more satisfying or fulfilling as he/she manages his/her symptoms of panic and continues normal responsibilities.

B. The client identified many ways in which his/her life will be more satisfying as his/her symptoms are managed and these changes were supported and reinforced.

C. The client has struggled to identify ways in which his/her life may become more satisfying and fulfilling in the management of his/her symptoms of panic and was provided with tentative examples in this area.

38. Schedule a Booster Session (38)

A. The client was scheduled for a booster session between 1 and 3 months after therapy ends.

B. The client was advised to contact the therapist if he/she needs to be seen prior to the booster session.

C. The client's booster session was held, and he/she was reinforced for his/her successful implementation on therapy techniques.

D. The client's booster session was held, and he/she was coordinated for further treatment, as his/her progress has not been sustained.

SUICIDAL IDEATION

CLIENT PRESENTATION

1. Death Preoccupation (1)*

A. The client reported recurrent thoughts of his/her own death.

B. The intensity and frequency of the recurrent thoughts of death have diminished.

C. The client reported no longer having thoughts of his/her own death.

2. Auditory Command Hallucinations (2)

A. The client described his/her experience of auditory hallucinations that direct him/her to harm himself/herself.

B. The client described difficulty resisting the command hallucinations to harm himself/herself.

C. The client's reality orientation is significantly impaired, and he/she believes that he/she must act on the command hallucinations to harm himself/herself.

D. As the client's severe and persistent mental illness symptoms have stabilized, his/her command hallucinations have decreased in intensity and frequency.

E. The client no longer experiences suicide command hallucinations.

3. Suicidal Ideation without a Plan (3)

A. The client reported experiencing recurrent suicidal ideation, but denied having any specific plan to implement suicidal urges.

B. The frequency and intensity of the suicidal urges has diminished.

C. The client stated that he/she has not experienced any recent suicidal ideation.

D. The client stated that he/she no longer has any interest in causing harm to himself/herself.

4. Suicidal Ideation with a Plan (4)

A. Although the client acknowledged that he/she has developed a suicide plan, he/she indicated that his/her suicidal urge is controllable, and he/she promised not to implement such a plan.

B. Because the client had a specific suicide plan and strong suicidal urges, he/she willingly submitted to a supervised psychiatric facility and more intensive treatment.

C. The client stated that his/her suicidal urges have diminished, and he/she has no interest in implementing any specific plan for suicide.

D. The client reported experiencing ongoing suicidal ideation and has developed a specific plan for suicide.

E. The client reported no suicidal urges.

5. Recent Suicide Attempt (5)

A. The client has made a suicide attempt within the last 24 hours.

B. The client has made a suicide attempt within the last week.

---

* The numbers in parentheses correlate to the number of the Behavioral Definition statement in the companion chapter with the same title in *The Severe and Persistent Mental Illness Treatment Planner,* 2nd ed. (Berghuis and Jongsma) by John Wiley & Sons, 2008.

C. The client has made a suicide attempt within the last month.

D. The client denied any interest in suicide currently and promised to engage in no self-harmful behavior.

6. Suicide Attempt History (6)

A. The client reported a history of suicide attempts that have not been recent but did require professional and/or family/friend intervention to guarantee safety.

B. The client minimized his/her history of suicide attempts and treated the experience lightly.

C. The client acknowledged the history of suicide attempts with appropriate affect and explained the depth of his/her depression at the time the suicide attempt occurred.

D. The client indicated no current interest in or thoughts about suicidal behavior.

7. Family History of Depression (7)

A. There is a positive family history of depression.

B. There is a positive family history of suicide.

C. The client acknowledged the positive family history of depression or suicide and indicated a concern as to the impact of this tendency on himself/herself.

8. Extreme Impulsivity (8)

A. The client displayed an extreme level of impulsivity due to his/her mania, psychosis, or other severe and persistent mental illness symptoms.

B. The client displayed impulsive thoughts about committing suicide.

C. The client has a history of acting on his/her impulsive thoughts due to mania, psychosis, or other severe and persistent mental illness symptoms.

D. As the client has stabilized his/her severe and persistent mental illness symptoms, he/she has decreased his/her level of impulsivity.

9. Increased Depression and Stress (9)

A. The client displayed a significant increase in depressive symptoms, coupled with a recent increase of severe stressors.

B. The client displayed a bleak, hopeless attitude toward life.

C. The client has encountered significant losses, relationship problems, or other crises.

D. As the client's depressive symptoms have stabilized, he/she has begun to cope with recent severe stressors.

E. The client's severe depression has lifted, and he/she is no longer a suicide risk.

INTERVENTIONS IMPLEMENTED

1. Ask about Suicidal Ideation (1)*

A. The client was asked to describe the frequency and intensity of his/her suicidal ideation, the details of any existing suicide plan, history of any previous suicidal attempts, and family history of depression or suicide.

---

* The numbers in parentheses correlate to the number of the Therapeutic Intervention statement in the companion chapter with the same title in *The Severe and Persistent Mental Illness Treatment Planner,* 2nd ed. (Berghuis and Jongsma) by John Wiley & Sons, 2008.

B. The client was encouraged to be forthright regarding the current strength of suicidal feelings and his/her ability to control such suicidal urges.

2. Perform a Risk Assessment (2)

A. A suicide risk assessment was performed, including evaluating the nature of the client's suicidal statements, specific plans, access to the means of suicide, and the degree of hope for the future.

B. The impact of the client's other severe and persistent mental illness symptoms was considered as a risk assessment was performed.

C. The risk assessment conducted regarding the client's suicidal ideation indicated no significant risk for suicide, and this was told to him/her.

D. As the client's risk assessment has indicated a significant risk for suicide, additional intervention was warranted.

3. Arrange for Psychological Testing (3)

A. The client underwent psychological testing to evaluate the depth of his/her depression and the degree of suicide risk.

B. The Suicide Lethality Scale and the Beck Scale for Suicidal Ideation were administered to the client.

C. The psychological test results were shared with the client, and the results indicate that his/her depression is severe and the suicide potential risk is high.

D. The psychological test results were shared with the client, and the results indicate that his/her depression is moderate and the suicide potential risk is mild.

E. The psychological test results were shared with the client, and the results indicate that his/her depression level has decreased significantly and the suicide risk is minimal.

4. Request Feedback from Support Network (4)

A. The client's family members, friends, and caregivers were asked about his/her level of suicidal ideation and symptom intensity.

B. The client's support network indicated significant suicidal ideation, and further steps to stabilize him/her were facilitated.

C. Feedback from the client's support network indicated little concern regarding suicidal ideation and symptom intensity, and this was told to the client.

5. Obtain Clinical Supervision or Feedback (5)

A. Clinical supervision was obtained regarding the necessary reaction to the client's current status.

B. Clinical peers were contacted for feedback regarding the client's status and the necessary reaction.

C. The use of clinical supervision or feedback has assisted in clarifying the most appropriate response to the client's suicidal ideation.

6. Obtain Emergency Medical Care (6)

A. Emergency medical personnel were contacted regarding the client's suicide attempt in order to provide immediate care to him/her.

B. The client was assisted in obtaining emergency medical care for his/her suicide attempt.

7. Arrange for Hospitalization (7)

A. Because the client was judged to be uncontrollably harmful to himself/herself, arrangements were made for psychiatric hospitalization.

B. The client cooperated voluntarily with an admission to a psychiatric hospital.

C. The client was referred to a crisis residential program with 24-hour trained staff.

D. The client declined voluntary admission to a more secure setting, and he/she did not appear to qualify for involuntary commitment; the client was encouraged to use a crisis home or psychiatric unit.

E. Contacts were made with the appropriate court or legal entity to involuntarily admit the client to a psychiatric unit until his/her suicidal crisis is alleviated.

F. The appropriate court or legal entity has declined to involuntarily admit the client into a psychiatric unit, and this was told to him/her.

G. The appropriate court or legal entity has decided that the client is in need of involuntary hospitalization, and this was told to him/her.

8. Develop a Crisis Care Plan (8)

A. A crisis care plan was developed, including supervision from caretakers, friends, and family.

B. As the client appears to be in a suicidal crisis, his/her crisis care plan was implemented.

C. The client was encouraged to voluntarily move forward with his/her crisis care plan.

D. The client has declined the use of the crisis care plan, and closer monitoring of his/her safety was arranged.

E. By using natural supports, such as the client's caretakers, friends, and family, his/her suicidal crisis has been averted.

F. The client's natural supports do not appear capable of providing the level of safety that he/she needs, and a more structured environment was obtained.

9. Remove Lethal Weapons (9)

A. Significant others were encouraged to remove firearms and other potentially lethal means of suicide from the client's easy access.

B. Contact was made with significant others within the client's life to monitor his/her behavior and to remove potential means of suicide.

10. Recommend Medication Removal (10)

A. It was recommended to the client's family and caregivers to limit the amount of available medication to a less-than-lethal or harmful dose.

B. The client was advised that his/her medications have been removed from his/her access.

C. The client's medications are being dispensed by others on a daily basis.

11. Develop a Suicide Prevention Contract (11)

A. A suicide prevention contract was developed with the client that stipulated what he/she will and will not do when experiencing suicidal thoughts or impulses.

B. The client was asked to make a commitment to agree to the terms of the suicide prevention contract and did make such a commitment.

C. Verbal and written directions were provided to the client and his/her caregivers about where to call or go if the suicidal ideation persists or increases.

D. The client was directed to contact the clinician or a 24-hour, professionally staffed crisis hotline if his/her suicidal ideation increases.

E. The client declined to sign the suicide prevention contract and was told that arrangements would be made for commitment to a psychiatric facility or other supervised setting.

F. The client was directed to go to an emergency room, local police unit, or other appropriate place should his/her suicidal ideation persist or increase.

12. Reinforce Positive Focus (12)

A. The client was reinforced for his/her more positive focus and hopeful statements.

B. As the client has been reinforced for his/her more positive focus and hopeful statements, he/she has been increasing such statements.

C. It was noted that the client's suicidal ideation has decreased as he/she has continued to develop a more positive focus.

D. The client did not display a very positive focus regarding his/her future and was provided with additional encouragement in this area.

13. Develop Structure (13)

A. The client was directed to develop structure to his/her time, scheduling his/her activities for the next several hours or days.

B. The client's specific plan for the next several hours or days was reviewed.

C. The client has not developed structure to his/her time by the use of scheduling the next several hours or days and was redirected to do so.

14. Nurture Life-Affirming Part of Self (14)

A. The client was reminded to focus on the portion of himself/herself that wants to go on living.

B. The client's interaction with the clinician was noted as evidence that a part of him/her wants to go on living.

C. The client was supported as he/she focused on the part of himself/herself that wants to go on living.

15. Verbalize Context of Suicidal Ideation (15)

A. The client's thoughts about suicide were identified as a common reaction to his/her current problem areas.

B. Emphasis was placed on the connection between the client's suicidal thoughts and emotional pain.

C. The client acknowledged that his/her suicidal thoughts and comments are related to his/her emotional pain and began to process his/her emotional pain.

D. The client was taught the importance of distinguishing between his/her thoughts of suicide and acting on those thoughts.

16. Talk Openly about Suicide Concerns (16)

A. Concerns about the client's suicidal ideation were brought up in an open and honest manner.

B. Emphasis was placed on the permanent nature of using suicide as a solution for a temporary problem or emotional state.

C. The client was reinforced for his/her decreased focus on suicide as a solution for his/her temporary problems or emotional concerns.

D. The client denied that his/her problems are temporary and does not see his/her way out of his/her current emotions; additional support, encouragement, and supervision were provided.

17. Discourage Denial of Suicidal Thoughts (17)

A. The client was discouraged from disregarding or denying suicidal ideation.

B. The client was reminded that disregarding or denying suicidal ideation generally leads to increased suicidal thoughts.

C. The client was supported as he/she talked openly and honestly about his/her suicidal ideation.

D. It is suspected that the client is continuing to deny his/her suicidal ideation, and he/she was encouraged to be more open and honest.

18. Acknowledge Control of Suicidal Activity (18)

A. The fact that the client is ultimately in control of his/her suicidal activity was acknowledged.

B. The client's idea of suicide as an inadequate solution to stressors that he/she temporarily views as intolerable was reinforced.

C. The client was supported as he/she acknowledged that he/she is the one ultimately in control of his/her suicidal activity.

D. The client tends to downplay his/her final responsibility for controlling his/her suicidal activity and was provided with additional direction in this area.

19. Provide Information about Treatment Options (19)

A. The client's caregivers, friends, and family were provided with information about available treatment options.

B. The client's family members were provided with feedback based on their concerns for him/her.

20. Provide Information about Suicidal Ideation/Concerns (20)

A. An appropriate authorization to release confidential information was obtained in order to advise the client's family, friends, and caregivers about his/her specific suicidal ideation/concerns.

B. Because the client's crisis state meets the legal requirement for breaking confidentiality to preserve life, information was provided to the client's family, friends, or caretakers without a written release of information.

C. The client's family members were reinforced for providing increased supervision and assistance to him/her as a result of being given additional information regarding his/her suicidal ideation.

21. Structure a Calm Environment (21)

A. The client's family or caregivers were directed to structure his/her environment in order to reduce the level of stimulation.

B. The agitated client was reassured about his/her safety and how the clinicians, family, and caregivers care about him/her.

C. As the client was provided with a calm environment and reassurance that he/she will be cared for, his/her level of agitation and psychosis has decreased.

D. Additional intervention was provided because the client remained quite agitated and continued to display symptoms of psychosis despite the more structured environment and support.

22. Refer to a Physician (22)

A. The client was referred to a physician for an evaluation for a prescription of psychotropic medications.

B. The client was reinforced for following through on a referral to a physician for an assessment for a prescription of psychotropic medications, but none were prescribed.

C. The client has been prescribed psychotropic medications.

D. The client declined evaluation by a physician for a prescription of psychotropic medications and was redirected to cooperate with this referral.

23. Educate about and Monitor Psychotropic Medications (23)

A. The client was taught about the indications for and the expected benefits of psychotropic medications.

B. As the client's psychotropic medications were reviewed, he/she displayed an understanding about the indications for and expected benefits of the medications.

C. The client displayed a lack of understanding of the indications for and expected benefits of psychotropic medications and was provided with additional information and feedback regarding his/her medications.

D. The client was monitored for compliance with, effectiveness of, and side effects from his/her psychotropic medication regimen.

E. The client was provided with positive feedback about his/her regular use of psychotropic medications.

F. Concerns about the client's medication effectiveness and side effects were communicated to the physician.

G. Although the client was monitored for medication side effects, he/she reported no concerns in this area.

24. Review Side Effects of the Medications (24)

A. The possible side effects related to the client's medications were reviewed with him/her.

B. The client identified significant side effects, and these were reported to the medical staff.

C. Possible side effects of the client's medications were reviewed, but he/she denied experiencing any side effects.

25. Identify Life Circumstances Contributing to Suicidal Ideation (25)

A. The client was asked to identify life circumstances that have contributed to his/her suicidal ideation.

B. The client was provided with support as he/she reviewed the life circumstances that have contributed to his/her suicidal ideation (e.g., the loss of a job or relationship, problems getting along with others, or hallucinations/delusions).

C. As the client has discussed his/her problematic life circumstances, he/she reported an increased hope for the future, and he/she was encouraged for this progress.

D. As the client has discussed his/her life circumstances, he/she continues to report suicidal ideation and was provided with additional support and supervision.

26. Inquire about Emotions (26)

A. The client was probed about his/her feelings that may be contributing to suicidal ideation.

B. The client was assisted in identifying how his/her feelings of hopelessness, anger, frustration, or sadness contribute to suicidal ideation.

C. The client was encouraged to share his/her feelings in order to reduce their intensity.

D. The client was supported as he/she vented his/her emotions and reported decreased suicidal ideation.

E. The client continues to be very cautious about expressing his/her emotions and was encouraged to do this at his/her own pace.

27. Identify the Emotional Effects of Mental Illness Symptoms (27)

A. The client was encouraged to identify the hallucinations and delusions that he/she experiences as a symptom of his/her mental illness.

B. The client was reminded that the emotional reaction that he/she experiences due to the hallucinations and delusions is not reality-based.

C. The client acknowledged that his/her hallucinations and delusions are symptoms of his/her mental illness, and the decreased emotional reaction that he/she experiences was processed.

D. The client maintains his/her hallucinations and delusions as being based in reality, continues to experience severe emotional reactions, and was provided with additional feedback.

28. Label Suicidal Behavior as Avoidance of Transient Emotions (28)

A. The client was presented with the concept of suicidal behavior as an avoidance of emotional pain.

B. The client was focused on the passing nature and changing severity of his/her painful emotions.

C. The client's experience was reviewed to identify his/her own use of suicidal behavior as an avoidance of emotional pain.

D. The client accepted that his/her suicidal behavior was his/her technique to avoid emotional pain, and alternative options were developed.

E. The client acknowledged that his/her negative emotions are transient in nature, and he/she was urged to tolerate the pain of these passing negative emotions.

F. The client denied his/her suicidal behavior as an avoidance of emotional pain and was given additional feedback regarding this concept.

G. The client refused to accept that his/her negative emotions are transient in nature and was provided with additional feedback in this area.

29. Externalize Suicidal Ideation (29)

A. The client was assisted in externalizing his/her suicidal ideation.

B. Emphasis was placed on the use of suicidal impulses as a warning sign that other issues need to be addressed.

C. As the client identified his/her suicidal ideation as a warning sign, he/she has become more focused on the underlying issues and was provided with assistance in processing these.

D. The client tends to deny and avoid his/her underlying issues and was encouraged to address these as he/she is able to do so.

30. Provide Clear Directives (30)

A. The client was provided with behavioral directives in a clear, straightforward manner.

B. The client was assisted in distinguishing between psychotic hallucinations/delusions and reality through the use of clear, straightforward information.

C. Philosophical discussions or "why" questions were avoided.

D. As the client has been provided with straightforward information, his/her ability to distinguish reality from psychosis has increased.

E. The client continues to experience his/her hallucinations and delusions as reality-based despite significant information and clear directives, and continued support and feedback were provided in this area.

31. Identify Hallucinations/Delusions (31)

A. The client was assisted in identifying the hallucinations and delusions that tend to prompt his/her suicidal gestures.

B. As the client discussed his/her hallucinations and delusions, he/she was provided with support and encouragement.

C. The client was reminded about the unreality of his/her hallucinations and delusions.

32. Explore Coping Skills (32)

A. The client's coping skills were explored that could assist him/her in decreasing psychotic thinking.

B. The client was taught a variety of interventions to decrease his/her psychotic thinking (e.g., reducing external stressors, implementing distraction techniques, and seeking a reality check with caregivers).

C. As the client has used his/her coping skills, it was noted that his/her psychotic thinking has decreased.

D. The client's psychotic thinking persists, despite the use of coping skills and other interventions, and he/she was provided with additional support in this area.

33. Identify Healthy Coping Practices (33)

A. The client was assisted in identifying healthy coping practices that support optimistic, upbeat thinking patterns.

B. The client was encouraged to implement his/her healthy coping practices (e.g., expressing emotions, social involvement, hobbies, or exercise).

C. As the client has used his/her healthy coping practices, he/she has experienced a more positive, upbeat thinking pattern, and this was reviewed with him/her.

D. The client tends not to use healthy coping practices and was urged to do so.

34. Monitor Sudden Mood Shifts (34)

A. The client's mood was monitored for sudden shifts from depressed and withdrawn to serene and at ease in spite of previously overwhelming problems.

B. A significant mood shift was identified, indicating that the client may have decided to pursue a suicide attempt rather than to fight the stressors.

C. The client seems to have decided to pursue the suicide attempt; therefore, he/she was provided with more intensive supervision.

35. Assign a Positive Letter (35)

A. During the client's period of stability, he/she was requested to write a letter to himself/herself regarding how positive and healthy his/her life could be.

B. The client's letter to himself/herself regarding how positive his/her life can be was reviewed.

C. As the client has decompensated into a suicidal state, his/her letter about how positive and healthy his/her life can be was read to him/her.

D. The client was assisted in processing the letter from himself/herself in a more positive time, and his/her suicidal ideation has diminished.

E. The client remains suicidal, despite the use of his/her own positive letter, and he/she was provided with additional support.

36. Develop Lists about Why to Go On (36)

A. The client was asked to focus on the positive aspects of his/her life.

B. The client was asked to develop a list of reasons why he/she should go on living.

C. The client's list of positive aspects of his/her life and why he/she should go on living was processed.

D. The client has failed to develop a list of positive aspects of his/her life and why he/she should go on living, and he/she was provided with additional feedback, support, and supervision.

37. Take the Reasons for Living Scale (37)

A. The client was requested to take the *Reasons for Staying Alive When You Are Thinking of Killing Yourself: Reasons for Living Scale* (Linehan).

B. The client's *Reasons for Living Scale* results were processed with him/her.

C. The client has developed a more hopeful attitude as a result of taking the *Reasons for Living Scale,* and this was processed.

D. The client has not developed a very hopeful attitude despite using the *Reasons for Living Scale,* and he/she was provided with additional feedback on this support and supervision.

38. Refer to a Support or Advocacy Group (38)

A. The client was referred to a support group for individuals with severe and persistent mental illness.

B. The client has attended the support group for individuals with severe and persistent mental illness, and the benefits of this support group were reviewed.

C. The client reported that he/she has not experienced any positive benefit from using a support group but was encouraged to continue to attend.

D. The client was encouraged to become involved in local awareness and advocacy groups and functions.

E. The client's involvement in local awareness and advocacy groups was processed.

F. The client has not used the support group or advocacy group for individuals with severe and persistent mental illness and was redirected to do so.

39. Assess/Treat Substance Abuse (39)

A. The client was evaluated for his/her use of substances, the severity of his/her substance abuse, and treatment needs and options.

B. The client was referred to a clinician who is knowledgeable in both substance abuse and severe and persistent mental illness treatment in order to assess accurately his/her substance abuse concerns and treatment needs.

C. The client was compliant with the substance abuse evaluation, and the results of the evaluation were discussed with him/her.

D. The client was referred for substance abuse treatment.

E. The client did not participate in the substance abuse evaluation and was encouraged to do so.

40. Teach Problem-Solving Skills (40)

A. The client was taught problem-solving skills through modeling and didactic training.

B. The client was taught specific problem-solving skills (e.g., focusing on the positive, negotiation, evaluating the pros and cons of alternatives, and practicing assertiveness).

C. The client was provided with positive feedback as he/she displayed increased understanding regarding his/her use of problem-solving skills.

D. The client continues to struggle with understanding problem-solving skills and was provided with additional feedback in this area.

41. Teach Social Skills (41)

A. The client was taught social skills through the use of modeling, role-playing, and behavioral rehearsal.

B. The client was referred to a group training program for social skills.

C. The client has developed increased social skills, and the benefits of this were reviewed.

D. The client has not developed increased social skills, and he/she was urged to place more emphasis in this area.

42. Monitor Possible Crisis (42)

A. The client was monitored more closely at possible crisis intervals (e.g., change in clinician, periods of loss).

B. The client was provided with additional support and supervision as he/she is experiencing possible crisis periods.

C. The client reported that he/she has been able to function well in his/her crisis situation due to the increased support that he/she has received.

D. The client has decompensated, despite being more closely monitored and supported, and an increased level of service was provided.

43. Develop a Long-Term Plan (43)

A. The client and his/her family were assisted in developing a long-term plan for dealing with stressors/symptoms contributing to his/her suicidal ideation.

B. Specific long-term plans for monitoring and supporting the client were developed.

C. The necessary portions of the client's long-term plan for support and coping with his/her stressors were coordinated.

D. It was noted that as a result of the long-term plans, the client has decreased his/her pattern of suicidal ideation.

E. A plan was developed to gradually taper the supervision of the client to a maintenance level.

F. The client's other therapeutic needs are cared for; therefore, the level of contact with him/her has been tapered to a maintenance level.

44. Develop Personalized Crisis Cards (44)

A. Personalized crisis cards were developed for the client, including a brief description of relapse prevention techniques, encouragement, and crisis contact numbers.

B. The client was provided with personalized crisis cards.

C. The client has used the personalized crisis cards and was encouraged to continue.

D. The client has not used the personalized crisis cards and was redirected to do so.

45. Identify Suicidal Gestures Impact (45)

A. The powerful responses that others have to a suicidal gesture were reviewed with the client.

B. The client was assisted in identifying and listing healthy ways in which he/she can have his/her need for attention and affirmation of caring met, without eroding trust or acting in a dangerous, suicidal manner.

C. The client received positive feedback as he/she has decreased his/her suicidal gesturing.

D. The client was reinforced for identifying a variety of ways in which he/she can attempt positive attention.

E. The client has not decreased his/her suicidal gestures, and was provided with additional feedback, support, and supervision.

46. Decrease Secondary Gain (46)

A. A specialized treatment plan was developed to assist in decreasing secondary gain from suicidal gestures.

B. An appropriate authorization to release confidential information was obtained in order to share the secondary gain treatment plan with other agencies that may be involved with the suicidal gestures (e.g., local emergency room).

C. The client's secondary gain for his/her suicidal gestures has been decreased, and he/she was focused on being more direct in order to meet his/her attentional and affirmational needs.